OXFORD STUDIES IN
SOCIAL AND CULTURAL ANTHROPOLOGY

BORN AND BRED

OXFORD STUDIES IN SOCIAL AND CULTURAL ANTHROPOLOGY

Oxford Studies in Social and Cultural Anthropology represents the work of authors, new and established, that will set the criteria of excellence in ethnographic description and innovation in analysis. The series serves as an essential source of information about the world and the discipline.

OTHER TITLES IN THIS SERIES

Sea Hunters of Indonesia
Fishers and Weavers of Lamalera
R. H. Barnes

Nationalism and Hybridity in Mongolia
Uradyn E. Bulag

The Heat of the Hearth
The Process of Kinship in a Malay Fishing Community
Janet Carsten

The Culture of Coincidence
Accident and Absolute Liability in Huli
Laurence Goldman

A Place Apart
An Anthropological Study of the Icelandic World
Kirsten Hastrup

Shamans and Elders
Experience, Knowledge, and Power among the Daur Mongols
Caroline Humphrey with Urgunge Onon

The Pastoral Continuum
The Marginalization of Tradition in East Africa
Paul Spencer

Dancing through Time
A Sepik Cosmology
Borut Telban

BORN AND BRED

Idioms of Kinship and New Reproductive Technologies in England

Jeanette Edwards

OXFORD
UNIVERSITY PRESS

OXFORD
UNIVERSITY PRESS

Great Clarendon Street, Oxford OX2 6DP

Oxford University Press is a department of the University of Oxford.
It furthers the University's objective of excellence in research, scholarship,
and education by publishing worldwide in

Oxford New York
Athens Auckland Bangkok Bogotá Buenos Aires Calcutta
Cape Town Chennai Dar es Salaam Delhi Florence Hong Kong Istanbul
Karachi Kuala Lumpur Madrid Melbourne Mexico City Mumbai
Nairobi Paris São Paulo Singapore Taipei Tokyo Toronto Warsaw

and associated companies in Berlin Ibadan

Oxford is a registered trade mark of Oxford University Press
in the UK and certain other countries

Published in the United States
by Oxford University Press Inc., New York

First published 2000

British Library Cataloguing in Publication Data
Data available

Library of Congress Cataloging in Publication Data
Data applied for

ISBN 0-19-823394-9

Typeset by Best-set Typesetter Ltd., Hong Kong
Printed in Great Britain
on acid-free paper by
TJ International Ltd., Padstow, Cornwall

For my

MUM AND DAD

'Where, then, is truth?' declaimed Bedap . . .
'In the hill one happens to be sitting on,' said Tirin.

Ursula le Guin

Only the ignorant and unwise could hold that the past is dead and forever separated by an impenetrable wall from the present.

Ivo Andrić

Everything has already begun before . . . The lives of individuals of the human race form a constant plot, in which every attempt to isolate one piece of living that has a meaning separate from the rest—for example, the meeting of two people, which will become decisive of both—must bear in mind that each of the two brings with himself a texture of events, environments, other people, and that from the meeting, in turn, other stories will be derived which will break off from their common story.

Italo Calvino

ACKNOWLEDGEMENTS

My largest debt of gratitude in the long making of this book is to residents of Bacup: to co-conversationalists and acquaintances, some of whom are now friends of the enduring kind. Reasons of privacy, caution, and anthropological convention prevent me from naming them here but my debt to them not only remains but grows. I want to thank the people of Bacup, warmly and sincerely, for their interest and unstinting generosity. I offer this in the memory of Mrs Margaret Edwards, Mr Arnold Hargreaves, Mrs Ellen Hargreaves, and Mr Harold Stevenson.

There is something slightly awry in having Bacup residents remain anonymous and yet naming colleagues without whom also this book could not have been completed. Despite the temptation to thank many individuals profusely and wordily, I extend but a large, single thank you to colleagues at the Universities of Keele, Manchester, Salford, Berkeley, and Barcelona who have provided, during the various drafts of this book, intellectual stimulus and space.

The bulk of the manuscript was prepared during 1993–4, in the Department of Anthropology at the University of Manchester, under the aegis of a Leach/RAI (Royal Anthropological Institute) Fellowship. I am grateful to the RAI, the Esperanza Trust, and the University of Manchester for their support. Financial support was provided by the Economic and Social Science Research Council (ESRC), initially for my doctoral research and then for a collaborative project, with Sarah Franklin, Eric Hirsch, Frances Price, and Marilyn Strathern (award number R000 232537). It was a great pleasure working with such fine 'collaborators', and I am grateful to them for teaching me a great deal.

Penny Harvey, Celia Lury, Sharon Macdonald, and Marilyn Strathern read earlier drafts and, with characteristic insight, commented, questioned, and advised. I thank them for that, and for much more. The flaws that remain are mine and are due, in part, to my not taking all their apt and incisive advice. I am indebted to Pattie Peach for her work on the index, to Patrick Crozier for past, pertinent, and unrelenting criticism of my written English, and to Andrew Lawrence for preparing the maps. Anne Ashby, Sylvia Jaffrey, and Dorothy McCarthy at Oxford University Press have been more than helpful, as have the Press's readers. I have benefited enormously from comments and questions of students and colleagues in conferences, seminars, and conversation. The power of a good question, like a good idea, is that when you try it on, it fits. I am grateful to those, too numerous to mention, whose questions and ideas I am wearing.

Marilyn Strathern was my Ph.D. supervisor and has given me unstinting encouragement, of all kinds, over the intervening years. Her intellect and integrity (professional and personal) continue to inspire me and for that, and more besides, I am *very* grateful. I am also indebted to David Turton, Roy Murphy, Ronnie Frankenberg, Jennie Popay, John Law, Jean Lave, and Verena Stolcke who, at crucial moments, supported my work with trust. I am fortunate to have been cushioned by the patience and humour of amongst others Rebecca Boden, Ben Campbell, Lorien Garth Edwards, Liz Edwards, Hassan Etemadi, Peter Gow, Sarah Green, Penny Harvey, Iris Jean-Klein, Sharon Macdonald, Pattie Peach, Frances Price, Nigel Rapport, Ursula Sharma, Tony Simpson, Pat Smith, and Helen Watson who have all, in their own inimitable way, been 'rooting' for me; as have my mother and father, Jean and Len Edwards, who deserve more than words.

CONTENTS

LIST OF PLATES

LIST OF FIGURES

LIST OF MAPS

LIST OF TABLES

NOTE ON TYPOGRAPHY

The study highlights commonly used Bacup idioms, particularly of kinship. They are marked in the text in italics. There is, however, an awkwardness in constantly highlighting culturally significant expressions in English when English is also the language of analysis. For ease of reading usually only the first occurrence of each such term has been italicized.

No typographical distinction has been made between quotations and passages of autobiographical detail; the difference will be clear from the context.

PART 1

In Social Anthropology

1

Familiar Places

BACUP is at the head of the Rossendale Valley, in the north of England. It is surrounded on three sides by higher moorland, which means that to travel in any direction from the town centre, except west along the valley, is to travel uphill. The road to the west meanders along the valley floor to Rawtenstall, the seat of local government, while to the east it climbs over the moors into Yorkshire. To the north, the road travels over the moors past the source of the river Irwell before descending onto the Burnley plain, and to the south it climbs to cross the border between the counties of Lancashire and Greater Manchester. A ribbon development of dwellings punctuated by shops, public houses, and small factories lines the radial roads and it is difficult for the untutored eye to discern distinct localities sometimes named by residents as if they were separate villages and at other times as if they were neighbourhoods of Bacup. When one travels north through the sprawling conurbation of Greater Manchester and looks down on Bacup from its southern boundary, it appears to be discrete and self-contained. I imagined initially (and naïvely) that its perimeter, or at least some of it, being discernible would contain the study, providing, as it were, its own limits. But the English are adept at conceptualizing boundaries, and where they locate them, and what and whom they enclose within them, depends on the view taken and the purpose for taking it.

An Unfamiliar Home

After paying a visit to the two estate agents in the main street (the only businesses flourishing in the town, I was told on many an occasion after that day, are estate agents and building societies), I went to the Teapot, one of several cafés in the town centre. My idea was to have something to eat and sift through the papers I had collected which I hoped would contain, amidst the hype, pertinent and relevant detail about suitable accommodation in Bacup. The front door of the café opens onto the main road and its back door onto the market. It is self-service. The menu is written in chalk on a large blackboard mounted on the wall opposite the counter and cash-till, where customers place and pay for their order before finding a table. I realized on subsequent visits to the café that the high level of noise is partly due to the way in which friends and relatives aid each other by dividing between them the labour of securing a table and ordering at the counter (it is no mean feat to negotiate shopping bags, infants, and pushchairs around fixed formica tables with attached chairs), so that questions and responses are shouted backwards and forwards across the

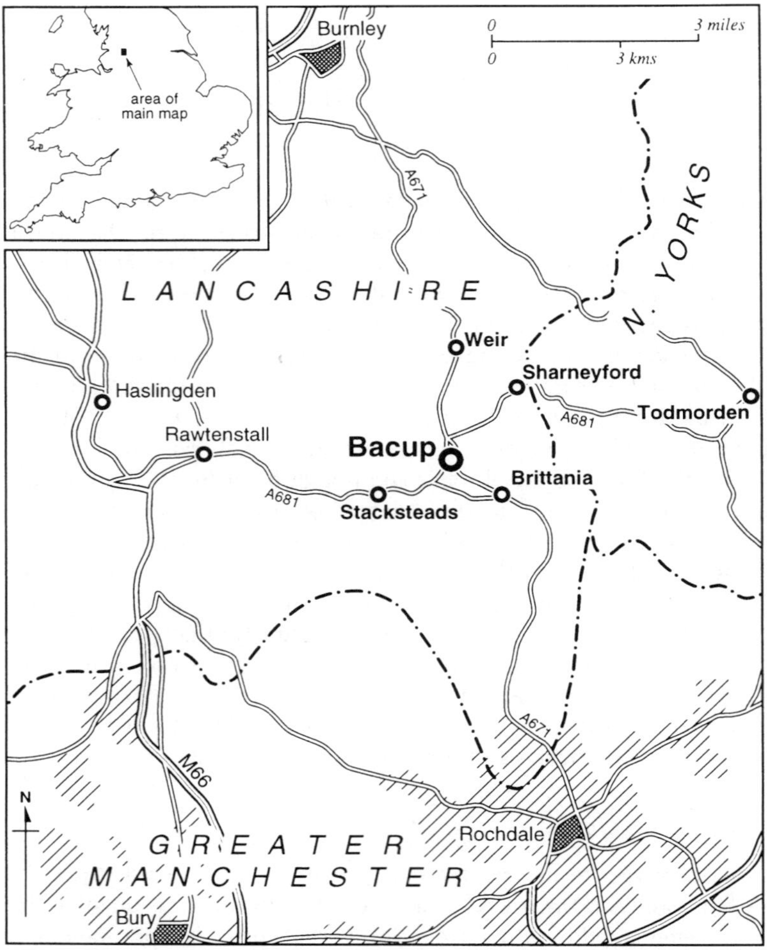

Map 1. Bacup and satellite villages

café between table and till. The blackboard is covered in writing which presents different combinations of all the items that constitute a full breakfast (eggs—poached, boiled, fried, or scrambled—bacon, sausages, tomatoes, toast, black pudding, fried bread, mushrooms); a variety of pies and puddings with or without peas, gravy, and potatoes (chips or boiled); a selection of sandwiches (toasted or not); tea or coffee (in a mug or a cup) and various cold drinks, including Vimto (in a glass or a can).[1] Two elderly women greeted me when I

[1] A sweet, blackcurrant-coloured cordial, without the flavour of fruit. Original Vimto is diluted with water, but a more recent version has it in a can and carbonated.

walked into the Teapot and, as I waited at the counter to be served, one recommended the steak and kidney pudding, which I ordered with peas and gravy and a mug of tea. I thanked the woman for her recommendation and she assured me I had made the right choice. She and her companion watched me as I spread the house advertisements out on the table and read them as I ate. After a while, the same woman asked me where I was from. I told her I lived in Manchester and that I wanted to come and live in Bacup for a while. She said she and her friend were *Bacup born and bred*[2] and they always had their dinner together on Thursdays, which was why they were there.[3] After telling them I was trying to find a house and, in a somewhat tentative and vague manner, explaining my intentions—'to study and write about Bacup'—the other woman, who had thus far said nothing, remarked: 'We used to live in back-to-backs'. She looked at me and, after a pause, went on: 'You probably don't know what they are, do you?'

In that one question, an assessment was formulated of my age and the social class from which I hailed: I was deemed both too young and too 'posh' to have lived in a back-to-back. It also marked, although I did not realize it at the time, a distinction between what is perceived as an idiosyncratic Bacup and a bland metropolis (a similar distinction to that sometimes made in anthropology between the societies it studies and the societies from which its readership is mainly drawn). This woman's comment on back-to-backs was as much a strategy of differentiation as a statement of fact.

The women, Mrs Marion Downs and Mrs Hilary Hardcastle, went on to describe back-to-backs.[4] They spoke of streets of them, such as those found in an area of town called Plantation Back, which had been three dwellings high with the basement row below ground level and built into the hillside. These streets, like those in other areas of town such as the Irish Back were like 'warrens', they told me, overcrowded, dark and narrow with 'piles and piles' of houses all on top of one another. They described rows of 'one-up-one-down' dwellings which had two rooms: 'one-up' for sleeping in and 'one-down' for everything else, and I was told that working members of many of these households used to have to go to bed, like they went to the factory, in shifts. Finally they described how the toilets were located at the end of these rows and the way in which they were cleaned, in turn, by women (sometimes children) from each house.[5]

[2] I place common Bacup idioms in italics at the first occurrence; see preliminary Note on Typography.

[3] I retain the Bacup (and more broadly English working-class) designation of a meal in the middle of the day as dinner. Tea is eaten in the early evening, and supper is a snack before bed.

[4] Back-to-backs in this part of Britain comprise terraced (connected) houses which have adjoining back and side walls. Consequently each dwelling, apart from those at the end of each row (where communal toilets were originally located), shares a dividing wall with the dwelling to the back and to each side and has a front entrance only (see also Dennis, Henriquez, and Slaughter 1956; Frankenberg 1966).

[5] The cleaning, or not, of communal toilets was a publicly available indicator of the moral worth of each household and women were, and still are, the moral guardians of the house and its relationships.

Mrs Hardcastle rightly surmised that I had neither lived in a back-to-back nor knew what one was. Her Bacup identity is secured in her own knowledge not only of what back-to-backs are but also in her experience of having lived in one. Yet despite the pride she expresses in this knowledge, in late-1980s Bacup back-to-backs are neither coveted nor prestigious dwellings. The coy descriptions of them as cosy and desirable 'cottages'—a favourite idiom of estate agents—allure only *incomers* (such as me) and leave Bacup people unmoved. Nevertheless, over the time I spent in Bacup, back-to-backs came up frequently in conversation (despite there being few still standing), as did particular neighbourhoods such as Plantation Back and Irish Back (despite their having been cleared and renamed in the 'slum-clearance' programmes of the 1960s). I had to rethink my initial image of back-to-backs as an obsolete form of housing belonging to the past and therefore irrelevant to the contemporary anthropological exercise, not least because they feature prominently on the present-day conceptual landscape. They bring to mind an industrial past and a harsh environment which is said to have *moulded* a particular and idiosyncratic Bacup character. Back-to-backs act to differentiate between a unique Bacup with contours, and a bland metropolis without features.

As a postscript to my pre-fieldwork encounter with Mrs Downs and Mrs Hardcastle, I bought a small back-to-back not long after our first conversation.[6] After I moved in, they came for tea. Back-to-backs did not come up in our conversation; they no longer served to differentiate Bacup folk from what are perceived to be middle-class incomers, or so I thought. But looking back, they made it clear they thought I had made a mistake and suggested I had bought a 'pig-in-a-poke'[7]—a sentiment echoed by a number of Bacup people, including many of my neighbours, during the next year. I was told over subsequent months, in no uncertain terms, that a Bacup person would not have bought that particular house. My interlocutors knew that only an ignorant incomer without any general knowledge about this kind of house, or any specific knowledge about this particular house, would have been tempted. They knew my putting in a damp-proof course was pointless, and my getting a local builder to knock a hole through a two and a half foot stone wall, in order to put in a window, was folly. Everybody, they told me, knew that this particular house had dry rot and had

[6] It was less expensive and easier for me to buy rather than to rent a house in 1987. There were several advertised for less than £7,000. These were small back-to-back houses, in relatively poor states of repair, and several housed squatters. There were comparatively few houses, and fewer flats or apartments, for rent. Many owners of back-to-back or terraced houses (some of which had been inherited) were unable or unwilling to invest in rendering them habitable for renting out. My intention was to put a habitable house back into a Bacup housing pool, without financial profit, after the completion of fieldwork. I was unaware, at the time, that few Bacup people, if they had a choice, would choose to live in a back-to-back.

[7] A pig in a poke (pocket): a blind bargain, as of a pig bought without being seen (*Chambers Concise Dictionary* 1988). However in Mrs Downs and Mrs Hardcastle's opinion, I clearly did not get a bargain.

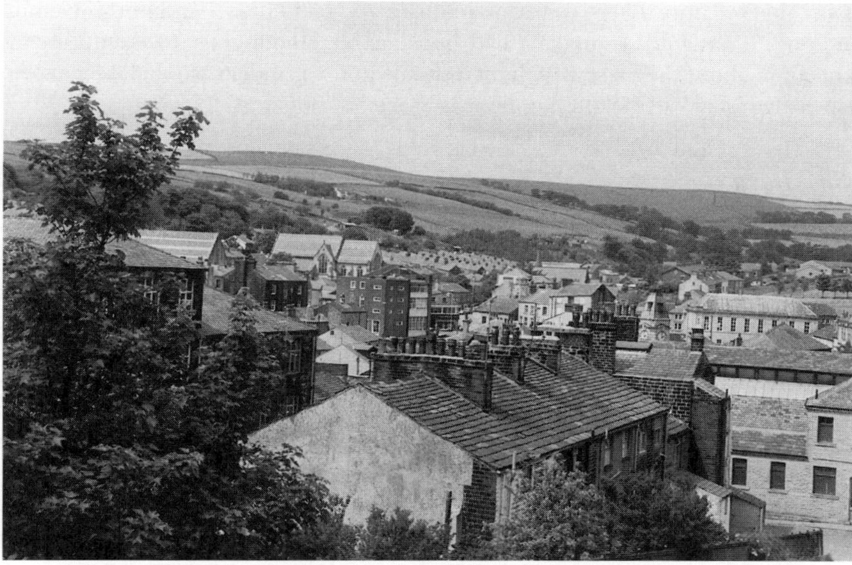

PLATE 1. Bacup

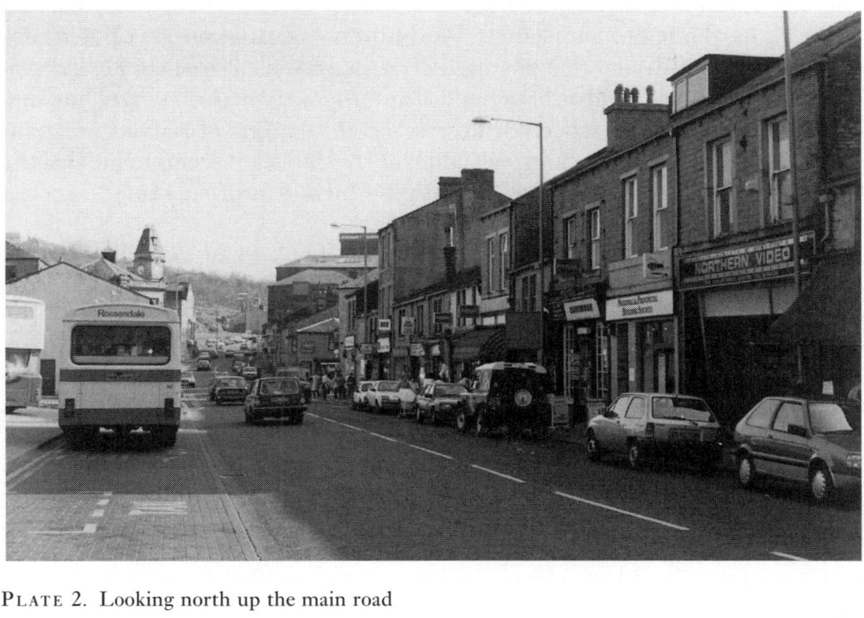

PLATE 2. Looking north up the main road

always been damp. There were good houses and bad houses, and nothing could be done, I was told, to make a bad house good. 'Belonging' to Bacup means 'knowing' about the place which includes its houses, and, as we shall see, expertise is a corollary of belonging, be it to places or persons.

Why Bacup?

I am often asked, 'Why Bacup?' A question which requires me, I always think, to identify some significant or special feature that makes it a suitable focus for anthropological interest. The accidents and vagaries of why would-be social anthropologists come to work in the places they do are often filtered out of written accounts. Fieldwork outside Britain might generate a similar kind of curiosity among non-anthropological audiences; perhaps the question, 'Why Papua New Guinea?' is asked, but it seems peculiarly irrelevant to anthropologists. Non-Western localities are deemed axiomatically of anthropological interest and legitimate arenas of study. If such a question is asked of the student, say of Papua New Guinea, then it seems to require an answer which relates the locality to theoretical concerns of the anthropologist. Further criteria explaining why Deri, Ocongate, or Mulungushi, for example, are appropriate places in which to carry out anthropological fieldwork need not be provided; that they exemplify, represent, or constitute particular Papua New Guinean, Peruvian, or Zambian cultures is sufficient. Perhaps this bias reflects a particular view of what ought to be the legitimate subject for anthropological attention. But it also exemplifies a world-view that not only acknowledges but also celebrates a diversity of social worlds. And although social anthropology may no longer buy into the idea of discrete and separate cultures, and the dangers of reifying and concretizing the concept have been well and truly rehearsed, it seems to me that the question, 'Why Bacup?' requires an answer which identifies a claim to special status.

I usually point to the accidental and adventitious when describing how I came to work in Bacup and emphasize that I knew little about the town before living there. My initial proposal for postgraduate research was to work in the north of England in an urban, post-industrial region. I was led to Bacup partly through pragmatism in the sense that housing was available[8] and it was close enough to Manchester to allow for a flurry of visits to secure accommodation and a school place for my son, who was 9 years old at the time.[9] But there are

[8] Nigel Rapport (1993: 55), in his evocative account of communication among residents (including himself) of Wanet, not too many miles from Bacup, writes of wanting to work in south Lakeland or the Forest of Bowland but of how he could not find affordable rented accommodation in a village which was not one of the many 'dormitory cum second home retreats, emptied of an indigenous population, inhabited by urbanites and deserted in winter'. His 'luck', he says, changed when he found Wanet.

[9] My very first visit to Bacup was with two sociologists at the University of Manchester who were carrying out research to the north of the city and who generously offered to show me around the area in which they were working. Looking at the map, I asked them to return to Manchester via Bacup. I am indebted to Liz Stanley and Fiona Poland for ferrying me on that first occasion to Bacup.

overriding intellectual and political concerns generated at particular historical moments which make the need for certain kinds of research apparent. Hence, while I might point to pragmatism and accident in going to work in Bacup, neither are devoid of history.[10]

Ronald Frankenberg (1990 [1957]: 166) writes of the accidental and unpredictable series of events which led him to carry out research in North Wales, and argues they coincided with theoretical concerns of social anthropology at the time.[11] Theoretical questions generated within the discipline itself, he writes, required the study of 'industrial society in its spatial residential aspects', consequently anthropology itself needed, at that point, to 'come home'. Such reasoning might be considered as no more than retrospective legitimation, but I want to argue that we are, for different reasons, at another point in the development of British social anthropology when it needs to come home, although it could be said it never left.[12] The pervasive and relentless reflexive exercise, often characterized as a feature of postmodernism, but with obvious antecedents (e.g. Bowen 1954; Powdermaker 1966; Briggs 1970; Favret-Saada 1980), has seriously and fruitfully scrutinized the way in which anthropological knowledge is itself generated. The enterprises of, for instance, writing ethnography (e.g. Clifford and Marcus 1986), doing anthropological fieldwork (e.g. Rabinow 1977), or inventing culture (e.g. Wagner 1975), have become an integral part of the anthropological subject of study (and see contributors to James, Hockey, and Dawson 1997). But a reflexivity which only scrutinizes the practice of anthropology itself is hardly broad enough. Cultural perspectives which generate the enterprise of social anthropology are revealed in the anthropological scrutiny of Britain: Brazilians doing anthropology in Brazil may, as George Marcus and Michael Fischer (1986) aver, be doing a different anthropology to the British in Britain but, as Marilyn Strathern (1987: 31) remarks, whether they are 'at home' or not depends on whether they share with those they study the same techniques of organizing 'knowledge about themselves'.

[10] My own desire to carry out anthropological fieldwork in Britain was fuelled by the fact that I had lived for the most part outside Britain between 1973 and 1981 and by a conviction that if social anthropology were as productive and illuminating as I had begun to imagine then this would be demonstrated in its insights into post-industrial, class society.

[11] In the second edition of *Village on the Border* Frankenberg gives a description of how he came to work in Wales in the early 1950s. He describes with wit and candour, how, in an era fraught with acute anti-Semitism, he was unceremoniously refused entry to St Vincent and then deported from Barbados after ten days under surveillance in a beach hotel. He was back in Manchester within six weeks of leaving, four of which had been spent at sea. He was dispatched first to South Wales, where relatives of his wife lived, and then to North Wales, where his supervisor could keep an eye on him and where he could find a Welsh-speaking village. For Frankenberg his being 'sent home' from the West Indies is of scant significance to the fact that anthropology needed at that point to 'come home'. Time has rendered the story safe enough to tell, as it has also mitigated the need to disguise the village.

[12] A flurry of anthropological studies in Britain during the 1950s including Firth (1956); Firth, Hubert, and Forge (1969); Frankenberg (1990 [1957]); Bott (1957 [1971]); and Young and Willmott (1957), has been followed by a small but steady flow: e.g. Emmett (1964); Ennew (1980); Strathern (1981); Cohen (1987); Rapport (1993); Macdonald (1997); Green (1997).

A scrutiny of anthropology as itself a cultural exercise, while exciting some scholars (e.g. Herzfeld 1987; 1992), is regarded with scepticism by others (e.g. Gellner 1992). One concern expressed is that the ability of the discipline through detailed and sustained fieldwork to describe and analyse the minutiae and intricacies of everyday lives is compromised in a stubborn focus on reflexivity. Such a concern is of course well founded if, by making explicit cultural concepts which inform the anthropological exercise, or in focusing solely on the cultural activity of creating ethnography, the richness and complexity of everyday life of those under study is, if not obscured, at least demoted. But this is not an inevitable outcome, nor is it the prerogative of a so-called postmodern reflexivity. A recognition that anthropologists and those they study share certain understandings of the social world in which they find themselves and which they constantly refashion, need not detract from analysis of the imponderabilia of everyday life and the political, economic, and historical trajectories in which it takes place. Scrutiny of Western social life, albeit one version of it, has the ability to shed light on the anthropological enterprise itself, just as a focus on premisses which inform the anthropological exercise has the ability to reveal wider cultural preoccupations.[13] Ethnography of Britain has the potential both to add to an understanding of the social milieu it studies and to reveal preoccupations that inform a British tradition of anthropology.[14] It implicates rather than ignores the richness and complexity of everyday life.

If an ethnographic study in Britain is also potentially a study of the premisses which have informed British social anthropology, then it is also a study of the process whereby conceptual connections are made by anthropologists and non-anthropologists alike. I was reassured (albeit temporarily) by a Bacup which appeared to be separate from the nearby conurbation, and I imagined that being able to see the physical boundaries of Bacup would help provide conceptual boundaries to the study; these illusions together with the question, 'Why Bacup?' draw on cultural understandings which this book addresses; cultural understandings which applaud distinctiveness and crave interconnectedness. My interest is in the ways in which the two are held together. I wish to trace resonances between ways in which Bacup residents at the end of the twentieth century and I myself, born in Liverpool, a resident of Manchester, and a British-trained social anthropologist, order and create the social worlds we share.

[13] Okely (1996) argues that anthropologists have too readily used the idea of a unitary and monolithic West in order to create a contrast for their 'micro-field study abroad'. The 'West' in these constructs reflects either their own childhood and educational experiences, or an uncritical ideology which ignores diversity. I do not wish to ignore diversity, difference, or specificities, but I am interested in the similarities in processes through which diversity and similarity are elicited.

[14] In the words of Herzfeld (1987: p. x), 'an anthropology that makes an ethnographic problem of itself offers pragmatic insights into the social worlds that it examines and to which it belongs' and, 'Taking anthropology itself as an ethnographic object is both a logical consequence and a valuable tool of a discipline that claims above all to be comparative' (ibid. 3).

At Home in Anthropology

With its sustained focus on a particular locality or social group over time, anthropology explicates connections between different spheres of social life. This is no less true whether the society under study is far from or near to the place of origin of the anthropologist. I do not intend to add more to the debate on, or defence of, anthropology 'at home' which, to my mind, has generated enough words. Needless to say, I disagree with those who adhere to a notion that anthropology at home is an oxymoron because anthropological knowledge is generated, by its nature, through epistemological unfamiliarity.[15] For the anthropologist in an unfamiliar setting, so the argument goes, it is through learning to participate (becoming sociable) that cultural understandings are learnt. The recording and the recalling of the process of becoming sociable is the raw material that, reworked and recontextualized, becomes the ethnography. The anthropological endeavour has been defined, crudely, as representing the unfamiliar (other) in terms that can be apprehended by a predominantly Western readership (us) (Marcus and Fischer 1986; Clifford and Marcus 1986). But this suggests that an anthropology of the so-called West is always about the familiar; which is of course far too simple a caricature (see also Shanklin 1985) and it begs the same old question of what is to be counted as (un)familiar, and for whom (Powdermaker 1966).

To participate in a shebeen in Manchester and then a game of croquet on a lawn in Windsor would require, for many of us, an adaptation in behaviour and language with a sensitive negotiation of appropriate manners.[16] Each context requires, at the very least, its own forms of etiquette, terms of endearment, appropriate dress, expressions, and vocabulary of enjoyment. Each of us may be socially inept in an unfamiliar social setting, say and wear the wrong thing at the wrong time, act indiscreetly, often unintentionally and sometimes despite ourselves, whether we consider ourselves to be 'at home' or 'abroad'. Gaucheness is neither a privilege of fieldwork nor does it only occur at cultural boundaries (see also Wolcott 1995). There is something unhelpful, it seems to me, in perpetuating the notion that there is an anthropology at home, which then requires, as its counterpart, an anthropology elsewhere. We need to focus attention instead on the way in which certain items of information come to be of anthropological interest—to tease out some of our reasons for homing-in on certain things and not others—and this requires more than a methodological reflexivity. This book presents ethnographic detail about a small town in the north of England. It focuses on idioms of kinship as they emerge in conversation about such things as the past, local government, new

[15] See e.g. Bloch 1988.

[16] Travelling with Traveller Gypsies, Okely (1996: 42) experienced what she calls 'a profound alienation' when moving along familiar roads, visiting towns she knew, and speaking with people of what she identifies as her own background and social class.

reproductive technologies (NRT), and *trouble.* And anthropology is at home in kinship.

Indigenous Experts

I began fieldwork before the self-conscious activity of doing research began.[17] From Bacup perspectives, I was an incomer, ignorant and requiring certain services. In the process of finding somewhere to live, I was helped and advised and, at the same time, assessed and evaluated. My very first meetings and conversations in Bacup foreshadowed and contained many of the themes which I address here (which is perhaps why I remember them); at the time, however, I considered many irrelevant to the task at hand. What appeared to be Bacup residents' overriding concern with the past—their memories of back-to-back houses, their stories about *th'owd characters*,[18] their insistence I speak with the local historians as 'they know all there is to know about Bacup'—seemed to me, then, to be marginal to what was truly of anthropological interest. Yet while much of the information given to me at that time only attained its salience in retrospect, incidents and conversations are vivid in my memory. My first meeting with Mrs Downs and Mrs Hardcastle, who were to become my friends and associates, is but one example and it highlights the difficulty in recognizing what is of ethnographic interest when anthropologists turn their attention to people and places which are to a lesser or greater degree familiar.

When I moved to Bacup in August 1987, tradespeople, shopkeepers, builders, workers from the gas, electricity, and water boards, as well as neighbours and mothers at the school gate, told me what I should know about the town. They told me where to go and where not to go; who to speak to and who to avoid. While I explained, in varying degrees of detail, my intention (to write about Bacup), my interest (in services[19]) and described, more or less explicitly, what I wanted to do (talk to people) and what I was hoping to achieve (a Ph.D.), people made sense of my endeavour in all kinds of different ways. They decided for themselves where my interests lay, and provided me with unsolicited information on those things they thought useful. They formulated their own ideas about what specific things I might be interested in, for example, trouble, unemployment, local politics, the past. Many reconfigured my role as 'finding out' about Bacup: an idiom which connotes a process whereby its true nature, through work, can be revealed (a point to which I return). At the same

[17] My sense is that the growing genre of texts on how to do research and in particular those with a focus on ethnography, attempts to purify the process and encourages an underestimation of information offered and received (and sometimes ignored) before and after research 'proper' begins and ends.

[18] The old characters (see Ch. 6).

[19] I defined services broadly, thinking initially of things like housing, education, health, and social services. Bacup residents defined and talked about services both more broadly and more specifically and they included formal and informal organizations and those things thought to belong to Bacup such as its public houses, churches, and factories.

time the people with whom I spoke expressed different degrees of interest and incredulity over my project. At times, I felt a palpable suspicion that I was connected to some sort of bureaucracy responsible for some sort of surveillance, while at other times I felt an obvious uninterest in my motivation as a researcher but a keen curiosity about my personal relationships and family history. Bacup residents with whom I worked expressed either positive interest or criticism of the enterprise of being a student or a social anthropologist, and if they appeared uninterested in that aspect of my identity, they were often interested in another, for example, my status as an incomer, from Liverpool, a single parent, or just single.

I joined the Bacup Natural History Society (known locally as the Nat), and went to the Unemployed Workers' Centre (UWC), as advised. I attended and participated in meetings of local branches of the Women's Guild, the Labour Party, and Greenpeace. I visited the Conservative Club, the Working Men's Club, and the Baptist church. I accompanied my son to his school, to his recently made friends, to the swimming baths, and, when he could be persuaded, to cub-scouts. I was an avid attender of jumble sales, bazaars, church fêtes, and the blood donation sessions at the Leisure Centre. I hung around the youth clubs, and was invited, and invited myself, to pubs, clubs, and dart matches. I journeyed with residents to hospitals and supermarkets as well as on out-of-town visits to their friends and relatives, and I spent a great deal of time in people's homes, drinking copious amounts of tea, and in pubs, drinking too much beer.

In a list of activities, fieldwork appears a fairly mundane series of events, possibly a little manic and maybe somewhat orchestrated. But the lives of the people who feature in ethnography are far from mundane. Fieldwork, in whatever part of the world, allows glimpses of lives lived. The intrigue and complexity of social relationships, people's humour and anger, as well as their hospitality and antipathy, are missing from inventories of research activities. A list of methods, or an account of the way in which data is recorded, or a reflection on the anxieties of representation, contribute little on their own to a discussion of the way in which anthropological knowledge is generated; which is not to say they are worthless activities but that reflexivity is as much a theoretical as a methodological issue. If we take seriously the idea that information is generated through and in social interaction, then a further move to tease apart shared concepts and ways of knowing the social world is required. When anthropologists and their informants frame their social worlds in similar ways, whether those worlds are, in terms of certain social identities, thought to be commensurable or not, it behoves us to reveal how observations that come to be seen as information are generated. In making explicit the process whereby the familiar is construed as such, as well as the way in which the familiar is then garnered to the anthropological enterprise, the process of knowing becomes central to ethnographic description. In this sense, it is the process by which the fieldworker comes to know which provides grist for the anthropological mill, rather than that which is eventually known which is always contingent and available for all to know.

I carried a notebook with me everywhere and eventually overcame, although not always, an initial reluctance to take notes during my conversations in Bacup. I was acutely self-conscious, particularly at the beginning of fieldwork, of what I imagined to be the intrusive nature of writing about people I met daily, in their presence. Yet many of the people with whom I worked regarded note-taking as an appropriate activity for a researcher. They expected me to take seriously, and therefore record, what they were saying. While they may have agreed, however, that their own observations were relevant, they would not necessarily have thought the same of mine. Part of the problem, as I perceived it, was that no matter how explicit I was about my role as anthropologist and no matter how explicable it was to Bacup residents that I should be interested in Bacup and consequently take notes, my notebooks recorded not only what they said (partially), but also my observations on what they said and on the settings in which they said it—they already contained an analysis, however rudimentary.[20] My co-conversationalists could not know what I was writing.

I gradually came to feel less anxious about taking notes,[21] but my discomfort returned when I started to write up the research. I was writing for an audience which included those about whom I was writing and who, again, could not have predicted what I might write. They were also likely to have their own interpretation of events which would not, necessarily, tally with mine.[22] In the meantime, several Bacup friends had already engaged in their own critique of social anthropology: wondering out loud, in my presence, why an anthropologist would want to study Bacup, and asking me, provocatively, whether I thought 'the natives' interesting. Marilyn Greaves, a Bacup woman in her mid-fifties, looked up anthropology in a dictionary which defined it as 'the study of humans zoologically'; she vowed never to speak with me again. Fortunately her friend intervened and told me why Marilyn had lost interest, and I scrambled to discredit the definition and the impression she had formed of anthropology.[23]

[20] This has interesting and important implications for research with colleagues that crosses disciplinary boundaries where different ideas about the status of data and the uses to which they can be put are brought to bear. In an era when data is coded as information and thus transferable, we need to be increasingly explicit about the status of fieldnotes.

[21] Mostly, of course, because of the kindness shown me in Bacup, and the assertion people made that they were helping me not the research.

[22] This reminds me of the discussion about carrying out anthropological research in a terrain already covered, dissected, and written about by scholars in other disciplines. It is suggested that this makes the anthropological task easy (Bloch 1988) or that it makes it difficult (Okely 1996) but, whichever it is (if either), the voices of other scholars are 'troubling presences' (Strathern 1991: 22).

[23] I like to think I succeeded as Mrs Greaves started a part-time evening class in sociology the following year and told me she would have chosen social anthropology had it been offered.

I returned to Bacup in the autumn of 1990 to carry out further fieldwork,[24] this time with an explicit interest in new reproductive technologies (NRT).[25] 'Things like egg and sperm donation, surrogacy, *in vitro* fertilization (IVF)', I explained. Initially I visited people I already knew. I spoke first with friends I had maintained contact with over the intervening two years and resumed contact with other residents I had not seen since leaving the town in 1988. In Bacup I was passed on to those who it was thought could help me and I was introduced to relatives, friends, colleagues, and neighbours in the process of fieldwork. In my second fieldwork, I already knew many of the people with whom I spoke and we shared a certain knowledge about the town and about each other. We drew on this knowledge, leaving certain things implicit and building on what we perceived to be shared assumptions. Many people with whom I spoke seemed intrigued by NRT, they raised their own questions and talked at length about implications of, and possibilities presented by, technological intervention in conception. They did so with reference to their own lives and relationships as well as to what they knew about Bacup and its people, and to what they knew about me. In talking about NRT, Bacup friends and acquaintances drew on ideas they assumed we shared about, for example, how children are conceived and grown, and families created and sustained. They talked, amongst other things, about biology, genes, and roots, and told me about what constitutes a mother, a father, a parent, and a child. In thinking about NRT, they explored ways in which intimate social relations are forged and broken and how persons are related not only in the present but also to pasts and futures. Again they talked about the past: a past which included back-to-backs, factories, pubs, hills, churches, and other things perceived to belong to Bacup and to have moulded a particular Bacup character. My aim in what follows is to combine two different studies, carried out at different times, with ostensibly different foci, and to show how similar preoccupations emerged in both. My point is that new reproductive technologies can no more be plucked out of the social milieu which informs them and, in turn, is informed by them

[24] This was part of a collaborative research project with Eric Hirsch, Sarah Franklin, Frances Price, and Marilyn Strathern, funded by ESRC award number R000 232537. Selected findings from this research can be found in Edwards *et al.* (1999 [1993]).

[25] I use the term 'new reproductive technologies', or NRT, as shorthand for techniques of medically assisted conception, some of which are hardly new and some of which require little in the way of technology (see e.g. Stolcke 1988; Pfeffer 1992; McNeil 1993; Price 1994; Bateman Novaes 1998). It includes donor insemination (DI), *in vitro* fertilization (IVF) with or without donor gametes, and maternal surrogacy arrangements. My interest is not in an analysis of NRT in and of themselves, and others are better qualified than I to assess critically the impact of medical and/or technological intervention in conception on a specific population (see, amongst others, Stanworth 1987; Spallone and Steinberg 1987; Rapp 1987*b*; Spallone 1989, 1992; McNeil, Varcoe, and Yearley 1990; Inhorn 1993; Ragone 1994; Daniels and Haimes 1998), or to analyse textual and popular representations of NRT (e.g. Franklin 1990; Balsamo 1996; Hartouni 1997), or the ethics of reproductive medicine (e.g. Whiteford and Poland 1989; Bromham, Dalton, and Jackson 1990; Bromham *et al.* 1992; Purdy 1996). My interest is in the way in which people with no vested interest in technologies of assisted conception can talk about them. What understandings do they mobilise in order to explore their implications?

than any other social phenomenon. In order to understand the ways in which people make sense of innovation, in this case in human reproduction, we need ethnography.

Selected Pasts

Arriving in Bacup, I did not find myself alone in an unfamiliar setting but in the offices of estate agents, discussing the pros and cons of particular neighbourhoods as places to live and struggling to assimilate the hyperbole which constructs—I use the word advisedly—every dwelling in the lowest price bracket as a haven of cosiness and taste. I found myself pondering over the health of the housing market, and wondering what a 'buyer's market' meant. I sat in cafés drinking mugs of tea, poring over printed descriptions of 'attractive' and 'desirable' dwellings, while dreading the sight of yet another almost derelict house described on some glossy A4 sheet as 'in need of slight renovation'.[26] I found myself in primary schools asking teachers about their policy on bullying and special needs, to learn they have neither: neither, that is, a policy or bullying, nor indeed special needs. I found myself on the street talking to builders about the cost and necessity of putting in damp-proof courses which, they told me, were unlikely to eliminate damp but were as likely as not the only route to a mortgage, or about whether this or that house could survive without a new roof, new windows, or new wiring. But to an extent my narrative of arrival renders the familiar heroic. I differentiate myself from both those already there and those absent. Perhaps the genre of arrival story is itself a strategy of differentiation—to arrive, you have had to leave somewhere. By arriving you are not to be mistaken for those already there nor for those you left behind.

It has been argued that the 'arrival stories' which introduce ethnographic accounts of anthropologists serve to make explicit the authority from which they speak—'they were there' (Pratt 1986). Bacup residents also narrate stories of arrival; they speak of the arrival of themselves or their ancestors in the town and they do so in ways which make explicit their place in Bacup today: the position from which they speak. Many Bacup residents, often unsolicited, told me about when they or their family first came to the town and from where. In so doing they located themselves in Bacup both in time and in terms of social class. Through narratives of arrival they made explicit the social class from which they came. In telling me where they or their ancestors came from, when they arrived, and why, people created contexts which gave their subsequent ideas meaning.

A recent focus on anthropology and autobiography has fruitfully examined

[26] I dreaded even more the possibility of a repetition of being shown around a house by a gushing estate agent with an unenthusiastic owner saying little, only to discover later that the building society was about to repossess the house.

the relationship between personal histories and the kinds of project upon which anthropologists embark (see e.g. Okely and Callaway 1992; Hastrup 1995; Behar 1996; Edgar and Russell 1998). It is clear that aspects of social identity such as ethnicity, social class, gender, sexuality, and age play a part, to a lesser or greater degree, in the kinds of social relationships anthropologists forge (or not) in the field. Such social attributes, it is also assumed, will influence the questions they pursue and the conclusions they reach (see also Okely 1996). The bits of autobiographical detail with which I was presented in Bacup were integral to, and made up the background for, what people wanted to say about, amongst other things, the town, its people, its services, and NRT. It was both beside the point—the context for the 'important bits'—and the point itself. In snippets of autobiography people advised me on the authority from which they spoke and the vantage point from which their ideas about all kinds of things would make sense. While autobiographical detail might reveal aspects of social identity and provide clues as to why people are interested in the things they are, of interest are the bits of the past, like the bits of social identity, which get selected as relevant.[27]

I am the eldest of six children born within eight years of each other to working-class parents who were both born in Liverpool, as were their parents. My mother traces her grandparents on *one side* to Yorkshire and on the other to Ireland, and my father traces his to Wales and Ireland. My mother was the youngest of five children and my father the eldest of seven. My mother's father was a coal merchant, a supporter of the local Orange Lodge, and a man who inspired more fear than affection from his wife and daughters. He spent a great deal of his time and money in the local pub, which caused my grandmother a great deal of distress, and eventually led to the bailiffs requisitioning the horse and cart with which he delivered coal. My grandmother took in washing to make ends meet and coped with what by all accounts was an oppressive domestic life. In 1939, my mother was 9 years old, her sisters were working, her eldest brother was in the Air Force and her other brother had been evacuated out of the city. Over the next four years, my mother attended school occasionally—in between air-raid warnings, helping her mother with the house and her father collect the coal money.

My father was born on the other side of Liverpool. His mother was Catholic, and according to all who mention the fact, devout. Her religion meant as much to her as it had done to her own mother. She had two ambitions that I know of: one was to visit Lourdes, and the other to live long enough to see the opening of the new Catholic cathedral in Liverpool. The first she managed, bringing back from Lourdes a phial of holy water which sustained her in the face of her husband's agnosticism and antagonism (my grandfather, it is said, refused to allow the priest to set foot over his doorstep), but the second eluded her and she died just months before the new cathedral was

[27] If autobiography is selective, biography must be doubly so. Biography, writes François Zonabend (1984), only yields its true meaning if it is placed in the social, economic, and historical context from which it springs The isolated life, she continues, not backed up by ethnographic enquiry, is like an empty shell. For Donna Haraway (1989), 'biography is woven into and from a social and political tissue'.

officially opened, although she could see it, almost finished, from her hospital window. As the eldest son, my father was drilled harshly on his responsibilities and duties by a father who was equally harsh on himself.

Both my parents left school at the age of 14, worked forty-eight hours a week in their first jobs, and presented their mothers with unopened pay packets on Friday evenings. They met each other in their early twenties and, despite stiff opposition from my mother's family, in particular her father and brothers, and little support from my father's family, they married. One major ambition of theirs, which they achieved against all odds, was to have a house of their own and to move their children (before we reached adolescence) out of the city. They accomplished both these things by moving to a town half-way between Liverpool and Manchester where housing was affordable and where they imagined their children would stand a better chance of not getting into trouble. They were more than aware of the stigma attached to big families. At 11 years of age, I thought the place to which we had moved the epitome of provincialism and spent most of my teenage years planning an escape.

Such snippets of autobiographical information do not explain why I am interested in the things I am. They do say something, however (albeit minimal), about my origins. Like many Bacup people with whom I worked, I too choose to make explicit my *background* in terms of social class and I do so in a narrative which dwells on the hard work and tenacity of my parents. I too desire to participate in the identity of my parents.[28] In the following chapters, I include autobiographical detail that Bacup residents think pertinent. They provide certain items of autobiographical information in order to establish the authority from which they speak. In telling me about themselves, they contextualize their ideas about, for example, Bacup, or NRT, or local services. They tell me about their origins and their ancestors, their residential and occupational histories, and their childhood. They theorize from what they know and make connections across different domains of social life; my interest is in trying to preserve some of the analogies they make. I do not intend to hive off certain narratives as 'personal histories' or 'life stories' to be analysed in their own right, but I do present selected and potted biographies to show the way in which Bacup residents ground their ideas in their own lives. They use themselves to create the context in which their ideas about Bacup, or the past, or NRT make sense.[29] I present some of the autobiographical detail they presume is relevant and attempt to re-present it in ways which reflect the language and manner in which it was told (see also Denzin 1989; Rosenwald and Ochberg 1992; Finnegan 1992; Personal Narratives Group 1989). It is inevitably selective. Autobiography is made up from permutations of accessible symbols, and biography is doubly permutated. The anthropologist of necessity makes further selections; transforming somebody else's autobiography in the light of her own preoccupations.

Autobiography is selective and people position themselves when they make

[28] I am grateful to Marilyn Strathern for this felicitous formulation of kinship.

[29] I am grateful here to Judith Monks (n.d.) who has made a sensitive and detailed analysis of the way in which people talk about their diagnosis of multiple sclerosis.

explicit certain connections and not others. The connections they make are not only to other people but to entities, such as factories, public and private houses. Selecting from all the elements that could constitute a past, a present, and a future, means not selecting others. There are not, however, infinite possibilities. The past may be reformulated when certain connections to kin, friends, lovers, colleagues, neighbours, and enemies are narrated, but that past is not infinitely plastic.

This book is predominantly, then, about people, places, and pasts by way of what people say, but in an attempt to include the ebb and flow and the aesthetics (Herzfeld 1987) of everyday life, I have attempted to place Bacup ideas in the context in which they arise. The following chapters are replete, then, with Bacup narratives: narratives about, for example, the past, origins, occupations, and intimate social relationships. Narratives, retold and reformulated, with recognizable and repetitive elements, and which include the bits of autobiographical detail that conversationalists think I should know. Narratives fashioned in interaction, often with the ethnographer, but not exclusively so (Abelman 1997).

The different perspectives, within Bacup, are organized through my perspective as an observer with an anthropological training and interest (see also Loizos 1992).The version I organize does not supplant, nor is it imposed upon, those versions it attempts to describe, but rather is produced for a different purpose (Holy and Stuchlik 1981; Gudeman and Penn 1982; Strathern 1987). Even if I reiterate the subjectivity of my account, I cannot deny that it is also an anthropological version of events. Anthropologists do not usually embark on fieldwork without prior preparation. Moreover, no matter how subjective their account, they draw on particular social science concepts to order and interpret the social phenomena with which they are faced; an anthropological interpretation is never purely the product of an idiosyncratic mind. In the same way, each interpretation of the social world that Bacup residents make, and within which they locate themselves, is informed by and draws on an archive of cultural knowledge, not in itself an entity but the raw material from which entities are conceived.

Culture: Too Much and Too Little

Britain in the 1990s is suffering from an overload of culture. The concept is used synonymously with 'lifestyle' and 'custom'. It can be attached to any social group or category to signify what are deemed to be characteristic practices and codes. Sunday newspapers devote sections to 'Lifestyle and Culture', and the culture of perhaps British Telecom specifically, or organizational culture generally, coexist with what are said to be minority or majority cultures.[30] At the time of writing this, a flyer was posted through my door advertising a care

[30] A phenomenon not confined to Britain: '[North] American society has become culture-conscious, almost to the point of a "culture cult" in civic society' (Eller 1997).

agency catering 'for the special needs of Ethnic Cultures'. An equation is constantly being made between a diversity of forms (be they bounded by variables such as class, ethnicity, or occupation) and a plurality of cultures. The ubiquity of the concept of 'culture' in contemporary British life, thereby, masks similarity (between) as well as difference (within) socially defined categories of person.[31] At the same time, scholars across different disciplines are wary, for good reason, of imputing the notion of culture to what they perceive as the diversity and plurality of British society, unless it is to reiterate its *multi*cultural nature, or to note the existence of a variety of subcultures, or perhaps to distinguish between working-class culture and middle-class culture. Yet each of these examples appears to be formulated from a position marked by the absence of culture: from an acultural baseline.

Bacup, thirty miles north of Manchester and, according to many residents, the heart and start of the industrial revolution, is often described as if it were remote—'the back of beyond', 'a backwater', 'cut off'. Those same idioms are used by Bacup people to describe satellite villages within its municipal boundaries, or a neighbourhood, or a cluster of streets. The idea of remoteness is as equally available to residents of Bacup as it is to residents of Manchester or Edinburgh, and it can work from inside as effectively as it can from the outside. And while clearly not all viewpoints are disseminated equally and some voices are louder than others, there is equal access to, and availability of, remoteness as a cultural concept. This concept is mobilized for particular reasons and acts as a means of differentiation. The idioms of remoteness that, for example, residents of neighbouring towns deploy to differentiate themselves from Bacup, are also mobilized within Bacup. Such means and processes of differentiation are not generated, then, within the confines of a particular locality nor in the confines of a particular mind. The process of inclusion and exclusion is an ongoing process, it is a 'constant cultural exercise' (Dening 1988) of the English. Ideas about distinctive cultures (e.g. working-class or gay), or distinct and distinctive communities, or unique persons, do not fix people in a community or a culture but themselves formulate communities and cultures.[32] They are models. The sense of differentiation imaged within and between communities constantly defines and redefines

[31] 'Of what, then, and how is this pressing sense of heterogeneity composed?' (Strathern 1992*a*: 30). And could it be that 'the apparent ubiquity of the emphasis on "cultural distinctiveness" highlights a cultural commonality' (Macdonald 1997: 9). There is a danger that the anthropologist with 'culture' as stock-in-trade and also carrying out fieldwork in a Britain that perceives a plethora of cultural forms conflates the indigenous model with the unit of analysis. It is clear that the idea of diversity itself, its reproduction and its greater or lesser emphasis, requires attention.

[32] I am reminded here of earlier attempts to conflate 'culture' with 'communicative community'; e.g. Michael Agar's study of the activities and language of urban heroin addicts in the United States rejects the notion of subculture, but argues that members of a communicative community 'communicate with each other in a manner not understandable to an outsider' (Agar 1973: 130). Language is but one, albeit a central, aspect of culture, in the same way as being a heroin addict is but one (albeit extremely significant) aspect of a person's life. Yet it seems to me likely, or at least possible, that the heroin users

'insider' and 'outsider', but who is an insider and who an outsider shifts according to the reason for delineating the distinction in the first place. Categories thus formulated are fluid and contingent, but congealed for particular purposes. From any partisan position, it is possible to concretize one possibility, or to solidify one set of connections.

If Bacup is hardly peripheral or remote to what is thought of, problematically, as 'mainstream' British culture',[33] it is none the less constantly described as if it were. I am interested in how to address the fact that similar preoccupations appear to emerge in Bacup as in, for example, the Western Isles (Ennew 1980), Wanet (Rapport 1993), or the Scottish Highlands (Macdonald 1997). Residents of all these places appear to be drawing on similar conceptual resources to categorize their immediate, but quite different, social worlds. What are we to do with the fact that similar idioms appear to link, however tenuously, people as seemingly disparate as Irish farmers (Arensberg and Kimball 1940), Welsh villagers (Frankenberg 1957; Emmett 1964), inhabitants of London (Firth, Hubert, and Forge 1969; Wallman *et al.* 1982; Wallman 1984), and its suburbs (Willmott and Young 1960)? What conclusions are we to draw from the observation that similar items of ethnographic interest are revealed in studies of localities as diverse as Ballybeg (Harris 1986 [1972]), Elmdon (Strathern 1981), and Whalsay (Cohen 1987)? Are we merely witness to what Ennew (1980: 121) describes as the imposition of a 'bland version of British culture'?[34] Whatever else Bacup is, it is not bland, and while I would not wish to deny or play down its idiosyncrasies and uniqueness, it is not peculiar either, despite what people say.

Cultural Critique?

The 1980s witnessed a call for cultural critique within anthropology, which although not original has been highly influential (e.g. Marcus and Fischer 1986). There is, to my mind, something slightly awry in this call which seemed to suggest that some cultures might be more open to critical analysis and

described by Agar are able to switch linguistic codes (or in Agar's term 'argots') when talking to non-heroin users, say their mothers, and using heroin is unlikely to encompass all aspects of identity. As Hymes (1974: 202) cogently observed over two decades ago: 'There is no way to analyse speech acts adequately without ethnography: no language is a perfect metalanguage for the acts that can be performed in it . . . For appropriateness is not a property of sentences and contexts. This holds a fortiori for the property of creativity, whether saying something new in a familiar setting, or something familiar in a setting that is new. At every turn, it almost would seem linguistics is wrestling with phenomena, and concepts, which turn out to entail relationships, only one pole of which is within linguistics' usual domain'.

33 David Schneider's (1997: 272) North American counterpart is 'mainline culture'.

34 Ennew (1980: 121) locates her study of Lewis, in the Western Isles, in the context of Britain as a multinational state within which 'distinct cultural forms coexist'. She argues that the consequences of not acknowledging the cultural specificity of the islands will result either in further depopulation, or in their assimilation into 'some bland version of "British culture"'.

available to suggested amendments by anthropologists than others. It seems that from some anthropological perspectives only certain, and certainly not all, cultures are a legitimate if not an obligatory focus of critique.[35] Is the development and maintenance of a critical awareness of the exploitation and abuses of power (not least in the academy itself) the same as sanctioning or somehow disallowing cultural understandings put to work by those who are the focus of anthropological study?

Some months after I completed my first fieldwork in Bacup and had returned to Manchester, I visited the Nat and took with me a video recording made during the last weeks of fieldwork.[36] On the video was film of an informal meeting of society members which showed members, including myself, sitting around the edge of the meeting-room drinking tea and chatting. One member recited a dialect poem and another told a story about one of th'owd characters, others reminded me of things they thought by now I ought to know, and others teased me about still not having gained access to a men's-only drinking club. I protested with blustery predictions that one day I would, and was told (with tongue in cheek) that even the Granada crew (all men) who had also been filming at the Nat had not been invited, and (still with tongue in cheek) perhaps I would get an invitation after I had lived in Bacup for twenty-five years. There is a great deal of laughter and a lot of talk on the film, but then there usually is at these weekly informal meetings. After seeing the film, Joe Smedley, a committee member whose self-appointed role over the past year had been to keep me in check and to remind me through gentle ridicule of my place as a junior in the society, commented (not harshly but with some admonishment) that I and my friends had probably had 'a right laugh listening to us local yokels'. I felt uncomfortable and unjustly accused. I was embarrassed by what I perceived to be a misreading of my motivations, and assured him that this was not the case.

Mr Smedley's remark bothered me and his comments, as they often did, made me think. I liked the film, not because it was a 'good ethnographic documentary'—it was not—but because I thought the footage flattered those it portrayed. I thought it had captured the warmth of people with whom I had worked: their humour and their eloquence. Mr Smedley's comment is partly referring to the distinctive Bacup dialect, obvious on the recording and which was, in fact, being celebrated and emphasized with pride on the film, but his remarks focus on what he knows, and on what he knows I know, to be the relationship between local dialects and social class in Britain. He suggests implicitly that I and my friends are middle class and will find the quaint ways of the working classes an amusing spectacle. Over the years since this incident, and

[35] So that when Bacup ideas, for example, and those of, say, academics (perhaps in the field of NRT) do not match, as co-cultural participants each assumes it their prerogative to question the other.

[36] In collaboration with, and with thanks to, Paul Henley at the Granada Centre for Visual Anthropology, Manchester.

after presenting papers and talks to different audiences both anthropological and non-anthropological, I understand better the response of Mr Smedley and my own duplicity. My rendering of Bacup does play up the wit of its characters and it does reveal the contradictions with which its residents make sense of their social worlds, but which are interpreted (as much by them as others) as idiosyncratic. I tap the rich seam of Bacup humour partly in my desire to captivate an audience. At the same time, I place comments and events from different times and different places alongside one another and reveal contradictions not apparent in the day-to-day run of events. As social anthropologists, we are warned and warn ourselves of the dangers in 'exoticizing' others. Trained to observe practices (religious and secular) performed by cultural participants, we listen to, watch, and read interpretations of, amongst others, teachers, journalists, colleagues, and students. We are taught to assume that people's activities have meaning, even if it is hidden or opaque. The people who feature in the narratives of anthropologists might be humorous and witty, but there are implicit rules about how to laugh with, not at them. Yet when it comes to those with whom we share ways of ordering the social world, in this case members of so-called mainstream English society, those rules are bent. Maybe there is an idea at play that people in non-Western societies think and act the way they do because of the influence of something tangible and worthy of study such as culture, whereas Englishness is an unmarked category: the baseline from which otherness is defined. There is a danger that we laugh at the ideas of, for example, Bacup people, or royal watchers (Rowbottom n.d.), or villagers of Wanet (Rapport 1993), because we think they are idiosyncratic, and as co-cultural participants we assume the prerogative of agreeing or disagreeing with our compatriots. But this begs the question again of what it is that makes some cultures and not others appropriate targets of anthropological critique.

The Bacup residents whose ideas I borrow theorize from what they know. They link different arenas of social life, drawing on one to explain another. My theorizing has also meant making analogies, but they are not always, or necessarily, the same ones my co-conversationalists would make. Mine are models of their models. The residents of Bacup whose theories I explore will, I think, agree with some and disagree with other of my interpretations. Different people will take issue with different things I have written, and more significantly with the topics and people I have selected to write about. My hope is that our engagement is couched in familiar Bacup ways, which means that no matter how vehemently we disagree on some things, there will be other things on which we just as vehemently agree.

2

Why Kinship?

MY original interest in carrying out anthropological fieldwork in the Lancashire town of Bacup was to study 'communication between providers and users of services'.[1] Given a diet of arid, turgid, and unpeopled kinship systems as an undergraduate student, I imagined kinship was the least of my interests, and was not, I have to admit, looking for it. But I was looking for social class; convinced I would find miscommunication at the interface of what I then crudely conceptualized as middle-class service-providers and their working-class clientele.[2] In 1987 and 1988, many Bacup residents seemed keen to talk about services, particularly with reference to local government. The already diminished manufacturing industry in the region was shrinking further and the weekly local newspaper reported, in almost every edition, the closure of one small business after another with its attendant job losses. There was little building going on in the town: a few new houses were being constructed but with private rather than state sponsorship; they were said to be affordable only by middle-class commuters moving to Bacup from 'the city'. The introduction of an iniquitous Poll Tax was imminent and many residents were thinking ahead to the hardship it would cause in an area of the country where the rateable value of property had until then been low, as had wages. In thinking about services, Bacup residents in the late 1980s talked about education, housing, health, and social services; they also talked about factories, shops, buses, churches, roads, public houses, informal organizations, and each other. They told me about Bacup: about its people and landscapes (past and present), its histories and geographies. I found class but not, of course, in the form of a simple reified opposition. Instead ideas about social class were contradictory, couched in euphemism, and, more often than not, implicit rather than explicit. In late-1980s Bacup, social class seemed to move in and out of focus. It was both relevant and irrelevant to the issue in hand. The same is true of kinship.

[1] My aim was to combine two pieces of research: one in a community in the north-west of England and the other in a public-sector organization in the city of Manchester. Rather than a study of communication between providers and users of services what emerged was a study of the way in which both providers and users of services draw on similar conceptualizations to order their different social worlds. The study ended up focusing more on similarity than on difference (Edwards n.d.; 1994).

[2] It could be said that serendipity led me to Bacup and to the Manchester branch of Shelter (a voluntary-sector organization providing housing advice and campaigning against homelessness), but to put it all down to chance would ignore the guidance, support, and push (sometimes in the opposite direction) of friends and mentors (both academic and non-academic) along the way.

Kinship: Absent or Absented

There has recently been a resurgence of interest in kinship from several anthropological perspectives. This rekindling of an old flame is partly inspired by the attention being paid to the enterprise of anthropology itself and, in particular, to the way in which it produces and legitimates its accounts of other cultures. It is argued that while kinship has featured large in the anthropological study of non-Western society, it has been relatively muted in studies of the industrialized West, and in particular of those societies in which social anthropology, as an enterprise, originated. Mary Bouquet (1993: 82), for example, notes that 'middle class' social anthropologists have been 'mainly indifferent to their own kinship', but have been 'fascinated by that of other people'. And Joan Bestard-Camps (1991: 9–11) writes:

> The anthropologist not withstanding the very sophisticated and developed theories of kinship which exist for other kinds of society will usually find that the study of kinship in our own society has been considered marginal and extraneous to the analysis of social organisation . . . The dichotomy which places kinship at the centre of theoretical analyses of 'primitive societies', but relegates it to the margins of the private domain in modern ones, can be regarded as an ideological prejudice rather than a positive anthropological science.

Kin connections in the West were all too often allocated and confined to personal and private domains of social life. Located in households and houses, they were said to pertain to domestic relationships which, in turn, were considered to be minor and marginal aspects of society. Confined, some might say relegated, to the home and the domestic sphere, kinship was perceived to be irrelevant to social organization. 'Kinship was seen as simultaneously dealing in (interior) primordial relations and as insignificant in its (exterior) social dimension . . . Kin connections did not seem sufficient to carry the entire imagery of social relations. They became internalised as "family"' (Strathern 1992*a*: 133). When kinship is regarded as a system in itself, and pertaining only to 'the family', it is also identifiable by what it is not and, for the English at least, 'the perspective of society seems to make kinship disappear' (ibid. 135, emphasis omitted). Indeed when anthropologists *had* turned their attention to kinship in England, it had proved elusive. A seminal study of middle-class kinship in East London (Firth, Hubert, and Forge 1969) confirmed Robin Fox's (1967: 14) earlier assertion (in the language of the 1960s): 'It is in the less conservative and more mobile middle classes that kinship now seems to be of little relevance beyond the level of parent-child relationships, and even these have a looseness about them which would shock many of our primitive contemporaries.' Other commentators on British society also took the view that, as a means of forming alliances in a hostile world, kinship was slowly but inexorably disappearing. And its demise was perceived to be further advanced amongst the English white middle classes than in white working-class, black, or otherwise ethnically identified communities. The social class which generated British social anthropology was the class for whom kinship was least relevant.

If studies of kinship in England tended to focus on 'the family' or 'the household', or on kin obligations and expectations, there were notable exceptions. Strathern (1981) analysed the way in which, in the Essex village of Elmdon in the 1960s, local discourses about kin connections and belonging (or not) to 'the village' provided an indigenous model of social class. Residents were identified and identified themselves as, amongst other things, 'real' Elmdon families or 'commuters', and such categories presented an image of immobility and mobility, respectively: 'The concepts of "villager" and "outsider" . . . bring together within one frame an association between geographical immobility, family and class, on the one hand, and on the other, mobility, personal networks and the individual who can alter social status' (p. 203).

Furthermore, a model of an immediate social world comprising discrete social classes fixed hierarchically in relation to one another, and with individuals who move up and down and between them is not, as Strathern (1981: 200; 1982*a*; 1982*b*; 1984) remarks, confined to Elmdon. It is a model found in wider society, as is the preoccupation with social class itself. For present purposes it is useful to think of this society as English (with all the caveats such a designation requires), and make note of its parochial and hegemonic status (see also Strathern 1993). But Bacup, while in England, is not only English. Its inhabitants trace their origins to places further afield than England, and preoccupations that emerge in Bacup are not exclusively Bacupian.[3]

Recent anthropological studies in Britain have tended to focus on kinship as one aspect, amongst others, of individuals or locally organized groups. Thus Anthony Cohen's evocative account of Whalsay, in Shetland, shows the way in which close association between islanders is maintained in the 'matrix of kinship, neighbourhood and crew' (1982: 38; 1987). And in acutely observed conversations between residents (including himself) of a Cumbrian village, Rapport (1993) highlights the numerous personae (one of which may be mother, father, spouse, or son) social actors mobilize in their everyday and daily interactions. I think it fair to say that it has been issues of identity, belonging, and local conceptualization of boundaries which have emerged as theoretically significant in recent ethnography of Britain, and indeed of Europe (Macdonald 1993). But kinship, I want to argue, is implicated in all of these. Identity and belonging, to both people and places, are aspects of persons which mobilize, and are mobilized by, kinship thinking. A view which identifies the dissolution of kinship in contemporary British society can only be

[3] The concept of Englishness itself, in both its inclusive and exclusive guises, emerges from the particular kind of kinship thinking that this book addresses.

maintained if kinship is perceived as a separate and discrete sphere of sociality, to be studied in its own right as a particular and domestic domain of social life.[4]

Kinship embraces connections people trace to each other through notions of shared substance, be it blood, genes, flesh, or bone; at the same time it places a greater or lesser emphasis, at different historical moments and in different parts of the world, on the creation and maintenance of social relationships through intimacies of care and effort. This is a potent combination with which to imagine relations of all kinds, not just the family kind. My interest in kinship is in the way in which it reckons relatedness not only to persons but also to places and to pasts. It is a mode of thought which orders and organizes immediate social worlds, and as such can neither be hived off as a discrete sphere of social life, nor be treated as one aspect amongst many of social organization. Instead it needs to be understood as modelling, and itself modelled on, cultural understandings of ways in which connections are made and unmade which permeate all domains of social life. This book addresses the tenacity of kinship at a time when, and in a place where, it is said to be disappearing.

Born and Bred Kinship

David Schneider's work has been significant in making stick the idea that the concept of kinship with which anthropologists have often worked cannot be universally applied (Schneider 1968; 1984; Handler 1995).[5] In the same year that *A Critique of the Study of Kinship* (Schneider 1984) was published Alan Barnard and Anthony Good (1984: 175) remarked: 'Since their own "emic" view of kinship is based upon a "biological" model, Western anthropologists have often found it hard to free themselves from its conceptual straightjacket.' More recently Ladislav Holy (1996: 144) reminds us that anthropologists were 'able to talk about kinship in different cultures as a system of social ties based on the acknowledging of relations resulting from engendering and bearing children because we projected onto them our culturally specific conceptualisations of what are universal "natural" facts with which all cultures have to cope even

[4] The same critique has been applied to reproduction (see Gonzalez Echevarria 1994). A. F. Robertson (1991: 3) writes: 'It is very difficult to observe objectively a process in which we are all so personally involved, which extends through and beyond our own limited lifespan, and which involves the private activities of masses of individuals. As a result our view of reproduction tends to be both very subjective and inert.' But the difficulty is perpetuated if reproduction is yet again confined to domestic domains and private activities.

[5] While not underestimating Schneider's contribution in interrogating what has constituted the anthropological analysis of kinship and in particular its grounding in biological facts (and see Bouquet 1993; Carsten 1995; 1997; Franklin 1997), it is profitable to recall other self-critiques of the anthropological notion of kinship, and in particular what Barnard (1994) refers to as 'the great debate' which focused on the relationship between biological and social kinship (see Needham 1971; Gellner 1973; Barnes 1973; and Barnard 1994 for a concise overview of the positions taken; and Kuper 1983 [1973] for Levi-Strauss's position). I focus on a culture which mobilizes a distinction between the biological and the social.

if they impose different cultural meanings on them'. My own interest here is in a society which mobilizes a distinction between the biological and the social, and which includes both in its delineation of relatedness. Rather than being *based* on the biological, however, the kinship on which I focus requires both the biological and the social: it emerges from an interplay between the two, rather than from the social elaboration of natural facts.

For Schneider, American kinship comprises both a normative and a symbolic system: it is made up of code of conduct (what people do and say they ought to do) and ideas of shared substance (symbolized in idioms of blood and increasingly genes).[6] He identifies a key distinction between the biological (derived from sexual intercourse) and the social;[7] and this distinction, he argues, is deployed in both Western indigenous thinking and in anthropological analysis. But how universally Western is the kinship he describes as American? It is clear from Bacup that what might be readily identifiable as biological and social are part of a kinship repertoire. That is, relatedness between persons is traced and symbolized in ways that might be described as belonging to the realm of the biological and the realm of the social; there are both given and forged elements in kin relations. But one (the biological) is not the substratum on which the other (the social) is constructed. Hence borrowing a Bacup idiom, but one not exclusively Bacupian, I call it Born and Bred kinship. This idiom juxtaposes what is perceived as an immutable place of birth, for example, with the effects of a variable upbringing.[8] To be born, say, in a particular place, does not axiomatically confer the status of belonging to that place, one also needs to be brought up in a particular way. In the same way as being biologically related to a person does not axiomatically make them kin. A claim of belonging (to persons and places) can be made through upbringing as much as birth. The juxtaposition of being born and being bred allows for kinship to be conceptualized through both or through either. A variety of ways, then, based on birth and/or breeding are mobilized in a constant process of including and excluding persons from social categories which are, in turn, reproduced in the process. To be born *and* to be bred, two interlinked and inseparable strands of the particular version of English kinship with which I

[6] Sylvia Yanagisako (1985) refuses to separate the symbolic from the normative, arguing that kinship relationships are structured by symbolic relationships and serve symbolic functions as well as social ones. For her, 'the material of cultural analysis is not the mental stuff through which individuals alone make sense of the world. Because it is an abstraction of discourse *among people*, a cultural system of symbols and meanings is no more located in people's heads than a social structure is located inside people's bodies' (p. 20, emphasis added). I have to agree with Yanagisako's emphasis on discourse and on meaning generated in the processes of social life, but agree with Strathern (1993: 3) when she writes: 'There is more to what people say than the view they are expressing. But there is also more to a cultural view than the analysis of genres.'

[7] And see Ingold (1990) for a commentary on the shift that has occurred in what the biological encompasses.

[8] I am grateful to Penelope Harvey and Celia Lury who prompted me to be more explicit about the unresolvable, and to Sharon Macdonald who made me think about the paradox of alternatives.

am concerned, each contain both symbolic and normative elements.[9] On the one hand, affective ties between kin develop, it is said, through the experiences of growing up, and growing up in a particular place, at a particular time, with particular people *moulds* a specific character. On the other hand, the facts of human conception (knowledge of the origins of gametes and the fixed genetic inheritances with which a person is born) are integral to the formation of a new individual. To be born and to be bred is to be constituted of relationships that are both affective ties *and* abstract connections between persons. In using the well-worn anthropological concept of kinship, I wish to go beyond a narrow dichotomy between shared 'natural' substance and affective ties, and to include connection with or without what are conceptualized as blood or genetic links (Edwards 1993; 1995; and see Carsten 1997).

My focus is on the way in which residents of a town in the north of England, who are predominantly white and, for the most part, trace their ancestors to other parts of the British Isles, put kinship to work. There is something arbitrary about linking the cultural understandings with which I am concerned here to an artificially created and bounded nation state. But at the same time it is not self-evident how generalizable such understandings are beyond England—to Britain, never mind Europe or the West. I am as reluctant to call it Western kinship, as I am English kinship.[10] If Born and Bred kinship is universally Western, it needs to be investigated rather than assumed. However, I hope that naming it Born and Bred rather than, say, English kinship deflects attention from the specificity of the locality and mitigates a tendency for the anthropology of Britain to focus on specific communities, sometimes at the expense of wider cultural generalization. To make my focus Born and Bred kinship is to acknowledge that my interest is in a particular, and some might say hegemonic, formulation of kinship which draws heavily on a model which includes the social and the biological and which is not confined to a geographical place—England—nor a population—the English—but appears to be a feature of what is loosely thought of as Western, or perhaps Euro-American thought.[11] This book is about the way in which certain sets of connections are

[9] I find it difficult to sustain Schneider's distinction between normative and symbolic systems. Since his formulation of this dual nature of (North) American kinship, a growing body of work has taken issue with his insistence on the separation of the normative and the symbolic in social life and, in particular, his suggestion that the symbolic system is located in the realm of cognition. He answers his critics in the additional material to the second edition of *American Kinship* by noting that 'there is always a social component, always a psychological component, always a biological component and always a cultural component in any social act' (1980: 126). Amongst others, Christina Toren (1993), in her continuing work on children's socialization, takes issue with theories of cognition which separate knowing from living. She argues that biological, cognitive, affective, and social processes are aspects of one another and, more important, aspects of active social persons (and see Irgold 1986).

[10] The first is too general and the second too specific.

[11] Bouquet (1993) writes of the differences between Portuguese and English kinship ideas. Hers has been one of the few attempts thus far to discern similarities and differences in kinship thinking across different European contexts, a task well overdue.

made visible while others are screened out, and the ability and tendency of 'the English' to conceptualize themselves as British, European, or Western, or not, and both to include and exclude their *roots* in, say, Ireland, Pakistan, or Jamaica as both relevant and irrelevant, are examples of this.

Assisting Kinship

In the title of this section I have two things in mind. First, NRT not only play a part in the creation of new individuals, they also create kinship; technologies of assisted conception assist kinship. Second, when the anthropological focus is on NRT ideas about kinship are elicited. Thus kinship is assisted (made explicit) by questions posed by the research.

All too often ways in which 'lay people' respond to NRT are likened to resistance and explained from certain perspectives as stemming from, at best, inadequate information and, at worst, ignorance.[12] From such a point of view if 'the public' were to be provided with more information, of the right kind, they would better understand procedures and imperatives of NRT and hence be less anxious about them.[13] A parallel argument is that, with time, 'ordinary people' will get used to technological innovation in human reproduction, and it is merely the new and novel that bothers them.[14] The birth of a child reproduces not only a new human being but also significant social relationships. Children are born (in English kin terms) as daughters, sons, brother, sisters, grandchildren, nieces, and nephews, they also create parents, grandparents, uncles, and aunts. They are also born to neighbours, townsfolk, colleagues, and friends. Human reproduction is always about more than conception, pregnancy, and birth, it is also always about wider social relationships, of family, places, and pasts. It has been argued cogently by anthropologists that culturally specific conception stories and theories are relevant to a society's ideas about itself (e.g. Malinowski 1929; Leach 1966; Delaney 1986; Martin 1987;

[12] There is a widely held assumption that 'the public' are more likely to approve biotechnology, for example, if given accurate and detailed scientific information about it (Douglas 1992).

[13] Bruno Latour (1987: 184–5), writing of more general distinctions made in science between what counts as belief and what counts as knowledge, puts it this way: 'Now the picture of non-scientists drawn by scientists becomes bleak: a few minds discover what reality is, while the vast majority of people have irrational ideas or at least are prisoners of many social, cultural and psychological factors that make them stick obstinately to obsolete prejudices. The only redeeming aspect of this picture is that if it were only possible to *eliminate* all these factors that hold people prisoners of their prejudices, they would all, immediately and at no cost, become as sound-minded as the scientists, grasping the phenomena without further ado. In every one of us there is a scientist who is asleep, and who will not wake up until social and cultural conditions are pushed *aside*.' In his inimitable style, Latour caricatures 'the scientist' as the scientist does 'the believer'. And even if an individual scientist is not recognizable in his critique, a position (a genre) from science certainly is.

[14] The flurry of publicity, for example, which attended the revelation that scientists in Edinburgh were studying the possibility of using eggs from aborted foetuses and cadavers, included the observation by one researcher that 'the public' were not quite ready for this development yet; he implied that, as with anything else, in time the public will get used to the idea.

1991; Hauser-Schaublin 1989; and see Franklin 1997 for a recent overview). It is therefore of anthropological interest to look carefully at narratives of conception revealed in the medical assistance of conception.[15] But this is not enough. People do not merely tell stories. They generate meaning in social interaction, and it is in social interaction that they formulate theory and apply conjecture. Furthermore, they theorize about specific practices, events, places, or persons without necessarily having been there or without necessarily having a technical knowledge of them. Bacup residents with whom I spoke theorized about the social implications of NRT without necessarily knowing a great deal about the techniques that the shorthand NRT covers. While techniques of assisted conception might enlist only a small number of people directly, its social resonances are not restricted to them. NRT present another vantage point from which the reproduction of human beings and social relationships are configured; from which connections and analogies are made. In telling me their thoughts about NRT, residents of Bacup in 1990 talked, amongst other things, of conception, gestation, feeding relationships, and love. They told me about ways in which intimate relationships of all kinds are forged, how they require effort to sustain in an appropriate manner and how easy it is to disrupt them. NRT problematize taken-for-granted premisses and, in this sense, they act as an ethnographic window through which notions of what constitutes relatedness, which usually remain implicit, can be discerned. In forcing an explicitness about elements that make up cultural understandings of the reproduction of persons and relationships, they affect us all and not only those with a vested interest in the technologies (see also Strathern 1992*b*).

Kinship Expertise

Knowledge about kinship, like knowledge about places and pasts, is said to stem from experience. From different perspectives, different people are said to be more knowledgeable about kin relations than others, and kinship expertise is thought to be distributed unequally. I have described how, when I first moved to Bacup, I was told by residents what I should know about the town and its people: particularly to whom I should speak, and whom I should avoid. I was

[15] e.g. Shore (1992) argues that anthropological interest in NRT has thus far not addressed the 'real' subject of these technologies, 'infertile couples' themselves. While this might be true, it misses a crucial anthropological question, namely: if doubts, anticipations, affirmations, ambivalences etc. which emerge in discussion of NRT reveal cultural understandings of the creation of persons and kin relations, what, then, is the 'real' subject of NRT? Perhaps the experiences of those requiring fertility services are missing in anthropological discussion of NRT (as are, one could argue, the voices of gamete donors, children born through *in vitro* fertilization (IVF), laboratory technicians, and so on), but such a criticism suggests that only those with a vested interest in NRT are touched by its possibilities, which is patently not the case. To suggest that only by collecting a variety of user perspectives can we begin to understand the cultural implications of assisted conception reminds me of the tendency for the anthropology of Britain to focus on discrete communities with an attendant reluctance to say something that cross-cuts them.

passed on to people who had lived all their lives in Bacup and to those who had only recently arrived; to those who provide local services and to those who are critical of them. I was referred to indigenous experts whose expertise has been gained through the experience of living in Bacup. Two years later, I told Bacup friends, acquaintances, and people I met for the first time that I was now working on a project about NRT. Those who knew me appeared readily to make a connection between my previous interests and this. They were not surprised that I should move from an interest in Bacup to an interest in what many of them glossed as 'test-tube babies'. I was passed on, and again to people who it was thought would be helpful. I was advised to talk to those perceived to have different kinds of knowledge about creating and maintaining family relationships: perhaps because they were men rather than women (or vice versa), or because they were older or younger, single, married, or divorced, living with or without children, or with step- or adopted children, or because they 'belonged' to large, *tight-knit* families or because they did not. Patty Cooper, for example, insisted I speak with her friend who, she explained, is *quite* different (from her): she is younger, getting divorced, and 'has no kids'. Patty was sure she (her friend) would provide me with a different point of view and it was clear to Patty that for me to find out about NRT I needed to solicit as many points of view as possible. She also urged me talk to her husband who, 'being a man', was bound to think differently about these things. Marilyn Greaves expected there to be a difference between the views of older and younger women, while Pamela Watson thought the major contrast would be between Socialist and Tory outlooks. One Bacup woman told me it was 'no good' talking to her as, having had only one child, she was 'not very reproductive'. A friend of Judy Wilder was convinced I ought to talk to Judy; she explained that her varied life, numerous relationships, four children with different fathers, and a chequered occupational history would make her well qualified to talk about such a topic. Judy agreed with this assessment of her expertise. I was passed on again to experts. This time to experts in kinship; to people who gained their expertise through their experiences of intimate social relationships.

In certain social arenas, however, a description of my new enterprise was received with unforthcoming silence, notably in forums where lively and rich discussion about Bacup and its residents, past and present, had previously been generated. At a meeting of the Nat, for example, I described my interests enthusiastically to four men in the library in response to the question: 'What are you doing now, then?' An uncharacteristic, noncommittal silence ensued which was eventually broken by one of the men asking: 'How's your son doing?' The subject was decisively changed, and while tangentially connected, in so far as we were on the topic of offspring, it was clear we were not going to pursue the specifics of NRT, at least not there and then.

Around about the same time, a Bacup friend and former neighbour, Mrs Jones, had her ninetieth birthday and a party was arranged by her daughters,

Evelyn and Barbara, in her home. There were thirty-five guests, many of whom I had met during previous fieldwork in the town. The newly elected mayor, whom I had not met before, decked in his chain of office and accompanied by his chauffeur, attended briefly. He sat with Mrs Jones for a while, talked with several of the guests, and ate sandwiches, sausage rolls, and cake, brought to him from the buffet table by Barbara. I was pleased and honoured to have been invited, and it was a pleasure to meet friends again and to catch up with acquaintances. Several people who knew me asked what I was doing now and I explained. It became obvious, however, that those who had been more than willing to talk with me in the past were not going to talk about NRT, at least, not there and not then. My reply to their question about what I was doing now was followed by a swift change of subject, not necessarily to one less controversial or unrelated, but to one deemed more appropriate for the setting.

The inappropriateness of NRT as a topic of conversation in certain social forums might be attributed to their association with sex and bodily substances. It could then be argued that, amongst other things, gender, age, and religion will play a part in whether people deem it appropriate or not to talk about, and when, where, and with whom. My co-conversationalists in the Nat and at the birthday party were predominantly over 50 years of age, many of the party guests Baptist, and members of the Nat male. It could be argued that I was being crass to raise the topic in such gatherings, and that its associations with taboo subjects could have been predicted, as could people's silence on the matter. But this alone does not adequately explain the kind of non-conversations I had in Bacup about NRT. In other social contexts, neither age, gender, nor religion seemed to influence people's willingness to explore their implications. Many of the same people who did not pursue the topic in the forum of the Nat or the birthday party talked at length with me on a different occasion. While gender, for example, might be an obvious influencing factor[16] and while there might be differences between public and private accounts, it seems to me that its inappropriateness as a topic of conversation in certain social forums stems from what people know, and don't know, of each other's lives, including their reproductive histories, kin relations, marriages, and, to borrow a Bacup idiom, 'the skeletons in their cupboard'. The subject of NRT provokes analogies with, for example, adoption and adultery. It reminds people of the joys and heartaches of life in and out of families, as well as the distress of infertility. While most Bacup residents with whom I spoke about NRT were intrigued by the topic, were more than willing to talk with me about them, and were reminded of their childhood, their origins, their kinsfolk, friends, and neighbours along the way, there were forums such as those described above where the topic was an unseemly focus of discussion. It is both knowing people

[16] My sense is that broadly speaking men talk about NRT in a more didactic way than women do, but the content of what they say, the cultural resources on which they draw, are similar.

too well and knowing people too little, that is, knowing or not knowing of their intimate social relations, that makes NRT both an indelicate and fascinating focus of attention.

The context of NRT, with a focus on innovative and novel ways of achieving conception, led Bacup associates to draw and elaborate upon pre-existing narratives of conception and ways in which intimate social relationships are created and sustained. Like tourism in Formentera (Bestard 1991), incomers in Wanet (Rapport 1993), and migration in France (Rapp 1987*a*), to name but a few, NRT are a context of innovation in which kinship thinking is deployed. Moreover, it is kinship thinking itself which elicits notions of persons and places, and formulates categories of, for example, tourist, incomer, and migrant. Kinship is mobilized, then, in all kinds of contexts which do not 'look like' kinship.[17] It formulates relatedness to places and pasts as well as to persons. In talking about the past, or factories, houses, and pubs, for example, people mobilize idioms of kinship as much as they do as when they talk about families, or conception, or the birth of a child. Such idioms inform, and give form to, understandings of the ways in which people live together in towns no less than in homes, and are as salient in discussion of services and communication as they are in kinship and NRT. In the first study I might not have been looking for kinship, but was presented with it incidentally and along the way. It was inherent in the way in which people educated me about Bacup: whom to speak to, whom to avoid, what made it special, distinctive, troublesome, friendly; why I would like it there and why I would hate it. In the second study, taken-for-granted ideas of relatedness were problematized in the context of NRT. My co-conversationalists spelled out relatedness, and again they told me about Bacup.

During my second fieldwork in Bacup, residents suggested repeatedly that different experiences of family life and different reproductive histories will inevitably generate different views on the topic of NRT. In exploring NRT with me, they drew on their knowledge of Bacup, its people and its pasts, while at the same time recounting their own experiences and knowledge of life in and out of families. They provided me with elements of autobiography which exemplified not only the intimacy of kin relations, but also the difficulty in sustaining them in an appropriate manner. It is their experience of kinship which qualifies them to speak with authority about NRT, as it is their experience of Bacup which qualifies them to speak with authority about the town. This means that in order to talk about either Bacup or NRT they need also to talk about themselves. In both cases 'the self' is not merely the vehicle for that knowl-

[17] It was working on, and writing about Bacup ideas about NRT that made me realize just how much kinship there was in the first study. The process of combining the studies led to a particular kind of focus on the original data collected. In the light of subsequent effort they have come to cohere in a particular way. I remark elsewhere that the second study could only have been carried out in the light of the first (it drew and built upon its findings and relationships). But the second study provided a particular vantage point from which to explore the first. This enterprise, no less than any other anthropological effort, draws on comparison.

edge but acts as an exemplar—a metaphor for human relationships. Consequently in the following chapters I attempt to preserve some of the autobiographical detail I was presented with.

The Ubiquity of the Past

The industrial and manufacturing base from which Bacup grew no longer exists and throughout the twentieth century out-migration has surpassed in-migration. Bacup residents appear to be preoccupied with the past. They tell histories which reveal strands that link them to the past, and in doing so they pin down what they perceive to be a highly fickle present. The town, the moorland in which it rests, the absent cotton mills, and shared hardship are just some of the things said to have *moulded* a particular Bacup character. This character, tough and rugged, is brought into relief by comparison with the soft, nebulous qualities of city-dwellers who represent all that Bacup people are not. The constant indigenous re-creation of Bacup identity rests on a strategy of comparison similar to that of the anthropological enterprise which implicitly or explicitly compares its subject of study to the West.

In describing myself as somebody who wanted to write about Bacup, it was more often than not assumed my interest was in the history of the town. History is a recognized and legitimate focus of study, and many Bacup residents with whom I spoke referred me to people they considered well qualified, and perhaps better qualified than they, to provide me with the kind of information they imagined I required. I was told, almost daily, to go to the Nat. Identified as the town's experts, members of the Nat were said to know *all* there is to know about Bacup. On other occasions, I was referred to those considered to be somehow better attached to the town. I was advised to speak to those in prominent positions in local organizations or local government when they also had an attendant expertise which stemmed from being either born or brought up in Bacup. Hence, while I was referred to the ex-mayor who had lived and worked in Bacup all his life, and was deemed well connected to the town via links mediated by, amongst other things, family, factories, pubs, and houses, I was not referred to the present mayor who lived and worked in Haslingdon and who was not perceived to be connected to Bacup in the same way. Indigenous experts are thus because of their attachments to the town which are secured through a wide range of persons and entities that belong there.

I was also sent to the Unemployed Workers' Centre (UWC). Workers in the centre, both voluntary and paid, provide an advisory service on welfare benefits and information on education and leisure facilities in the region. The centre also houses adult education classes, a playgroup for pre-school children, and a toy library. The Nat and the UWC, two organizations prominent in Bacup perceptions of expertise, appear at first glance to be concerned with quite different arenas of Bacup life. The UWC claims an interest in the contemporary social and economic life of Bacup, while a commonly expressed view from the Nat is that they themselves know 'nowt about today'. A distinction between past and present is difficult to sustain, however. Those who participate in the UWC are as preoccupied with the past as members of the Nat, and both are concerned with the present. At first I was impatient (I hope not too obviously) with yet *another* description of Bacup at the turn of the eighteenth century, or another vignette about th'owd characters, or more memories of what it was like to live in a back-to-back. I recall making futile attempts at deflecting speakers away from their reminiscences towards what I imagined was my concern with the anthropological present. But the past, no less than the present, is constituted by and constitutive of a particular kind of kinship thinking; selections have to be made which means making certain connections and not others. The past, like kinship, cannot be hived off as a separate domain of social life to be studied in its own right; it not only permeates the present but also gives conceptual shape to it. One strand linking the chapters of this book is the way in which the past is put to work by Bacup residents; the present is formulated and ordered not merely with reference to the past but through a process which carries the past with it.

There has been a recent and fruitful emphasis on the centrality and interconnectedness of history and kinship (e.g. Gow 1991; Yanagisako 1985).[18] Bacup residents constantly refer to the past when they talk about the town (including its landscapes, inhabitants, and services). If the past is invoked in the present, it is also the case that the present is elicited in formulations of the past. It is not merely that narratives about the past act as vehicles for contemporary concerns, instead the past is fully implicated in the present. Present and past entail each other in a way that is irreducible to neither. Selection of pasts is of a piece with the selection of kin. Both present people with a problem: what to remember and what to leave out, and both require tracing certain connections and not others. Certain characteristics are said to have emerged from specific historical experiences, and the experience of being born and bred in Bacup fashions a character recognizable as Bacupian: idiosyncratic, resilient, and tough. A harsh environment and poverty are said to promote particular characteristics, and the experience of growing up in the town is thought to prepare one for life in a special way.

Part 2 of this book is replete with histories of Bacup. I focus first of all on the efforts of local historians who perceive their role as 'unearthing' and 'preserving' the past of Bacup, and rather than writing an initial chapter that purports to be a definitive history of Bacup I present their history-making: their

[18] For Yanagisako (1985), the cultural history told by Japanese Americans is central to their understandings of contemporary kinship. She explores the way in which constantly repeated idioms of 'traditional' and 'modern', and 'American' and 'Japanese', are used when Japanese Americans, in the 1970s, talk of familial expectations.

interests, preoccupations, and activities. It is not only local historians who are occupied with the past: most residents in talking about the town, themselves, and each other mobilize the past and many histories are told; I go on to look at the way in which indigenous ideas of expertise are exemplified in contestation about who and what should stand for Bacup. Part 2 also focuses on houses and homes, and cities and villages; how are distinctions between these things made and for what purpose? Bacup residents, like anthropologists, categorize localities with reference to different kinds of social relationships. Consequently, 'the village' is characterized by its interrelatedness, and 'the city' by its preponderance of single-stranded, utilitarian relationships (the simplex and multiplex relations of, amongst others, Gluckman 1955; 1965; 1969; Boissevain 1974). Idioms of 'born and bred' are put to work in the process of differentiating between cities and villages, and houses and homes.

In Part 3 I turn to what happens when people focus specifically on kinship. What cultural resources do Bacup residents draw on towards the end of the twentieth century when the presence of NRT impinges on them through, for example, the windows of mass media, the experience of family, friends, and neighbours, or through the anthropologist with an explicit interest in the topic?[19] They talk about NRT in familiar ways; in ways that resonate with how they talk about the town and its people. NRT is another context in which they make and break connections between persons, places, and pasts. In exploring the possibilities and potentials of assisted conception they draw on, and refer to, a knowledge of the kind of place Bacup was, is, and ought to be.

A tension between Bacup as a distinctive locality with a unique history, geography, and character on the one hand, and on the other as part of and exemplifying English culture—the same but different—is a powerful interplay of ideas. Kinship, in this English version, relies on a similar interplay: the unique and discrete individual is enmeshed in a network of unbreakable and enduring links between kin.[20] Furthermore, the image of the fixed and unchanging locality embracing networks of enduring and unbreakable social ties is not confined to England, nor is that of the mobile cosmopolitan perceived to have ties with no one place. The conceptualization of a discrete and bounded individual allows boundaries of both kinship and class to be breached—people are mobile, they have lives different from their parents and wish better things for their children. The idea of the individual moving around fixed classes in a bounded society (Strathern 1982*b*) has its counterpart in ideas about biological inheritance. Fixed inherited elements, located in discrete entities—genes, or in

[19] In Part 3 I present extracts from interviews and conversations in Bacup about NRT, and readers will take to them their own interests. They will read them from different vantage points and be led to alternative interpretations.

[20] A number of scholars have focused on an English notion of the individual (see e.g. Macfarlane 1978; Strathern 1981; 1992*a*; Handler 1988), and this is not the place to pursue this theme, except to say that it is generated by a particular kind of kinship thinking.

smaller and more precise molecules of DNA, are said to constitute a person and to influence the kind of person they are. But that is never the full story. A person's background—a particular upbringing, childhood experiences—plays a part in reproducing persons. Both genes and values perdure; they are passed on to children, and to children's children. The way in which these two aspects of kinship thinking—nature and nurture, ascribed and achieved, social and biological, fixed and fluid—are put to work in different domains of social life is the focus of the chapters that follow. They are about the way in which residents of Bacup towards the end of the twentieth century draw on cultural understandings of kinship in a variety of ways, with different emphases and slants, to make sense of the social worlds which they themselves mould and which moulds them, and upon which they reflect.

PART 2

In Bacup

3

Naming and Placing Bacup

MANY Bacup residents in 1987 and 1988 claimed an interest in the history of the region in which they lived. They suspected this was my interest also and if it was not then it ought to be. They spoke mainly of the town's industrial past and remarked that it was not a very attractive or healthy place in which to live during the heyday of the textile industry. They described a polluted, open river running through the town centre, factory chimneys belching smoke, and overcrowded, dark, and damp dwellings. They pointed to these as just some of the things responsible for poor health and high infant mortality. They agreed that Bacup was a much healthier and more pleasant place in which to live today, and some mentioned the slum-clearance programmes of the 1960s, and various Clean Air Acts (1956 and 1968) as having made a positive impact on the environment and on the health of the population. At the same time, those who have lived in Bacup through such changes expressed a longing for 'them days', and commented on the way in which improvements to the physical landscape had not necessarily resulted in a better 'way of life'. 'Them days' took on the quality of a mythological past, the narrating of which suspended for a moment the former harshness of life in the town which, at a different moment and for a different purpose, was emphasized. The past as resource was drawn upon by all Bacup residents, and the comparison between 'them days' and the present was not confined to those born and bred in Bacup. Residents who moved to the town from elsewhere and who thought of themselves (and were defined) as *incomers* also dwelt on social and economic changes that had occurred in their lifetime. They pointed to such changes as having occurred in the places they left behind and how it was they that prompted them to settle in Bacup. Younger Bacup people who had no recollection of Bacup as a 'thriving, industrial mill town' also mobilized the past; they recalled their growing up in the town and pointed to how things were different today.

An apparent English preoccupation with the past towards the end of the twentieth century has been analysed as nostalgia: a sentimental longing for coherence in a present-day fragmented world (see for example Wright 1985; Hewison 1987). It is argued that the present burgeoning interest in industrial heritage, for instance, has arisen at a time of great social change: at a time when the manufacturing industry in Britain has been decimated and when employment is precarious and insecure. In a post-industrial and post-colonial era, so this argument goes, we look with nostalgia to the past and such a backward glance epitomizes the insecurity of the present age. If this is true, then it follows that in another period of great and rapid social change, say in the middle of the nineteenth century with the rapid development of the textile industry in Bacup and the concomitant increase in the population and growth of the town, residents at that time would be looking back with nostalgia to non-industrial pasts. But nostalgia does not capture a Bacup preoccupation with the past, nor does it adequately describe the endeavours of local historians who are the focus of this chapter.[1] The pasts Bacup people compose towards the end of the twentieth century are neither unproblematically good nor unproblematically bad; they are tinged with ambivalence. The past, like kinship, presents people with a problem. It raises questions of what to recall and what to ignore; what to reveal and what to conceal. Some of the selections they make will be explored here.

An Industrial History

The region of England in which Bacup is situated is commonly associated with the manufacture of cotton during the nineteenth century. But the seeds of industrialization were, in fact, sown at a much earlier point in the history of the town. There is record of a fulling mill in the Rossendale Valley in 1611, and one in Bacup in 1713.[2] Prior to the nineteenth century the main subsistence activity in the region was sheep farming, but even then locally produced wool was spun and woven domestically by handloom, and many households supplemented small-scale cultivation with income from domestic cloth production. There was a steady immigration of individuals and families from rural areas of Britain and Ireland throughout the eighteenth century. And merchants and clothiers, mainly from Rochdale but also from other centres such as Manchester and Bury, 'put out' work in the Valley. They provided the raw materials and paid local spinners and weavers, by piece, for the end product. One historian estimates that by the early part of the eighteenth century 'half of the total population of Rossendale was dependent on the textile trade' (Tupling 1927: 178).[3] Domination of the industry by the 'Rochdale masters' continued through the second part of the eighteenth century with increasing numbers of households dependent solely on income from the woollen industry (Tupling 1927: 189). In 1751, a Dr Pococke wrote that Bacup was a 'large village at which they have a great manufacture of

[1] I use this term purposely to exploit the ambiguity it entails. Local historians are both historians resident in Bacup and historians whose expertise lies in the history of Bacup and its environs (and see Edwards 1998*b*).

[2] Fulling entails pounding, washing, and stretching woven wool cloth to produce a smooth surface.

[3] An extensive network of communications between Rossendale and other parts of the British Isles was in place by the beginning of the nineteenth century. Factory owners recruited labour through advertisements or through agents who both bought raw materials and sold finished cloth. Many labouring families, having heard of The 'Golden Valley', came in search of work from rural areas of Britain. Early immigrants came from the same places from which wool was imported, notably Ireland, the Midlands, and southern counties of England. Reports in newspapers cite Norfolk, Cambridgeshire, and Lincolnshire as places where many of the labouring families at that time came from.

woollen goods which they send white to London' (cited ibid. 184). By the end of the eighteenth century, manufacturing activities had shifted from domestic to factory production. Workshops (or loomshops as they were called) were increasingly being built to house labouring families[4] and centralize production.[5]

Early mills were built on the banks of the river Irwell and its tributaries so as to accommodate water-powered looms. But then steam from locally mined coal replaced water and photographs from around the middle of the nineteenth century portray a landscape dominated by smoking factory chimneys. In 1850 there were fifty factories operating in Bacup (BNHS 1987), and during this period the Rossendale Valley was referred to colloquially as the 'Golden Valley' and is reported to have been 'one of the wealthiest valleys in England' (Tupling 1927; Aspin 1983).[6] The cotton industry, given its reputed impact on this region of Britain, was surprisingly short-lived. By the late 1870s very few mills were working at full capacity, and during this period, with the availability of empty premises and trained labour, the manufacture of shoes began. The cotton industry was to recover briefly in the final years of the nineteenth century. Ross Mill was completed in 1912, had eight floors, and housed 72,000 spindles.[7] By the end of the First World War, however, the export of cloth had more or less dried up and the manufacture of cotton was at a standstill. Mills were demolished and those left standing were converted into smaller industrial units and given over to the manufacture of footwear.

The Slipper Works

In 1987 and 1988 the footwear industry was the major employer in Bacup. The industry was small and precarious and characterized by low pay and periods of short time.[8] Like a past which features cotton mills, the past of the footwear industry is also told in both oral and written histories of Bacup. Connections

[4] I use the term 'labouring family' because although many individual men moved to this area of England in search of work, many did so in families. And it is families which impinge more on a collective memory of who came to Bacup, when, and for what purpose, and it is often pointed out that frequently whole families worked in the same mill.

[5] In the home and later in the factories spinning was confined to women and children and weaving to men. A gendered division of labour continued through the cotton mills and into present-day shoe factories where 'clickers' who cut out shoe uppers tend to be men and sewing machinists predominantly women.

[6] Bacup was granted municipal borough status in 1882, with Haslingdon and Rawtenstall following suit in 1891.

[7] Ross Mill was demolished in 1981 amid some controversy over whether it should be preserved or not. Residents who remember it clearly recall that it was enormous and that it was unusual in so far as it was built of red brick rather than stone.

[8] The average wage in the shoe industry in 1988 was £78 per week before deductions. The union-agreed rate at the beginning of 1990 was £82 per week. Outworkers, working from home, are paid piece-rates, a flat rate per item which takes no account of the number of hours worked.

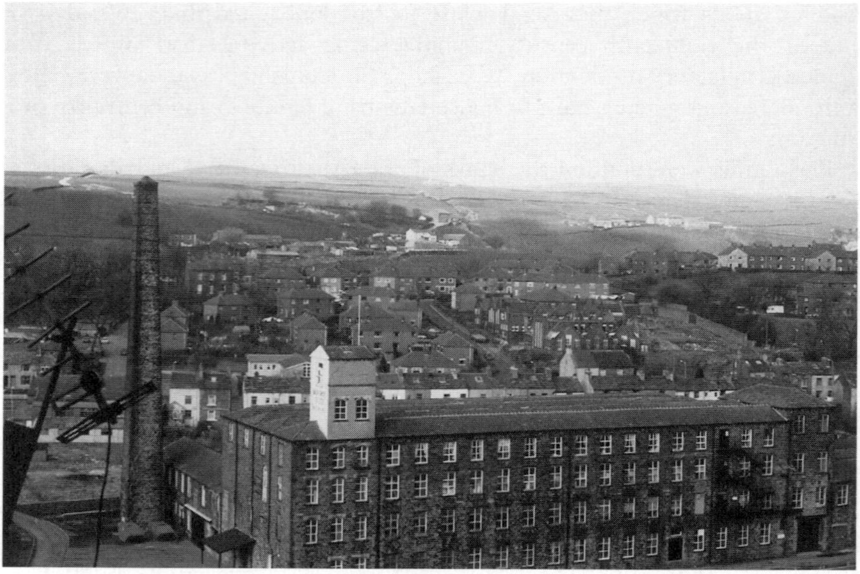

PLATE 3. Atherton Holme Mill: in 1988 it housed the Bacup Shoe Company

are traced between the *slipper works*[9] and other and former industrial activity in the region. It is reported that the manufacture of slippers gained its inspiration from block printers who worked in the cotton mills. In order to be able to walk over the cloth they were printing and to protect it they made themselves slippers out of felt which was readily available from waste material produced in wool-carding. After designing slippers for their own use, the block printers went on to make them for 'family and friends' and then as a commercial enterprise (Bowden 1972). The depression of the cotton industry in the last two decades of the nineteenth century, when empty premises and a trained workforce became available, provided the impetus for the development of the footwear industry. According to local historian Willie Hardman, in an article entitled 'The Beginnings of the Slipper Trade' (Bowden 1975), Mr J. W. Rothwell, a block printer of Waterfoot, was the first person to produce a batch of slippers as a commercial venture. These he sold to a Manchester retailer in 1874 for 'nine shillings a dozen'. Subsequently, in partnership with 'two other local men', he employed four assistants and

[9] The term 'slipper works' is a local idiom used for any kind of shoe factory, although slippers are a soft-soled version of indoor footwear (bedroom slippers) in which many Bacup shoe manufacturers specialize.

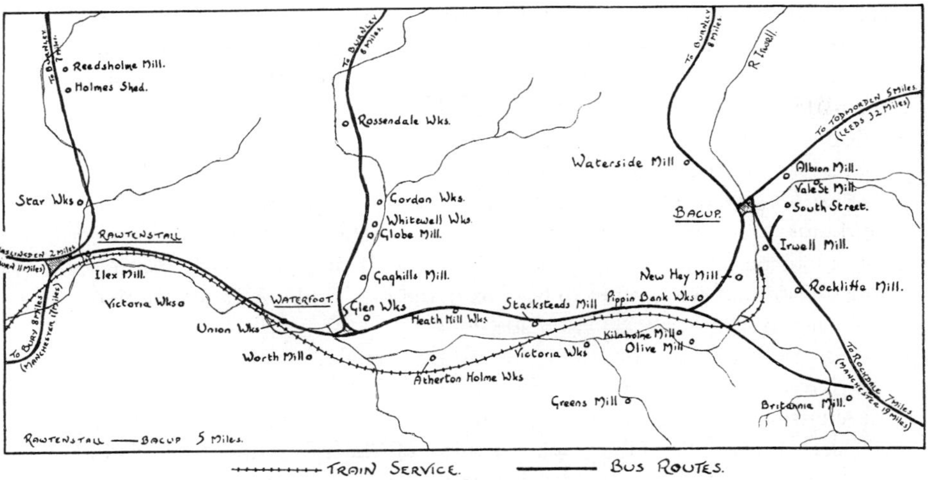

Map 2. Distribution of footwear industry in Rossendale Valley *c.* 1958

the first shoe factory was established. Hardman goes on to name two other 'founding fathers': Mr McClerie who was initially employed by Rothwell as a 'foreman fulling miller', and Sir Henry Trickett who, by 1895, employed over 1,000 people. Hardman describes how Trickett left school at 8 years of age and worked in a printworks. He is a prime example, Hardman suggests, of a 'local lad made good'. The fact that Henry Trickett was knighted and became a politician and a wealthy and successful businessman does not compromise his status as a 'real' Bacup person. His roots, background, and origins in a working-class occupation qualify him for 'proper' Bacup status. The short biography of Willie Hardman (1870–1940), attached to his article about Trickett (1857–1913) describes a similar background. Hardman also left school at 8 and embarked on formal education through night classes at the Mechanics' Institute while employed full-time in a mill, manufacturing wool. He too became a factory owner and was also, like Trickett, engaged as a local politician.

One thing striking in all descriptions of the early days of industry in Bacup is the credit given to 'ordinary working men' as innovators. The early textile industry, while initially controlled by Rochdale merchants, gradually developed a 'considerable measure of self-controlled organisation' (Tupling 1921: 201). One commentator, writing in 1795, notes that while previously workers had been 'chiefly employed by monied men at Rochdale', the trade was increasingly 'supported by capital acquired on the spot by the industry and enterprising spirit of the manufacturers' (Tupling 1921). Beatrice Webb, who first visited Bacup in 1883 and then again in 1885 and 1886,[10] was also struck by the success of working-class mill owners in Bacup: 'Class spirit hardly exists because there is no capitalist class; those mills which are not companies being owned by quite small men of working class origin and connected with working people' (Webb 1926, cited in Buckland 1986[11]).

Part of contemporary history has it that factory owners were mostly 'local lads made good' who, it is said, were 'ordinary folk' who through hard work and enterprise acquired wealth, prestige, and status. The steady in-migration of labouring families throughout the eighteenth and nineteenth centuries begs the question of who comes to be considered local and how; a question to which I return, but first, a local lad made good.

At the beginning of 1988 the largest remaining shoe factory in Bacup employed 420 people. It was opened by Tom B. Thompson in 1928, and I spoke at length with him on several occasions in the committee room of his factory.[12] A large rectangular table took up most of the room and framed diplomas and awards as well as local landscape paintings hung on the walls. Tea, in a delicate and ornate china teapot, was brought to us by the Director of the factory. Mr Thompson told me he is now just an honorary chairman and the factory is run by the Director and a committee of shareholders,[13] but that he nevertheless comes to work most days, knows the names of all the factory's employees, and still produces his annual Christmas newsletter which, amongst other things, records the marriages, anniversaries, and retirements of workers. It also noted the births to employees, and reviewed the previous year in the form of a poem. He said he started the newsletter in 1936 'for fun', making a joke about everybody (which, he said, was possible when the factory employed only fifty people). In the newsletters: 'I used to say "Lizzie does this" and "Bob does that", but as the years went by and we got to eight hundred instead of sixty I couldn't do it any more.' So now, he told me, he divided the newsletter into two parts: a general review of the trade as he saw it, and a separate section which carried details of 'activities

[10] She writes that her visits to Bacup were highly influential on her subsequent career (see also Walsh 1989): 'The Bacup adventure gave a decisive turn to my self-development. The die was cast, the craft was chosen. Through the pressure of circumstances and the inspiration of the time-spirit, I had decided to become an investigator of social institutions' (Webb 1926: 121). Her biographers write: 'It was entirely characteristic of Beatrice that after seeing the most splendid and the most picturesque cities of Europe and America without being moved by them personally she should lose her heart to this drab industrial small-town, set in an uninteresting part of the manufacturing north of England' (Muggeridge and Adam 1967). They go on to suggest Beatrice Webb's initiative in creating the London School of Economics (which she is said to have described as her baby) with money bequeathed to the Fabian Society stemmed directly from her Bacup experience.

[11] Theresa Buckland has carried out detailed studies of the Coco-Nut Dancers of Bacup (see Ch. 7) over many years, and I have benefited a great deal from our conversations.

[12] One of the conversations from which I cite was carried out in the context of our interview on film.

[13] He explained to me how all employees have a share in the company and how difficult it could be to negotiate fair and accurate settlements when people left the company.

The Chairman's Christmas Letter 1986

My Christmas Letter shall be one of hope
Throughout this year we had more scope
Our trading conditions were fairly calm
Not as many businesses suffered harm.

The weather was mild, damp and dull
In the parts when we expect sunshine full
We made footwear utility, not style glamour
There were no queues for the fashions clammer.

Full-time production was achieved as well
Many a story of factory loyalty I could tell
There is happiness within the factories, a bond of trust
To reward the staff when overtime is a must.

For we have a computer that is accurate and true
Ordering materials and programming work for you
But not yet have we found how we can undertake
The fast repeats of the popular styles we make.

Nor can we rapidly fill that vacant spot
When a football accident or the flu you have got
Our willing Trainees that are eager to learn
Step in with their skill, extra pay to earn.

There is opportunity in the factories to gain more skill
Carefully monitored with goodwill
People forsake us for family reasons or a Wedding Bell
Whilst of many, early retirements I tell.

Our Design Team are all on alert to make sure
That fashion will play its part and satisfaction endure
As the high street shops fill more and more from overseas
With copies of the designs we thought would please.

Machinery manufacturers seek less developed races
To install the latest attachments to machine places
With their labour and social insurance costs low
We could not compete if our reaction was slow.

So work hard, play hard, is our theme
Rather than twiddle our fingers and dream
We study the problem and search around
Then develop expertise on our own ground

Then say we thanks to one and all
Who have responded well to any urgent call
Customers have been pleased at what our response has been
When into their premises our products are seen.

Besides the haste of buying, making and selling
There is a happy spirit in the firm dwelling
The tragedies of life have been braved and met
Where sympathy and love a good response can get.

Our Engineers have played a full part
In keeping the plant up to the mark
Adaptations and adjustments make operations true
With less corrections for you to do.

The cleaning, tea-making, Canteen staff
Everyday thinks up something good for a laugh
And Foremen have not failed to notice too
That Cleanliness means less rejects from you.

A simple scratch or a stitch out of place
The customer's eyes and mind embrace
A call to pay less and profit goes down
Shoes must be attractive in the shops in town.

Now I must think of the many joys we have had
It has been a good year, we are not doing so bad
And meeting the targets we set ourselves
With happy customers emptying shelves.

Future prospects good as quality we maintain
Happy recruits in the factory, our people to train
Prompt deliveries from our suppliers depatch
Every day a new theme to hatch.

So let's say thanks to each other once more
To happiness in working, leave open the door
Difficult jobs that are bad to do
Quickly are mastered with success in view.

Let the Christmas message of hope in the land
Come nearer so that we too can understand
Industrial work is a great opportunity to say
We will do our best for the Lord of all today.

We shall share in practical sympathy and love
As we are directed by the Lord from above
We shall encourage each to develop more skill
And give support for recovery whenever we are ill.

We shall remember that happiness is the key to success
Find a joke or a bright spot when something is a mess
And give our best endeavour each day
And be glad of the privilege to meet you on the way.

We know full well that whatever we spend
Has to be earned on the repeat orders customers send
So in joy for a year's work well done
A Christmas gift, relaxation and fun.

Just a day older than yesterday
And yet I hear some folk say
Octogenarian, a ripe old age
It is to me a new development page.

There are new materials, new methods, new need
To develop processes with accurate speed
New time for opportunity to rejoice
And meet the future with welcome voice.

So we had a halt in the daily scheme
And spent a day just like a dream
Singing, cheering, in factories and store
And great excitement and much more.

Video cameras, press cuttings for news
Remarkable tributes in airing views
The footwear trade, an opportunity service to give
Parties, enjoyment, we did really live.

J.W.J. sold his house, a slow affair
Then decided the proceeds we must share
He gave £80 each to all employees
From hard earned tax paid fees.

He was glad of the pleasure to save
Now he returns thanks for thanks you gave
And looks forward to being one hundred and one
With happy enjoyment in whatever is done.

FIG. 3.1. The Chairman's Christmas letter, 1986

and worker participation'. For Mr Thompson the newsletter had become a forum for commenting on the past and the future of the business specifically and the shoe trade more generally.

Mr Thompson told me about himself. He selected and highlighted certain elements of his past with which to say something of his present and presence.

In turn, I select from what he told me, and for the moment ignore what others told me of his life and relationships.

Tom B. Thompson was born in 1904, one of nine children. His family lived on farming land on the outskirts of town. His father was a miner and his father's father married the 'widow of a felt maker'. 'Being a farmer's boy', he told me, he was 'grown up at 7'.

'We used to deliver milk and when you went out with milk you found a way of earning money. So I apprenticed myself, unknown to my parents, to a locksmith and decided I'd be an engineer . . . My father was a colliery engineer and he encouraged me when he knew. You see, he used to buy the things for the colliery company from the same firm and I was found out. You know, it always surprised me to find my father let me go to work at twelve years of age for 22*d*. a week for thirty-eight hours and they call it half-time, and my father at that time was a senior engineer, certificated and all that goes with it. And he was earning well over £6 a week—I have his wage books and I think "well nay—he could have let me go through technical school or the Grammar School because I had passed the examinations" [*laughs*]. But I didn't get a chance to go—so I set to work to earn money and anything that would earn money was added to my lot because one day, I said, I am going to do better for the family, and for the town than has been done before.'

So Tom B. left school at 12 years of age and, in 1928, after working in shoe factories for several years he went into business himself. He started making shoes and his business expanded and he bought several empty mills and converted them into slipper works.

Mr Thompson purpose-built a factory in 1974 and, despite fierce competition from imported footwear, particularly from the Far East, and the difficulties of seasonal fluctuations in demand, the factory continued to that day as a major employer in Bacup, despite periods of uncertainty and short-time. Mr Thompson presented me with a genealogy of the textile industry, within which he located his factory.

In the days of the factories when felt was the mother of the industry—that's pressed woollens—and felt goods were sold for all purposes throughout the country, it was an ideal place for felting. Having done that then it developed into using the wool: spinning, weaving and making yarns and after that we came to cotton, and through that times of great prosperity came and some of these wonderful buildings you have seen were built in the 1850s to 1890s period [when there was] no income tax to call anything and a lot of trained labour. Short of labour they brought people from Ireland and Cambridge and anywhere else that people would come from particularly with the potato famine in Ireland. Conditions of living were very low, but they were far superior to what they were in their own place. And its a common thing to go through Bacup even now and you'll find rows of houses where the petty or the necessary house, as it was called, was at the bottom of the street and anybody who wanted to go to the toilet would go down past twenty houses and queue at the bottom winter and summer. But of course now all that is gone and [*pause*] er, I should think that the last of that kind of thing was only as recent as 1920.

Mr Thompson's genealogy of industry in Bacup traced the emergence of cotton from felt. He went on to narrate the emergence of shoes from felt and cotton. Each industry contained the others and hybrids of combinations of raw materials, factory spaces, and skilled labour emerged. Mr Thompson narrated the connections between factories and houses, and between Bacup and other places in Britain. He linked up Bacup and its industry, not just internally but to places like Ireland and Cambridge. Listen to how he placed workers (including himself) in the landscape of factories and houses:

> Now against that background, people were used to work. They had nimble fingers. They were glad to work. They wanted the money . . . we went on to full-time which was sixty-four hours, later reduced to fifty-eight and then to fifty-four and forty-five and then to forty where we are now. The wages for me at 13 years of age was 50*d*. a week. If we worked overtime we didn't get paid but we did get fish and chips provided which you could buy in any chip shop, you know, for five pence and if you wanted black peas it were ha'penny extra.

Long hours and low pay, and recognition for overtime presented in fish and chips which, while inadequate financial compensation (after all you could buy them anywhere for fivepence), provided a shared reward. Mr Thompson concluded his tracing of industrial connections: 'Then mothers, fathers, grandfathers, and grandmothers all worked in cotton and shoes, and the nimbleness of the fingers has been our salvation.'

In 1988, apart from the slipper works started by Tom B. Thompson, there were numerous smaller footwear manufacturers in rented, industrial units which had been created from the partitioning of larger factory floors. In some cases, capital to start such a business came from the redundancy payments that had been made to workers when the factories in which they had been employed, sometimes for all their working lives, had closed down. Mr Whittaker, a Bacup man in his early sixties, and two colleagues set up their own business with their redundancy payments on the closure of the factory in which all three had worked for more than thirty years. They make ballet and other specialist dance shoes and, at the time of fieldwork, the business was 'ticking over'. Mr Whittacker told me 'it was better than being on the dole' even if it paid them hardly any more than they would have received in benefits. Many other small shoe factories set up in the late 1980s, however, were short-lived and skilled workers (clickers and machinists) moved around, like a peripatetic workforce, from one job to another. The smaller slipper works employed mostly women who tended to work shifts designed to fit in with the school-day. I met several women who at different times in their history of paid employment had been outworkers. They worked from home sewing slipper uppers with machines supplied by employers who delivered materials and collected the finished product. Outworkers are paid by the piece, and often at lower rates than in the factory. For many women, however, it provides extra income without compromising household commitments and without the cost of childminding.

Short time and redundancy are as much a feature of the footwear industry today as they were of the cotton industry 100 years ago. Fluctuations in both industries have meant a continuous movement of labour in and out of the town. It has always, in this sense, been connected to wider society and to a global political economy. The demise of the cotton industry in Bacup was linked to economic changes in trading countries and, I was told, never fully recovered from the aftermath of the American Civil War and subsequent scarcities of raw cotton. Tom B. Thompson impressed upon me the fact that fluctuation in the demand for labour in Bacup's footwear industry was directly linked to the availability of footwear imported from Asia and the East which was produced at a fraction of the cost. His ability to keep his factory going depended, he said, on being able to stay a step ahead of the competition by producing fashionable or novelty shoes quickly and in relatively small batches and selling them before they were manufactured elsewhere. The threads of the textile industry run through Bacup not only connecting it to the past and to rural areas and urban trading centres of Britain, but also to other parts of the world. Bacup is located and implicated in a larger world, and tales are told of family members who emigrated to the 'New World' as they moved into the twentieth century. The industrial history of Bacup told today portrays neither powerlessness nor passive acceptance of the whims of the world. On the contrary, a history which emphasizes hardship also portrays an indubitable spirit of survival. The industrial history of Bacup, generated and sustained within the town, explains the industrious and innovative character of former inhabitants despite filth, disease, and poverty. Local historians provide the context in which the emergence of resilient and resourceful inhabitants takes place. The history they tell renders visible, and celebrates, a strength of character which has, and will, survive.

Tom B. Thompson ended one of our conversations with a story about a man who came to Bacup from Rugby, but did not stay.

TOM B.: A gentleman—he'd right good ways—came up from Rugby to Bacup. He settled amongst us. We never knew why. We felt he must have had a grimy past. He'd been married three times anyhow and been married again while he was here. The pigeon club asked him would he be their president and when they went to him they said: 'Sir, would you like to be the flying club president?' 'Ooh! He'd be delighted since he was an insurance man for . . .'

JEANETTE: Why did they ask *him*?

TOM B.: 'Cause he was a newcomer and might add a bit of dignity and they were getting stale with chap that had it, you know? So this particular public house asked him to be the president for the pigeon club. But they didn't say that. They said: 'Will you be president of our flying club?' He said he would. 'Well, week next Friday we're having an inauguration meeting. Will you come?' He said he would: 'What time?'

'Eight o' clock'. 'Right, I'll be there,' and he was. So they were all sat—about fifty chaps in this room—and they were all looking forward and the chairman got up and he says: 'We've been fortunate in getting the services of a new president. He has come up from Rugby'. 'Oh!' everybody said 'Wonderful! New blood.' And he made a nice little speech, and in the middle of his speech it suddenly dawned on the chairman that he thought it were an aircraft club and he had to break the news that it were a pigeon club [*laughs*]. And he said to him, he said: 'Well if that's what it is, I'll still be president.' And he did, all honour to him. But he didn't stay in the town above another couple of years—we were too crude for him.

'Fragments ofFact and Legendary Lore'

The idea of human activity moulding a particular landscape, which in turn moulds a particular character, draws on pre-industrial evidence. *Grass Routes*, one of a series of locally published booklets, describes the region in prehistoric times.[14] It notes that the activities of prehistoric man made an ineradicable mark on the landscape of the Rossendale Valley and by 800 BC the topsoil of the moorlands had already been eroded due to the activities of 'semi-nomadic pastoral farmers'. Soil erosion, together with an extension of peat bogs due to climatic changes occurring during the same period, prevented a regeneration of the woodlands, and we are told that the poor soil and inhospitable environment of the moorlands deterred early settlement in the region. Until the time of the Norman conquest the area was predominantly unoccupied wasteland and it was not until the eleventh century, with the allocation of land to favoured Norman aristocrats, that the Forest of Rossendale appeared on the official historical map (Tupling 1927). By the end the eleventh century, Robert de Lacy, lord of Clitheroe, had been granted feudal rights over the hundred of Blackburn, which included the Rossendale Valley, and it remained under the jurisdiction of the Lacy family for the next 250 years. During this period much of the area was converted into a hunting chase, the preserve of which was jealously guarded by the successors of the Lacy family. Thomas Newbigging in his widely cited history of Rossendale notes that, before this period, the unoccupied wasteland of the Rossendale Valley was inhabited only by wild animals such as deer, boar, and wild cattle, and that after the area had been converted into 'Forest' (royal hunting grounds) responsibility for its upkeep was placed in the hands of a chief Forester who, himself not 'necessarily a resident', was helped by 'a few stray keepers of the deer' (Newbigging 1893: 51).

Newbigging (1833–1914), a historian of Bacup, is himself of historical interest. He was born in Glasgow and moved to Rossendale in 1857 as a manager of the Rossendale Union Gas Company. In 1864 he was secretary of the Bacup

[14] Published jointly by Rossendale Borough Council and Rossendale Groundwork Trust, The Changing Faces of Rossendale is a series of booklets illustrating major aspects of what they refer to as man's effects on the face of this region.

Mechanics' Institution and in 1886 ran, unsuccessfully, as the Liberal candidate for Rossendale. He first published his *History ofthe Forest of Rossendale* in 1868, and it ran into a second enlarged edition, published in 1893. He begins his historical treatise with the words:

> Some apology or explanation would seem to be due from me to those who will peruse the present Work, why I, who am no native of the Forest of Rossendale, should have presumed to write its History. I am aware that there are those residing in Rossendale who, by their antiquarian and genealogical acquirements and their longer acquaintance with the locality, are more fitted for the duty, and have access, probably, to more copious sources of information than those of which I can boast. (1868: p. vii)

He goes on to describe how his affection for the area and its inhabitants has influenced his decision to undertake this work even though, as he suggests in the quotation above, he considers other residents better qualified than he to compile 'their own' history. Newbigging legitimates his decision to undertake the task by underlining his length of residence in the area, noting that he has lived in the town for seventeen years. He draws on his 'affection' for the area as legitimate qualification. But overriding any qualms he may have of appropriating somebody else's history, there is a need to preserve what he calls the 'fragments of Fact and Legendary Lore' before they are irretrievably lost. The idea that they may be lost spurs Newbigging—a non-native—to attempt the work. He also points to the pleasure many people such as himself gain in learning 'more than they at present know of "the rude forefathers" who thinly tenanted its bleak hillsides or wandered centuries ago in its wooded cloughs; where instead of the noise of manufacturing Industry, the rush of the Red Deer through the leafy covert alone broke the prevailing stillness' (Newbigging 1868: p. viii).

Newbigging wrote these words in Bacup in 1867 and it is striking how they resonate with views put forward by present day members of the Nat about their own role as local historians. First, Newbigging assumes that being able to trace one's ancestors in Bacup, that is, being able to trace one's connections to the past through kin, provides credentials along which authority travels. Second, Newbigging's interest is in the preservation of a unique and idyllic past; not all past is necessarily history. There is an appropriate history with which to represent Bacup in the present. As autobiography is a selection of elements from the past which fashions the present, so elements of the past are shuffled and selected to serve the needs of history.

OfKey English Battles

In 1988, there was a lively debate amongst certain members of the Nat about whether Bacup was the site of the battle of Brunanburgh. Newbigging is convinced Bacup is the site of the battle waged in 937, during the reign of the

Saxon king, Athelstan. It is said to have been a crucial moment in Anglo-Saxon history, and secured the position of the Saxon rulers in the face of repeated Danish intrusions. A description of the battle is found in an Ode recorded in the *Anglo-Saxon Chronicle*.

On the death of the Danish king Sihtric, Athelstan king of Wessex annexed and assumed power over the kingdom of Northumbria. Sihtric's two sons were forced into exile. The eldest, Anlaf (or Olaf in some commentaries), fled to Ireland where, determined to regain control over Northumbria and to depose Athelstan, he organized support from 'the Scots, the Welsh, and his Danish kindred' (Newbigging 1893: 15). Members of his confederacy have been identified as Constantine, king of the Scots—believed to be the one described as a 'heavy haired warrior and the old and wily one' in the Ode (Whitelock 1961)—the king of Strathclyde, Owen of Cumberland, and the Danes of Northumbria (Freeman 1871; Plummer and Earle 1899). Anlaf launched an expedition from Ireland and it is at this point that Newbigging disagrees with most other writers on the subject who, he suggests, are of the erroneous opinion that Athelstan landed all his 'six hundred and thirteen vessels' at the mouth of the Humber. In his view this is unlikely. Anticipating his thesis (that the battle of Brunanburgh took place near Bacup), he surmises that most of Anlaf's ships landed in the estuaries of the rivers Mersey, Ribble, Wyre, and Lune. Hence the invading army advanced from the west across the Lancashire plain and the battle of Brunanburgh took place near Bacup which is where Anlaf and his 'league of warriors' met Athelstan and his brother Edmund.[15] The Ode of the battle of Brunanburgh describes a bloody fight with a great number of fatalities—'the field was slippery with the blood of heroes'. Five Danish kings, seven earls, and the son of the king of Scots were killed (Freeman 1871). Anlaf escaped and returned to Ireland. It is clear where Newbigging's sympathies lay. His support goes unquestionably to the victorious Anglo-Saxons and more specifically to Athelstan who he says was both kind and generous. Newbigging suggests the unsuccessful attempts of Anlaf—'the Danish invader'—to regain the throne were foolhardy and doomed to fail, and he blames what he says is Anlaf's ungracious acceptance of defeat and his continued life of piracy on his 'roving Danish propensities': 'It is probable, however, that Athelstan would have exercised clemency towards the brothers; for the elder, on surrendering himself some time afterwards, was received with kindness by the king, and might have lived in peace, had not his roving Danish propensities led him to renounce his quiet life, and assume that of marauder and sea-king' (1868: 14). Athelstan's victory over the combined forces is said to have been a turning-point in English history leading to the formation of a single kingdom of England. Where and how, then, does Bacup feature in this story? The site of the battle is not named in the *Anglo-Saxon Chronicle*.

[15] Edmund succeeded Athelstan as king of England in 939.

Commentators and historians have put forward a variety of suggestions which include: Bromborough on the river Mersey in Cheshire, Bramber south of the river Ribble in Lancashire, and Brough on the Roman road from Carlisle to York in Westmoreland (Plummer and Earle 1899). Newbigging (1868: p. ix) reveals his own inspiration came from a paper read to the Historic Society of Lancashire and Cheshire by Mr T. T. Wilkinson ('Esq. FRAS, of Burnley') and entitled 'The Battle of Brunanburgh and the probable Locality of the Conflict'. This paper convinced Newbigging that the battle took place not only in the vicinity of Burnley but on what is now Bacup's doorstep. So what was the evidence T. T. Wilkinson presented in 1818 which convinced Newbigging that Bacup was the site of the battle of Brunanburgh?

To the north of the town centre, on the lower slopes of the moorland which climb to Weir (and to the Deerplay Inn), there is an overgrown embankment. It is about 1,800 feet long and follows the curvature of the hillside. For much of its length it is about 50 feet wide and at its deepest 12 feet which, according to Newbigging, is the depth of the original excavation. The earthwork is known as Broadclough Dyke after the area in which it is located. Those who present an opinion on it appear to agree that the dyke was dug originally for military purposes. Whittacker believes it to be an unfinished and therefore unused British camp but thinks the iron arrowheads found on nearby hills were from deer-hunting rather than pitched battle. Newbigging (1868: 15–16), on the other hand, considers the iron arrowheads to be further proof of battle, and is persuaded the dyke played a decisive part in the defences of the Saxon armies: 'it is in the highest degree probable that one or other of the rival armies . . . forced, or attempted to force, a passage through the valley of the Irwell; and that here they were encountered by the confederated hosts intrenched behind the vast earthwork at Broadclough that commanded the line of their march'.

Newbigging, as a local historian, is clearly excavating a history of Bacup which conforms to and confirms its uniqueness. He emphasizes its special and distinctive place in the history of England. Many present-day members of the Nat are sceptical but others carefully study historical tomes and archival material with a view to finding further references which may associate the battle of Brunanburgh with Bacup. While a unique past has *moulded* a distinctive Bacup character, different elements of that past and, indeed, different elements of that character, are connected up according to the reason for doing the connecting in the first place. On the one hand, an idyllic romantic past is evoked: so, for example, beautiful moors and frolicking deer inhabit a pre-industrial landscape, while sociability and mutual support dominate the industrial landscape. On the other hand, it is the harshness and inhospitality of a landscape marred by violence, pollution, and ill health, which is brought to the fore. Ultimately, however, honest, resilient, clean, and humorous characters emerge from an unhealthy, unfriendly, and inhospitable environment.

'A Nice History'

The first recorded settlement in the direct vicinity of Bacup is a monastery in Brandwood, a neighbourhood of present-day Stacksteads. At the beginning of the thirteenth century, monks were granted grazing rights over land which they cleared and cultivated. According to one source, the farming activities of the monks 'set an example to the Lords of the Manor' and by the beginning of the fourteenth century (by which time the amount of game in the area had decreased considerably) eleven cattle-breeding farms or vaccaries were operational in Rossendale (Tupling 1927: 20): one such establishment was operational in 'Bacope'.

The many variations in the spelling of Bacup over time have given rise to extensive speculation as to the derivation of the place-name. The more popular versions of its etymology appear to ignore the oldest recorded spellings which feature 'cop' or 'cope', as in Bacope (above), as well as Bakcop, Baycope, and Fullbachope. Instead, in the early part of the nineteenth century, local historians appeared to be looking to and for a romantic past. James Hargreaves (cited in Newbigging 1893) rejected a current idea that the name of Bacup derived from Bay cop meaning 'red earth' on the grounds that the soil in the area was not generally red, but black. He went on to conjecture that, in some unspecified past, 'the deer in their excursions for pasture or play' ran down the valley from Deerplay Hill and, when they reached the place where Bacup now stands, turned and ran back up again—hence 'Backup'. Eventually the 'k' was dropped, changing the spelling to Bacup and the pronunciation to /Baekup/. Another historian of that period is also taken with the association between Bacup and red deer and claims 'Baycop' refers to the cop or hillock where the deer stood at bay (Whittacker, cited in Newbigging 1893).

Newbigging presents Hargreaves's hypothesis in detail but argues it 'lacks dignity'. He prefers an explanation which retains the association of 'bay' with 'red' and of 'cop' with 'land' (more specifically hill). Thus 'red hill', he suggests, refers to the 'large abundance of red deer frequenting the hillside' (ibid. 4). Other origins mooted for the place-name but not appropriated to the same extent by residents of Bacup (both past and present) have included Fulebach-hope—the break in the shut-in valley—and Back Cowpe referring to its location in the hills behind the village of Cowpe.

I was offered, unsolicited, the story about frolicking deer running back up the hill by several Bacup residents during fieldwork. Marilyn Greaves is a keen reader of local history and after relating this story to me, she mused 'we have a nice history'. Another Bacup woman, in her late twenties, discerning some scepticism on my part, insisted indignantly 'that's *really* where the name came from'. The veracity or otherwise of this etymology is, of course, beside the point. As in all origin myths, its meaning is as much in the telling as it is in the content and in this case what both women express is the idea that Bacup *and they* have a history and, furthermore, a 'nice history'. Those who define themselves as Bacup born and bred lay claim to Bacup's past; it is also their past, it belongs to them. The links they make between themselves and the town's past is of a piece with the links they make between themselves and their ancestors. Both require a selection of detail; a selection of what to make explicit and what to leave out.

The past as resource is not the prerogative of those who lay claim to the history of Bacup as their own. Judy Wilder, a resident of sixteen years, talked on many occasions of how she thought Bacup's past, embodied in its artefacts and edifices, could and ought to be exploited for the tourist industry. She pointed to 'the smallest street in Britain', the cobblestones, Bacup's Coco-Nut Dancers (Ch. 7) and the beautiful architecture of the derelict and abandoned market hall as evidence. However she insisted it was up to those who owned this past to do the exploiting. 'Bacup people should exploit what they got', Judy told me forcefully, 'because you can't *make* history.' In this, Judy concurs with ideas put forward by members of the Nat about what constitutes appropriate and relevant history: for the facts of the past can only be excavated not created; they perdure and are immutable.

As accomplished local historians, many members of the Nat carry out historical research, and they describe their work as revealing the facts of history. As one member said of his research, 'I'm digging up facts there, I'm digging up something which I want to verify (pause) a kind of authority. If I can get a

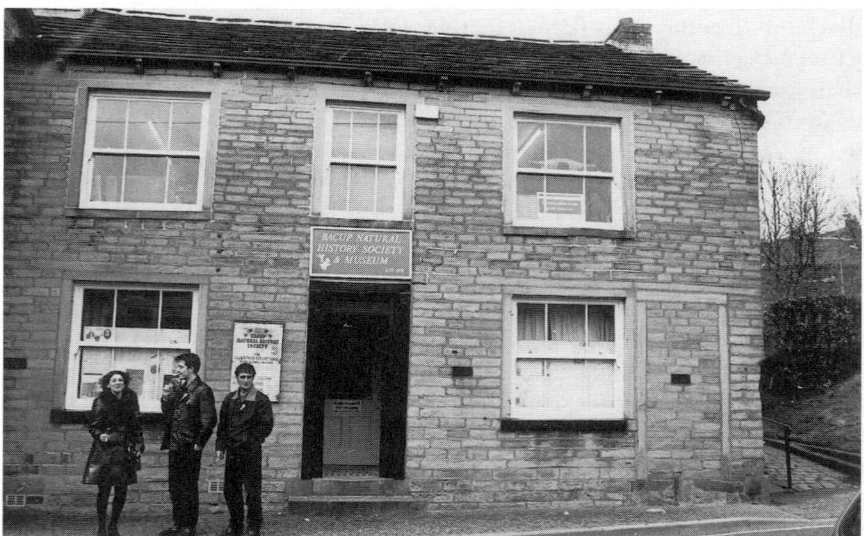

PLATE 4. Bacup Natural History Society

date for an event from a local paper, that seals it to me. It happened. That paper published it. That's a fact.'

But at the same time, there is a self-conscious process of making history. Judgements are made as to what counts as a proper history and there are decisions constantly being made as to what the future's history will be.

The origin story which features deer running back up to Deerplay Hill portrays an image of an idyllic and charming landscape which has disappeared. In insisting on this version, people lay claim not merely to Bacup's past but to a past which is charming as well as unique—'we have a nice history'. Likewise, they may point to the difference, minute to the untutored ear, between a Bacup dialect and that of a neighbouring town, and relate anecdotes which describe and embellish the idiosyncratic, and in some cases bizarre, behaviour of named inhabitants (past and present). It is the uniqueness of the dialect and the distinctiveness of individuals which is celebrated in the telling and retelling of these particular pasts.

The Nat: From Eggs to Artefacts

In 1988 there were over 100 paid-up members of the Nat, eight office-holders, and nine elected committee members.[16] I encompass all office-holders and elected committee members under the general rubric of 'the Committee', and it is they who best exemplify the constituency of the weekly meetings which are held on Thursday evenings between 7 p.m. and 9:30 p.m. The Committee comprises predominantly middle-aged and elderly men, many of whom define themselves as Bacup born and bred. Three women regularly attend weekly meetings of the Nat, one of whom, Maureen Doherty, is a committee member (the first in the society's history). Committee members trace their connections to Bacup through being born in the town, or through what is said to be a shared working-class background. They also share an endeavour of 'unearthing' history and 'preserving' culture. I recall Martin Firth, treasurer and well-respected local historian, who I had assumed was from Bacup, being teased on one occasion by a fellow member for being a *furriner* (foreigner). As if to reassure me of his credentials as a local historian, Mr Firth told me he had come to Bacup when he was 4 years old and that his father had been a printworker. He used both the length of his residence in Bacup and his father's occupation to mitigate his place of birth.[17]

[16] There were also eight named vice-presidents who had been nominated at various Annual General Meetings for services rendered to the society, but who did not usually attend meetings.

[17] The mayor talking of his origins at Mrs Jones's 90th birthday party in 1990 (see Ch. 2) made explicit his connection to Bacup via selected ancestors in an attempt to mitigate the fact he lived in Haslingdon. Being unconnected he could be seen as a 'furriner' and as such unqualified to serve and speak on behalf of Bacup.

The Nat is housed in a listed building in the centre of town. The building was formerly the Hare and Hounds public house and lodgings and has been occupied by the Nat since 1947. It was initially rented and then purchased from the brewery in 1951 for £375: one committee member informed me the society had put up £100 and an anonymous donor £275 in order to buy the property. Renovation of the building is currently being funded partly by National Heritage, and its upkeep from private donations, public collections, and fund-raising activities. Many committee members donate a substantial amount of their time and labour to maintaining the building, archives, and artefacts. There is a museum on the first floor, and on the ground floor a meeting-room where public lectures are held, a library where members of the society meet once a week, and a small kitchen. At the time of fieldwork another ground-floor room was closed but housed several large pieces of machinery taken from local factories. As well as the regular weekly meetings, a public lecture is given every Saturday evening during the autumn and winter and usually attracts a full house. The museum is also open to the public on Thursday evenings, but the curator also arranges for individuals and groups to visit the museum at other times, and he provides guided tours for, amongst others, school and church groups, voluntary associations, and visiting academics. The curator's talks are renowned for their wit and anecdote and the richness of historical detail.

At its inception in 1878 and up to the end of the nineteenth century the Nat was predominantly, as its name suggests, interested in natural history.[18] The founders of the Nat were collectors of the flora and fauna of the region at a time when mills were working and Bacup a busy industrial town.[19] The museum contains a reminder of this prior interest in natural history, and the shift in interest from natural to industrial history is evident in the fact that the geological specimens, stuffed birds and their blown eggs, caterpillar larvae, pinned butterflies, and small dead mammals, for example, now take a back seat in the museum. To the front are artefacts from an era of intense industrial development and two world wars. Machines, gadgets, toys, utensils, and ornaments jostle for space with footwear, clothes, gas masks, and commemoration pottery; intricate models made of matches, cigarette cards, and carved wood share cabinets with Victorian paraphernalia and obscure—and one hopes obsolete—medical instruments. Display cases are crammed full with clogs, typewriters, postcards, souvenirs, and tools from the textile industry, and all in all the impression is created of a veritable, as the curator put it, 'Aladdin's cave'.

[18] See Anne Secord (1994*a*; 1994*b*; 1996) for an excellent historical analysis of the early nineteenth-century pursuit of natural history by working-class men in north-west England (and see Percy 1991). Her exacting historical perspective is both stimulating and challenging and I am grateful for her comments to me on the origins of museums such as the Nat.

[19] There has never been full employment in Bacup, and for many of the working classes in this region of England employment has never been secure.

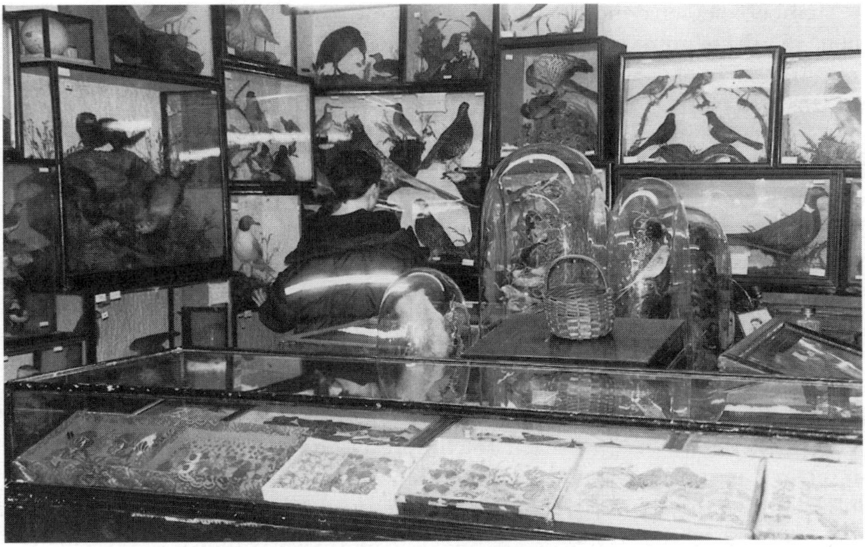

PLATE 5. In the Nat museum: a natural history collection

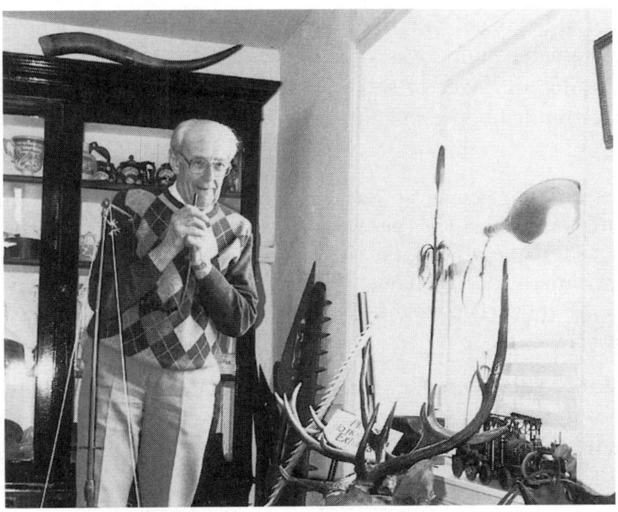

PLATE 6. In the Nat museum: demonstrating dentist's drill

Members perceive the Nat as preserving the town's 'culture', symbolized in their guardianship of its cultural artefacts. There is a library which houses a collection of books, photographs, and newspapers, and objects in Nat keeping are guarded with care and possessiveness[20] and rarely is a donation to the museum or library refused.[21] Most of the exhibits in the museum are seen to belong rightfully to Bacup, and the appropriation of certain items by Rawtenstall museum is a matter of controversy. For example, in the Rawtenstall collection there are pieces of furniture and paintings taken from Bacup Town Hall after the abolition of Bacup Borough Council. Some Nat members believe they should be returned to Bacup where they say 'they rightfully belong', others point pragmatically to the lack of space.

The Nat not only guards the town's cultural artefacts and archives, however, it also makes explicit the proper Bacup behaviour which is deemed central to the well-being and preservation of the town. In crafting a history of Bacup, Nat members make explicit their role in preserving 'tradition', and the Nat is an integral part of the history crafted. Hence the events they organize are not only about history but also about themselves as part of that history. The Nat of the past, as textualized by present members, is clearly linked to present-day concerns and preoccupations. For example, members emphasize the strength and character of individuals who, despite poor social conditions prevailing during the second half of the nineteenth century, succeeded in their quest for knowledge. They celebrate the fortitude of townspeople who were able to triumph, through self-help, over squalid conditions which existed at the time. The Nat promotes an image of self-reliance through particular readings of the past. A booklet published by the Nat in 1978 to mark the centenary year of the society notes:

> The great mass of the people of Bacup were either poor or practically destitute. Keeping a family on 12/- to 15/- per week must have been a struggle, and when short time came, as it so frequently did, the situation must have been desperate. The picture however, is not entirely gloomy. There were quite a number of people (rich and poor) who sought to rise above their surroundings, and became keenly interested in learning. (BNHS 1978: 11)

One stated aim of the Centenary souvenir booklet is to pay homage to founder members and it acknowledges the contribution and skills of many named members as it traces the changes that have occurred over the years in pre-

[20] While most things brought to the museum and library are accepted, for reasons of space selections are made as to which appear frontstage and which are stored backstage; there is also the occasional cull. One of the most difficult and divisive tasks undertaken by the librarian during the summer of 1988 was to take stock and relinquish certain books which he and others considered irrelevant to the present concerns of the society. What is of contemporary relevance to both the library and the museum is inevitably a matter of contestation.

[21] This also relies on those donating objects knowing what are appropriate or relevant items of Nat interest.

mises, membership, and preoccupations. The booklet also published a dialect poem by Bill o' Bows,[22] born Clifford Heyworth in Milnrow, near Rochdale, in 1910, which expresses pride in the Nat. Here are the first two verses:

> Th'owd 'Nat' has had its ups an' deawns,
> But stood time's changin' test,
> It's lived through laughs an' smiles an' freawns
> An' still con rank wi' t' best.
>
> Long live the Bacup 'Nat', an' so—
> Give service born to last,
> That generations all shall know—
> The history of the past.
>
> Bill o' Bows

Dwelling on the origins of the Nat, the authors refer to a letter published in the *Bacup Times* of 25 March 1878 and written by Mr James Holmes, who subsequently became the first secretary of the society. In the letter, Mr Holmes mentions a paper he gave to the 'mutual improvement class in connection with the General Baptists' which 'so stimulated the class' they held a series of rambles and invited Mr Henry Halstead 'a stonemason and local botanist of no mean repute' to lead them (BNHS 1978: 1). The Bacup and Rossendale Field Naturalists' Club was born and attracted those who were interested in 'the local flora and fauna'. Meetings are reported to have been well attended and 'a valuable source of education to those interested in natural history' (ibid.). By the time the club became the Bacup Natural History Society in 1879, premises were being provided by Dr J. H. Worrall, MRCS—'a wonderful instructor and generous friend' (ibid.). The first president of the society was Mr Henry Halstead who was replaced by Mr Thomas Aitken, JP, with Dr Worrall heading a list of vice-presidents six of whom were local doctors.[23] The authors of the booklet comment on how the Nat provided a means of escape from the squalid and dismal conditions prevalent in Bacup at that time. In 1888, as a result of a decline in membership, a general meeting was called inviting 'all who had any interest in the welfare of the town', and it was reported that 'many of the gentlemen of the town who attended promised their support, and urged the continuance of the Society' (ibid. 2). From that meeting the membership grew, the society flourished, and the mayor of Bacup was elected president. The collection of 'botanical, geological and ornithological' specimens was moved into larger, rented premises in the town centre in 1889. The official opening of the

[22] According to *The Second Bacup Miscellany* he moved to Bacup when he was 2 years old and, by 1937, had 'achieved great popularity' as a dialect poet (Bowden 1975).

[23] The secretary told me that vice-presidentship is no longer a significant role in the Nat. He explained that in the past the title vice-president was given to those who could be expected 'to put their hand in their pocket'; an honorary title for those who might be relied upon to donate cash in times of need.

new rooms was marked by a 'grand exhibition' organized by the society in the Mechanics Hall and reported to have been a great success.[24]

The history of the Nat, presented by the Nat, is striking in more ways than one; I am struck, for example, by the way in which the contribution of 'the gentlemen' of the town is emphasized; by the centrality of self-help in learning; and by the link made between the survival of the Nat and the welfare of Bacup.[25] According to the history of the society, reworked and rewritten by members, the benefactors and founding members of the Nat were 'men with a vision' who saw that the quality of life could be improved through self-education. Not only did they help themselves, but they also acted on behalf of other townsfolk and had the foresight and the benevolence to create something which could provide pleasure and education to others. Present-day Nat members in writing the history of the Nat connect past and present, and are thus seen as successors to the founders, being given, and taking on board, similar responsibility for the town's well-being.

As well as preserving the past in the form of archives, artefacts, and—as we shall see—information collected and stored by individuals, Nat members formulate a relevant and appropriate past. The museum collection configures not only particular pasts but also possible futures. Members foresee what will be historically relevant. In September 1988 a pair of shoes was donated to the museum. The shoes were described on the box in which they came as 'fashionable lady's court shoes', with 'man-made uppers', and 'rubber soles'. They were shiny patent leather with an acrylic bow attached to the front and had come off the production line that week. The factory which produced them had closed down the same week. Its closure was due, a spokesperson said, to 'increased competition from abroad'. All workers were made redundant and the machinery was due to be sold by auction. The curator catalogued and displayed the shoes as the 'the last pair of shoes' to be made in 'the first Bacup shoe factory'. He showed them to me and told me that if the museum only preserved old things then it would die. The Nat, he said, needed to be *making* history at the same time as preserving it.

According to historian Ann Secord (1996: 378), by the middle of the nineteenth century, when public houses had become exclusively the preserve of working-class men, artisan botany was thriving in Lancashire. Manual

[24] The contents of this exhibition are not detailed. A second exhibition was staged in 1928, to celebrate the fiftieth anniversary of the Society; this was a Science and Art Exhibition, and included 'items of scientific interest' as well paintings by local artists.

[25] One local historian insisted that there were only ever two landowners in Bacup. He was referring to landowners with inherited land, and one he named as James Maden Holt, who was rewarded with land by Henry VIII for his support in the pilgrimage of grace, an event associated with Henry's secession from the church. By contrast, the majority of millowners were, I was told, 'local lads made good'; often entrepreneurs who through hard work and thrift succeeded. My neighbour Mrs Jones also told me, on several occasions, that Bacup, unlike other Lancashire towns such as Wigan and Preston, where she said landowners were Catholic, never had a 'landed gentry'.

workers—predominantly artisans and operatives—formed natural history societies which met regularly in public houses. Secord (ibid. 391) comments that the role of such societies in the production and accumulation of botanical knowledge is difficult to determine and all too often ignored because the historical record is compiled from the 'literary traces of elite botanists'. The question of whether the origins of the Nat are to be found in the public houses of mid-nineteenth-century Bacup and in the activities of working-class botanists, as were other similar societies of the time and region, awaits further investigation. Present-day committee members are predominantly skilled and semi-skilled working-class men; many are retired, and were formerly artisans, machine operatives, and local entrepreneurs.[26] They, however, identify the society's founders as 'the gentlemen of the town': its clerics, general practitioners, and Justices of the Peace, and the shift from an interest in natural history to local history is not explicated in Nat reflections on their past.[27] It is recorded that a move of premises in 1889 was initiated because of the growing *natural history* collection and a shortage of space. It is also recorded that the president from 1896 to 1908, Revd J. S. Doxey, the vicar of Christ Church, was a 'keen collector of coins, old books and anything which could be called a curio' (BNHS 1978: 6). A shift in interest from natural to local history might reflect a change in the management of the society, and it is the case that individual interests of presidents and curators, for example, inevitably influence what is collected. At the same time, a shift from collecting local 'flora and fauna' to local industrial artefacts might also have been a means of making visible a history affirming and foregrounding working-class identity. But if we look beyond the management and control of the museum, to the social relationships contained therein, then we have to include donors as much as guardians. While a major Nat interest is in objects produced during an era of intense industrial activity, it is often relationships embodied in those objects which are the focus of discussion. Who made and used them? Who passed them on (donated them) and to whom? Nat members tell of such relationships and in so doing identify and locate Bacup's artefacts within Bacup. Present-day members perceive the Nat to have a responsibility for collecting and preserving 'Bacup's heritage' and they rarely refuse to accept an object brought to them. But this means other residents have not only to donate but also assess what is appropriate to donate; they have to know what is a relevant offering. Explaining the shift from natural to local history, Thomas Shields the curator of the museum told me people 'just started'

[26] I am grateful to conversation with Peter Crawley and Gordon Fyfe which prompted me to think about changes in the management of the museum, and to Peter Crawley for his enthusiasm about the topic.

[27] And, in fact, some members would disagree with my observation that there has been a shift in interest and argue that there are members today who are still interested in natural history (particularly in fossils).

bringing in different objects and the Nat *had* (had an obligation) to collect them. The collection emerges then from a reciprocal relationship. The things donated to the museum already belong to Bacup; they are not gifts, and local historians, who also belong to Bacup, are perceived to be appropriate guardians. The objects in Nat keeping act as mnemonics for relatedness in and between domains such as work, kinship, and neighbourhood. If the town's past is implicated in them, it is necessary to guard them for the town's future, and who better to do so than those who also 'belong' to Bacup?

Experts and Patrons

When I first explained my intentions to members of the Nat I stressed my interest was in present-day Bacup. Apart from a tongue-in-cheek comment that 'we know nowt about today', it was emphatically and eloquently pointed out to me by Charles Hardcastle that the present cannot be divorced from yesterday and for me to even *begin* to understand Bacup I needed to know about the past.[28] This was a view reiterated by other members of the society over the next year and it embraces a notion that Bacup is unique and its distinctiveness is partly due to what is perceived as its unique history. A character typical of Bacup folk is said to have been *moulded*, not only by the physical environment which itself is marked and created by the activities of past inhabitants, but also by the kind of industrious life they led. Nat members do not necessarily consider contemporary Bacup an appropriate subject of study. They claim an expertise on a Bacup upon which they themselves reflect but which does not, necessarily, include them. In conceptualizing their research as unearthing the facts of the past, members knew they were able to provide me with relevant information, armed with which I would understand contemporary Bacup life better. This view of the kind of relationship pertaining between the anthropologist and indigenous expert, whether self-appointed or ascribed, is not, of course, confined to Bacup and its local historians.[29] The Nat not only theorize about Bacup society, but also recognize the activity of research as a legitimate pastime (if not quite a proper job). They assume we are engaged in the same endeavour. But I could no more pretend to be unearthing the facts about Bacup

[28] I discovered, after knowing each independently, that Mr Charles Hardcastle was Mrs Hilary Hardcastle's brother-in-law—her deceased husband's brother. Mrs Hardcastle had been ill and had moved in with her brother, Leonard Pickering, and his wife. I went to visit her and was telling her about my visits to the Nat. She mentioned in passing, and appeared to attach little significance to the fact, that her brother-in-law was 'one of them' (that is, a Nat member). She allowed me to work out the connection, bemused I think by my enthusiasm, and she named their other siblings. Mrs Hilary Hardcastle died in 1990 and Mr Charles Hardcastle in 1991. They are missed, and I remember with gratitude their interest in my work and their kindness.

[29] Maryon McDonald (1987) writes of how members of the Brittany movement expected her to use their research as the baseline from which to understand rural peasants. And Okely (1983; 1987) reveals the way in which gypsy folklorists assume their version of gypsy history is not only correct but conclusive.

than I could leave out the Nat from the Bacup in which I am interested. My interest, unlike that of local historians, is not in the facts of history but in which elements of the past become history and the way in which they are put to work (connected up) to create contexts in which they then assume significance.

Most members of the Nat reiterate that their knowledge of Bacup is based on experience of the town gained through having lived there all or most of their lives. However, local historians of today and yesterday acknowledge that Bacup can also be known through study. On the one hand, expert status is gained through the experience of living in the town, and on the other, through study.[30] Rather than seeing these as alternative forms of acquiring knowledge (as different epistemologies), it is more useful, I think, to see them as aspects of each other. A notion that knowledge is acquired through study requires a counterpoint, in this case, that one can know through experience (and vice versa).[31]

Members of the Nat define their role as 'finding out about Bacup'. Some, at present, have gone beyond an industrial history of Bacup, contained in the collected artefacts and archives of the museum and library as well as in the individual knowledge of members, to a pre-industrial era. The unique and idiosyncratic nature of Bacup is verified in narratives which connect Bacup to the battle of Brunanburgh and Anglo-Saxon victors; or to the 'rush' of deer and the moors; or to idiosyncratic characters and characteristics. While research might involve unearthing facts, one's ability to find out about Bacup is enhanced by a knowledge of the town gained through experience, even though it may be the past before living memory which is being explicated. Hence, Newbigging acknowledges he is not necessarily, as an outsider, the best person to write a history of the region; a sentiment echoed by present-day Nat members who acknowledge that being born and bred in the town gives one a legitimate claim on it and the things that belong to it, including its history. But all is not lost if one is not born in Bacup because other connections can be traced; thus one can 'know' Bacup through length of residence (we are told the poet Bill o' Bows came to Bacup when he was 2 years old, the local historian Martin Firth when he was 4 years old, and Newbigging lived in Bacup seventeen years before he presumed to write about it), or shared class experiences (which include housing and occupational histories). Time and experience,

[30] I have elsewhere compared ideas put forward by members of Housing Aid, a voluntary sector organization in Manchester, and by members of the Nat about the ways in which knowledge is acquired (Edwards n.d.). Members of Housing Aid make a distinction between knowledge gained through formal means, such as education and training, and knowledge gained through experience. In certain contexts and particularly in conversations with me both as a Ph.D. student and somebody wanting to learn about the organization, they privilege knowledge gained through experience and argue that they understand the needs of their clients better than members of statutory agencies because they share a similar background.

[31] Similar to the way in which a notion that upbringing is influential on who a person becomes requires the idea that birth itself is.

however, are not necessarily adequate teachers, they require the addition of respect and affection for the town and its people in order to be effective.

Preserving Culture

> We have tried in a modest way to show how the 'Nat' has played a great part in the promotion of culture in Bacup over the past 100 years.
>
> (BNHS 1978: 10)

Nat members perceive themselves as preserving and promoting culture in Bacup.[32] The context created, in which this rendering of culture is significant, is a past comprising a squalid and 'God-forsaken' Bacup; where cotton mills dominated the landscape as well as the social relationships of a majority of inhabitants; where long hours were spent in factories; where dwellings were dark and overcrowded and children started work at the age of 12 or 13. Such a rendering of the past celebrates the fortitude of those townspeople who were able, through self-help, to triumph over the harsh conditions they faced. The past cannot be divorced from the context in which it is told. The evocation of a past in which people were more friendly, more honest, industrious, and generally more caring, firmly connects the speaker to that past and in so doing makes a statement about themselves and hence others in the present, and it is this process of constantly categorizing persons, in inclusive and exclusive terms, which is consistent.

While Nat members textualize a history of Bacup which includes the Nat, that history does not include themselves as individuals. They compose a past *on behalf* of Bacup. The accumulated knowledge acquired by individual historians collectively formulates and adds to the knowledge of Bacup, for Bacup. The excavation and preservation of the history of the town might be seen to further an understanding of the place but the point is that it is put to use. The preservation of pasts guarantees futures—to lose them would be to lose an integral part of present identity. And without the present, which requires presence, there can be no future. The indigenous exercise of writing history becomes, then, more than a reflection on present-day preoccupations; it becomes a transformation necessary for futures. It is in the light of this that we might want to understand Charles Hardcastle's exhortation that to understand today, 'we need to know about yesterday', and we cannot separate the past from the present.

As well as the museum, the Nat has a library which houses an ageing collection of reference books, newspapers, and photographs. My interest here is in the resource of knowledge held by members themselves. Each of the com-

[32] 'Culture' is loaded, an idiom of relatedness *par excellence*. It connotes, here, civilization and sophistication, and at the same time is conceived of as an entity—a thing which can be preserved and passed on, or destroyed and lost.

mittee members proclaims a specific area of interest and their expertise in that field is recognized and acknowledged by other members. On my first visit to the Nat, Maureen Doherty took me under her wing and pointed out and named various individuals: 'John Pickering is an expert in quarries', she said, 'Joe Davidson, an expert in mines', and 'James Howarth, an expert in buildings'. 'Charles Hardcastle', she went on, 'knows everything there is to know about churches and Martin Firth knows all about the mills.' When I asked Maureen in what area her expertise lay, she laughed and replied 'making the tea'. When pressed, she admitted an interest in Scottish history and a passion for Vikings; she commented wryly that the others had not yet disowned her for this idiosyncrasy. Two other female members also have their own areas of historical interest—one is particularly interested in a pre-industrial Bacup and the other in heraldry—but neither were identified on this occasion as experts. Depending on my questions over the next year, I was sent to different members of the society. With questions concerning religion I was referred to Charles Hardcastle, about mills I was sent to Martin Firth the treasurer, the museum was the preserve of Thomas Shields the curator, while information about the society itself was the province of the president.[33] Local history is carved up into separate domains of expertise, and expertise entails knowledge achieved in two separate but interrelated ways. First through experience gained, in this case, from living in Bacup. And second through study, that is, through careful research which involves unearthing 'the facts'. The discourse of knowing shifts between these two possibilities, and like 'being born' and 'being bred', they are each implicated in the other. One may be brought more into focus as the other is momentarily screened out, but they rely on each other. Knowledge is as much a hybrid as kinship.

During the winter months, from October to March, the Nat runs a series of weekly public lectures which are well attended, often attracting an audience of between thirty and forty people. They take place on Saturday evenings at 7 p.m., and comprise a talk given by an invited speaker. Lectures are often about a journey, in Britain or abroad, and usually take the form of a travelogue accompanied by slides. The first and last talk of the series focuses on Bacup in 'times gone by' and are entitled 'Owd Bacup' and 'Owd Stacksteads'.[34] At these talks, said to be the most popular of the season and always attracting a full house, slides from old photographs of the town and its former inhabitants are shown

[33] Joe Smedley, whose self-appointed role was to keep me in check, curbing my excesses and testing my loyalties, overheard me asking Martin Firth a question one evening. His response was swift and loud: 'Where, why, when, how, she never bloody stops!' It was he who suggested my friends and I would have 'a good laugh' at their expense (Ch. 1). Mr Smedley kept me on my toes; his comments were often challenging and discomforting and for that all the more helpful, not least in keeping complacency at bay.

[34] In the history of the Nat written by the Nat, it is recorded that these particular lectures were first given in 1928 at a Science and Arts Exhibition held in the Mechanics' Hall and organized by the Nat to mark its fiftieth year (BNHS 1978: 7).

BACUP NATURAL HISTORY SOCIETY FOUNDED 1878

and

CAMERA CLUB.

Illustrated Lectures.

1987 - 1988.

****

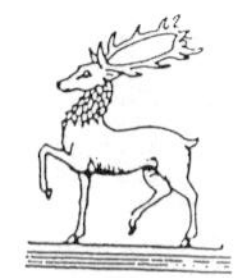

You are once again invited to our Saturday evening lectures during the coming winter season.

As you will observe from our Syllabus we cover a large part of the world, including Bacup & Stacksteads.

Much effort and skill has gone into the assembling of these lectures and we have the privilege of seeing the results of their work from the comfort of a Nat chair (!)

We hope you enjoy them.

Our Museum is open to the public every Thursday evening from 7.30pm.

You are very welcome.

Admittance to our Museum and all lectures is free.

Donations for the Society's upkeep are very welcome.

Groups and organisations can visit our Museum any day or evening by appointment.

Contact any of the Nat officials.

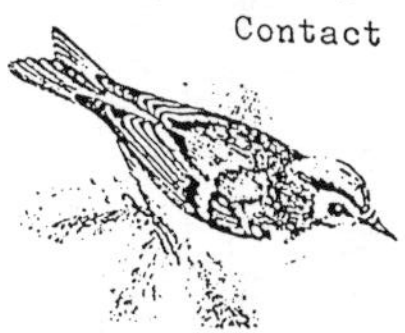

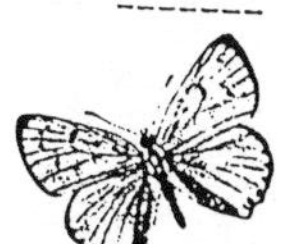

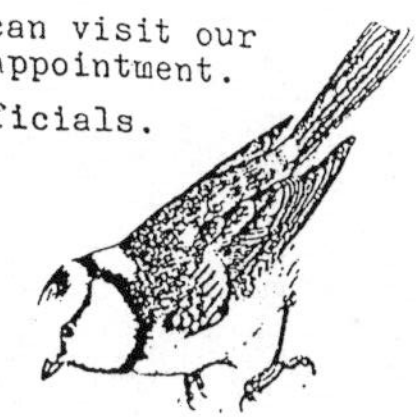

Bacup 'Nat' - - - - - Lectures.

Oct.24.	'Owd Bacup'	Mr.B.Ashworth.
" 31.	A Pacific Journey.	Mr.G.Woodcock.
Nov.7.	Days in the Highlands of Islands.	Mr.Joe Jackson.
" 14.	A Look at Natural History.	D.Tempest.
" 21.	The Lake District from Valley Floor to Mountain Top.	Mr.A.Tennant.
" 28.	The Orkneys.	Mr.H.Hemmett.
Dec. 5.	Through the Alps from Venice to Vienna.	Ron Jackson.
" 12.	American Holiday.	Mr.Brierley.
" 19.	CHRISTMAS PARTY.	
Jan. 9.	Ribblesdale.	Les.Hardman.
" 16.	Turkey.	Miss.L.Riley.
" 23.	Details Later.	Chris March.
" 30.	Peru & Bolivia.	Mary Davison.
Feb. 6.	Travels in Western Australia.	Ruth Pearson.
" 13.	Our Northern Heritage.	Mr.Hirst.
" 20.	The Natural History of the Yorkshire Dales.	Ron Freethy.
" 27.	Islay & Friends.	Mr.FJ.Sharpe.
Mar. 5.	Details Later.	
" 12.	A.Miscellany of Films.	Mr.& Mrs.Price.
" 19.	Recollections in Pendle.	Mr.Driver.
" 26.	'Owd Stacksteads'	Mr.A.Shelton.
May.18.	ANNUAL GENERAL MEETING.	

All Lectures commemce at 7pm.

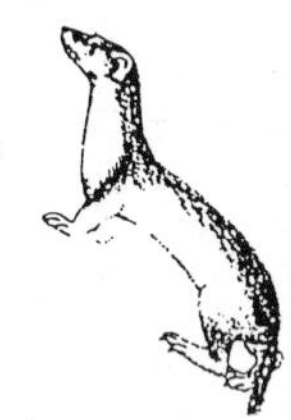

FIG. 3.2. Bacup Natural History Society programme of illustrated lectures, 1987–8

with a running commentary provided by a committee member, usually the president, sometimes the secretary, and occasionally the curator. Members of the audience participate in the commentary, identifying places and people, and offering memories of events and placing the people identified within their networks of family and neighbours, workmates, and political alliances. Connections are made, triggered by the visual reminders. In adding living detail to the images, participants express both their knowledge of the locality and their identity as Bacup people; they make manifest their connections to the past. The secretary Charles Hardcastle, who at the time of fieldwork was responsible for the planning of the Saturday night lectures and the task of inviting speakers as well as scouting for new talent, answered what he clearly thought a rather inane question on my part: 'What do I do it for? [*pause*] I suppose to bring to a lot of old folks who have never travelled a bit of experience of other places. There is also a bit of nostalgia involved in talks of old Bacup or Stacksteads.'

In a similar spirit, 'the best Christmas party in Bacup'—the opinion of more than one committee member—is organized by the Nat for themselves, their spouses, lecture-goers, and occasional visitors. Female members and wives of office-holders bake large 'tater pies'—potato with beef, and sometimes onion, cooked in a deep dish, with a thick pastry lid—and serve each portion with pickled red cabbage and onions. The men bring something to drink: perhaps wine, beer, soft drinks, or whisky.[35] Prior to the food being served, in 1988, the president had shown a series of his own slides depicting rural and mountainous landscapes in different parts of the British Isles. He accompanied the slides with a running commentary, identifying the localities and including details of geography and geology. Another popular annual event organized by the Nat is an Open Day held every Easter Saturday, known locally as Nutters' Day (Ch. 7). On this day the museum is open to the public, old photographs and maps are displayed, there is a raffle, and refreshments are sold in the meeting-room.

The building is also open to members on Sunday mornings when more contemplative activities are pursued by fewer people. It is Sunday mornings which best exemplify the curator's observation: 'the Nat is most of all a club.' An observation reiterated frequently in half-joking comments that the Nat provides 'an excuse to leave the wives behind'. This seems to bear little relationship to what 'Nat wives' actually do. For example, the Bacup Women's Guild also meets on a Thursday evening (attracting twice as many members as the Nat) and the wives of several Nat members play a prominent role in the organization. The committee of the Women's Guild arranges guest speakers as well as day-trips and fund-raising activities, and they also perceive themselves to be

[35] At the feast of 1988, I was the sole whisky drinker and the bottle, almost full, was taken back home by the man who brought it.

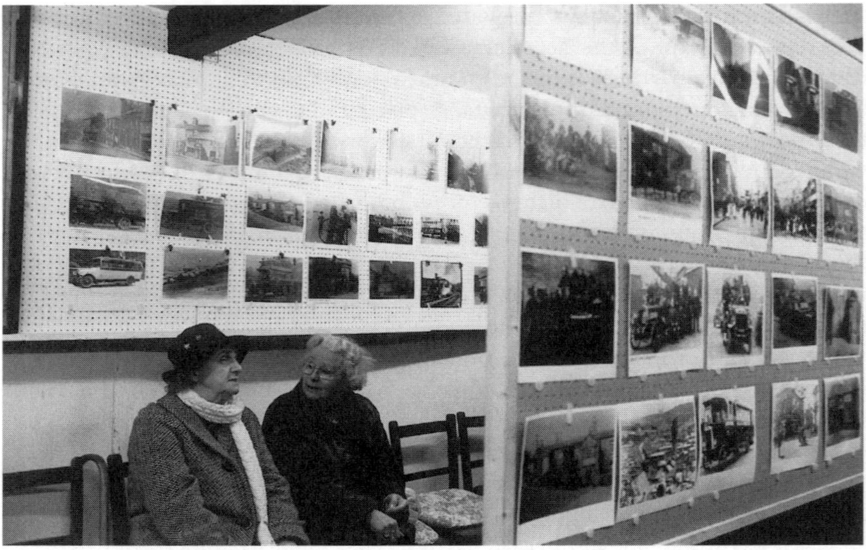

PLATE 7. In the Nat meeting-room: display of photographs of 'owd Bacup' on Nutter's Day

working on behalf of Bacup and its residents, providing a service which adds to the well-being and future of the town. There are many other formal and informal associations organized by and for women and some are affiliated with national organizations such as the Soroptomists and others with local churches and public houses. The Bingo Hall is also a popular venue for Bacup women. The support shown by the wives of Nat committee members at the Nat Christmas Party and Open Day are as much an extension of their own services to Bacup and its people as it is support of their husbands. The women both concur with their men (on behalf of Bacup) *and* diverge from them and which they do depends on the context they create in which it is relevant. In responding to general questions about Bacup, women acknowledge and emphasize the expert status of local historians; they referred me to the Nat, reasoning it was Nat members who *knew* all there was to know about Bacup. In such comments they place a claim on the Nat and its resource of experts, whom they entitle, in this context, to speak with authority on their behalf. However, when the same women address their own social activities, they suspend the connection between the Nat and Bacup. The Nat does not now stand for Bacup; and from this perspective it is not as active, as prolific, or as interesting as the women's organizations. It is, indeed, quirky. When I first explained my interest in Bacup to Barbara Jones, a neighbour and member of the Women's Guild, she, like many Bacup people, told me to go to the Nat. Several months later, I arranged

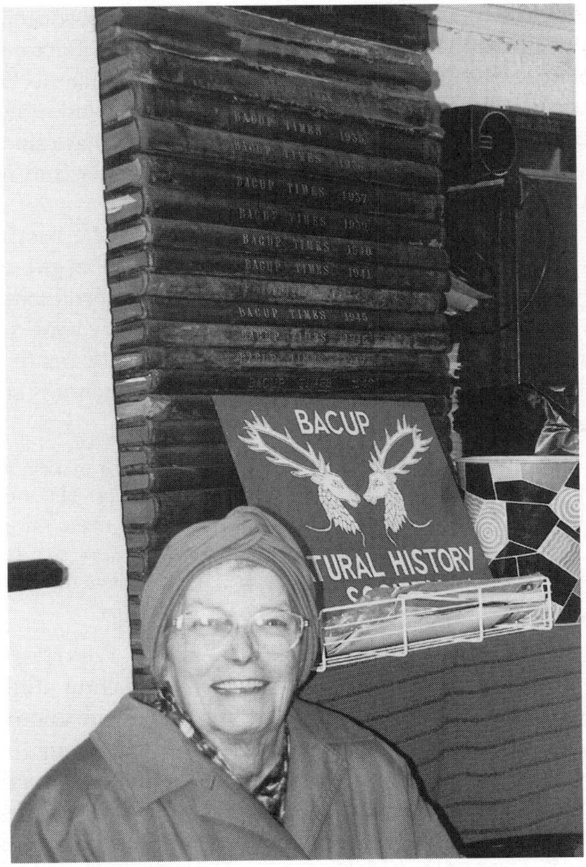

PLATE 8. The Nat collection of *Bacup Times*

to accompany her to a meeting of the Women's Guild and on the way I commented on its clash with the Nat. She gently admonished me: 'You don't want to go there, anyway,' she said. The same amused tolerance was shown by two other women that same evening for what they implied were the self-aggrandizing ideas of the men at the Nat. A similar kind of amused tolerance to that displayed by Nat members for what they imply are the infinitely less important activities of their wives.[36]

[36] Collusion is not a privilege of women. Between 1987 and 1988, Ann Summers parties were gaining in popularity in Bacup. Ann Summers is the brand name for a range of sex aids and lingerie and its sales strategy is based on a similar kind of model to Tupperware, where goods are demonstrated and sold at 'parties' in private homes with hostesses receiving a commission on goods sold. Ann Summers demonstrators are all women, and only women are invited and attend the parties. Women who agree

The history presented by the Nat reflects present-day concerns, and views expressed by Nat members resonate with those of other Bacup residents. But while members of the Nat act as critics of social change orchestrated from outside the town and perceive themselves as guardians and a reminder of the moral qualities necessary for the town's survival, they have no authority and not all residents consider the Nat to be the town's keeper, and if they do, not necessarily all the time.

From one anthropological perspective, textualizing the past takes place in the present and is seen to address issues significant to that present. If history written today reflects contemporary concerns of those producing it, and consequently it 'assumes its meaning from the contemporary context' (McDonald 1987: 129), it does more than recreate the past in the terms of today; it also constitutes the present, it creates its own context in which it is significant. For Greg Dening (1988: 2):

> History is all the ways we encode the past in symbol form to make a present. It is in this sense very vernacular. It is an everyday, every moment act. Making History is our constant cultural exercise. We express the past and by that make our social relationships and our social structures. We make boundaries of class, of sex, of age or role in our constant History making. We create change, we establish the status quo in our History making.

This begs the question: to which 'we' is Dening referring? A universal we perhaps; a we of humanity. Yet my history-making differs from the Nat's history-making and perhaps neither are what an anonymous reader of this book meant when calling for a chapter on 'the history' of the town. An apparent preoccupation with the past does address distinctions between then and now, as it addresses distinctions between categories of person, both past and present, but importantly it also projects a future. It is not merely an effect of nostalgia which prompts Bacup people to dwell on the past but an active fabrication of the links and connections which endure and which do not end in the present. The past is a domain in which relatedness is made explicit.

to host a party have to tread carefully in deciding who to invite; they need to avoid inviting a woman who might take offence, not only because they may 'spoil' the party by not participating in an appropriate manner, but also because they may judge the invitee negatively. Both those thought to be 'too posh' as well as 'too rough' are to be avoided. Only those who it is assumed will enter the spirit of the event and 'have a laugh' are invited. Most men I spoke with about these parties displayed the same kind of amused tolerance that some women expressed about the activities of the Nat. They also, however, collude with the women by including themselves in the sensitive negotiation of who may and may not participate. One morning, after an Ann Summers party at a neighbour's house to which I had been invited, the hostess's husband and I were hanging out our washing in the street at the same time. We greeted each other and he asked politely if I had enjoyed the party the night before. I was not expecting him to mention the party and was slightly flummoxed at his bringing it up. I said a few enthusiatic words (but not too enthusiastic), none of which I can recall. Thinking about it later, it seemed to me he had been making explicit his complicity in the event. Ann Summers parties, in this context, do not exclude men but 'the posh' and 'the uptight'.

In formulating particular pasts, people make explicit certain connections and screen out others and the links they make are mediated by particular persons and events. Pasts are construed by connecting up certain places, entities and persons—by making tangible relatedness. History, in the telling, constitutes the present and it draws on cultural premisses from which it is made. Wendy James (1988), writing of the Ebony order in Uduk society, says that knowledge is not 'secret or arcane'. For the Uduk 'authority has its source in the existing moral knowledge of people'. The Nat, in reflecting on the past in the present, draw on the cultural resources available to them. They tap into the existing 'archive of substantive notions' (ibid. 5), contextualizing them according to their concerns. And interestingly the way in which preoccupations are composed appears to have changed little over the past hundred years, despite the enormous social and economic changes that have taken place.

'A Bit of History'

One Thursday evening at the weekly meeting of the Nat the following story was told, partly for my benefit, but for everybody's amusement. The storyteller, Henry Frazer, is in his late fifties and a managing director of a Bacup shoe factory. He has taken an active interest in the Nat for many years and is the source of many an unusual artefact and many an amusing story. No particular area of expertise, such as Vikings, or religion, or mills, or mines, is ascribed to Mr Frazer, as it is to other members, but he is recognized as a skilled raconteur. While Maureen Doherty was serving the tea, Henry was asked by another member to tell me the story of the 'incomer and his cottage'. He allowed several other members to persuade him before telling us that if we were sitting comfortably he would begin. I recount his narrative here in a manner that only hints at the humour and wit with which it was delivered and received.

One Sunday afternoon, Henry Frazer and fellow Nat member George Parker were having a drink at the Deerplay Inn, up on Deerplay Hill. A man they knew—a local—was talking to another man whom they did not know. This man was clearly an *outsider* and, it turns out, somebody who had recently moved to a cottage not far from the pub in which they were now drinking. This man had been asking different people in the neighbourhood and in the pub whether they knew anything about his house. He was 'dying for a bit of history for his cottage', explained Henry. The local, spotting Henry and George across the room, told the outsider, 'If there's owt to know about that house they'll know it.'

Now Henry had already heard about this man and had already heard he was dying for a bit of history, so he guessed what was going on when he saw the man coming in their direction. The outsider introduced himself and had a bit of a chat before asking them whether they knew anything about 'them cottages' up on the hill. George and Henry looked pensive. After a while George shook his head, slowly, 'No, [pause] there's nowt much to tell about them places up there.' The man's shoulders drooped; he was evidently disappointed. The three of them carried on drinking their beer, apparently deep in thought. After a while Henry said, 'I did hear something once about two brothers', a pause, 'they were hung up there.' The man's shoulders perked up, he looked interested, he urged Henry to continue. Henry did: 'I think they were supposed to have lived in the second one from the top.' The outsider was now visibly excited. With the help of George, Henry provided some convincing biographical detail of two brothers—'Francis and Virgil Pugh'—they concluded their description of the two brothers with the information that both had been hanged at the gallows. 'What did they do?' asked the man. 'It is said', concluded Henry Frazer with a pause, 'that they rode with Dick Turpin.'

At this point Henry checked that I knew where the Deerplay was and then confided in us all that when he identified the house as the second one from the top, he knew it was the one the newcomer had bought. Furthermore, he told us, inspiration for the name 'Pugh' came from the alive and well John Pugh who was, at that very moment, sitting directly in front of them 'drinking his pint' and 'minding his own business'. Henry concluded that the man was 'delighted to have a bit of history' for the cottage he had acquired. A postscript to the story, which amused everyone (including me, although I did not understand why it was so funny, but like many other things, amusement is infectious—it can be passed on) was provided by a member of the audience who revealed that in the week following this encounter in the Deerplay Inn there had been an item in the local newspaper which described how Dick Turpin had drunk in the inn.

Deception or joke, the newcomer's interest in a 'bit of history' was not questioned, nor was the status of Henry and George as the appropriate providers of that history. It rendered visible the connections between Henry, George, the local, and the alive and well John Pugh, as well as making explicit a special, if not anarchic, past of Bacup and its environs. The story reiterates the distinction often made between *Bacup born and bred* and *outsider.* It displays the wit of Henry Frazer and George Parker at the expense of the newcomer's gullibility, but legitimates the ruse because in the end everybody is happy. But, not any old history will do; Henry and George were aware that a colourful and infamous history was required. Their story reveals the way in which distinctions between Bacup people and incomers are made and sustained and highlights a common recognition that the pursuit of a bit of history is an understandable and worthwhile activity.

Given the importance attached to the past by Bacup people, it can neither be ignored as irrelevant to the anthropological exercise, nor constrained within a chapter posing as a definitive history of the town. I find I cannot confine the past to the history of Bacup which I locate at the beginning of my account in order to contextualize what follows. There is no one social domain which provides the context for an understanding of others, instead analogies are made across different domains of social life which analytically appear to be concerned with different things. The past will emerge, then, in other chapters of this book which are not ostensibly about history at all. The past, like kinship, poses problems for Bacup people—certain items are to be selected while others ignored. I have focused, here, on Bacup's history by concentrating on the activities of local historians and by presenting some of the events, eras, entities, and persons upon which they dwell and which they connect up. The past is a forum in which relatedness is put to work.

4

In-Migration and Out-Migration

SITUATED, as many Bacup people claim, at the heart of the industrial revolution, Bacup's histories are full of industry. Industry has entailed, at different times, a need for labour—labour which has subsequently become surplus to requirements. A demographic history of the region shows successive waves of in- and out-migration since the beginning of the nineteenth century. In 1660, the population of the area covering present-day Bacup and its satellite villages is reported to comprise only 200 people, and in 1798, 1,426 people (Bowden 1972). No reliable figures are available, however, until 1851 when the census recorded a population of 10,313.[1] Table 4.1 shows a rapid growth between 1861 and 1881 and then a steady and continuous decrease in numbers until the present. The census of 1991 recorded a population of 14,706.[2]

During the second half of the nineteenth century there was a steady influx of labouring families and individuals to Bacup from rural areas of England and Ireland, but by the end of the century mills were closing and labouring families moving on. The second half of the twentieth century has seen a trickle of in-migration which seems to have stabilized the size of the population at about 15,000 people. Apart from recent immigration to the town by what are said from Bacup perspectives to be middle-class commuters from the city, two other categories of recent immigrant are indigenously salient. The first is young people evacuated during the Second World War who stayed, and the second is working-class families who arrived in the 1950s and 1960s in response to the availability of council houses. They formed a new category of incomer. Working class, they moved to Bacup because of the availability of council housing, and competed for local employment, which by that time was becoming more scarce. The historical emphasis on rural midland and southern counties of England as places of origin of real Bacup people, relies on an implicit comparison with alternatives such as Ireland, Scotland, and Manchester. The implication is that those who hail from the latter are not real Bacup people. But as we shall see, being a real Bacup person is a mixed blessing and is not necessarily, nor always, invoked positively.

Post-1970 immigrants to Bacup are perceived to be distinctive in particular ways (e.g. the type of houses in which they live and the occupations in which

[1] This figure excluded Stacksteads which was formally annexed in 1876.

[2] The introduction of the Poll Tax in 1989 had an enormous impact in Bacup where historically the cost of housing and local authority housing rates had always been low, as indeed were and are wages. It is my impression and that of other commentators that the predicted large increase in the cost of the Poll Tax compared to former levels of local authority tax based on the rateable value of property led to a significant under-reporting in this census.

TABLE 4.1. *Population of Bacup since 1851*

Year	Population	Year	Population
1851	10,313	1931	20,590
1861	10,395	1941	no census
1871	17,199	1951	18,374
1881	25,034	1961	17,295
1891	23,498	1971	15,102
1901	22,505	1981	15,116
1911	22,318	1991	14,706
1921	21,263		

Source: Based on the official census figures 1851–1991 (census of 1941 not carried out due to war), and taken from Bowden (1972).

they engage). But most residents trace their ancestors to places outside Bacup including those who define themselves as Bacup born and bred. Clearly there have always been incomers and many have stayed. This begs the question: when or how do they become Bacupian? It is not merely, I argue, a matter of time. This chapter explores what it means to be Bacup born and bred or to be an incomer. But to do so it also needs to explore the kind of place Bacup is perceived to be. In English thinking, different kinds of place (e.g. villages and cities) are associated with different kinds of social relationship. Hence the village is idealized as containing residents attached to the place by ties of kin, whereas the city is perceived to contain a more fluid and moveable population. The ambiguities surrounding the notions of village and city are mobilized by residents in their descriptions of the kind of place Bacup is, and the kind of place Bacup is emerges from the kind of social relationships said to characterize it. Place and person are juxtaposed, and either may stand for the other.

A Proper Place

One day, in May 1988, I was working at home. Michael, an 11-year-old neighbour, came to visit. He wanted my son, but made do with me for a while. He asked what I was doing on the computer and I told him I was writing about Bacup. He professed, offhandedly, to being bored with Bacup and not really liking it very much:

MICHAEL: There's nothing in Bacup. It's dead. There's no cinema. The nearest McDonald's is in Burnley. I'm going to move out when I get older.
JEANETTE: Where do you want to go?
MICHAEL: London [*pause*] or the country.

Michael perceives Bacup not to have those things, in this case a McDonald's and a cinema, which constitute a 'proper' place. It is neither 'the city' nor 'the country'. For Michael, either one or the other would be preferable to the limbo in which he perceives Bacup to lie. On the one hand, it is 'dead' because it does not have the facilities and entertainment associated with a cosmopolitan world, in this case, epitomized in London; on the other, it is hardly rural and by implication charming enough to be the country. The country and the city are, for Michael, equally exciting and seductive places, and Bacup is neither.[3]

Villages rather than cities are associated with the country, but are not confined to the rural. Hence indigenous English models of the city include the village.[4] Both the city and the village evoke a cluster of ideas which do not necessarily map on to a preponderance of either concrete (and a cathedral) or green fields (and cows), although they may include those things. This kind of ambiguity is nothing new. In 1848 Bacup's population was recorded as 10,000 (excluding Stacksteads), and it is reported, at that time, to have been 'scarcely more than an immensely overgrown village'.[5] The census of 1881 recorded a population of 25,034 (including Stacksteads), and at that time local historian, Edward Baines, commented that Stacksteads was a 'little town of itself' and 'a considerable manufacturing village' (in Bowden 1972).

OfCities, Villages, and Hamlets

One evening I went out with Maureen Doherty, from the Nat, and her husband Jim. Their friend, Brad, a folk guitarist and singer, was playing that evening in their 'local' and they were keen for me to meet him.[6] We drank our pints of beer and listened to Brad play some rock and roll and some folk-songs. While he was taking a break, I asked him about the words of one of the songs he had sung earlier. He explained that the tune was from a traditional folk-song called 'Rawtenstall Fayre' but that he makes up a verse or two himself. At the end of the night he passed me a slip of paper on which he had written out the words of one of the verses for me, complete with footnote (marked with an asterisk).

> Roll up! Roll up!
> See the tattooed lady,
> See the lovely lady
> All the pictures on her skin;
> In went the lads, and they all gave a cheer,
> 'Cos tattooed on her back were all the town o' lankysheer.[7]
> Thur wur Bacup City,

[3] See Gullestad (1992) for similar ideas in Norway.

[4] In Manchester, for example, Withington village is embedded in the urban sprawl and only two miles from the city centre. Recently an area of the city centre reclaimed from urban wasteland and with a thriving gay nightlife has come to be known as the Village, sometimes the Gay Village.

[5] *The Official Handbook to Bacup* (1958), 9th edn.

[6] Your 'local' is usually the public house closest to home and the one you frequent most often: the pub to which you 'belong' and which 'belongs' to you.

[7] Lancashire.

Rawtenstall Village,
Haslingdon hamlet,
The Broken Jaw* near the Square.
Thur wur Burnley, a' Bolton a' Ashton under Lyne,
The Coal Pit at Wigan were looking mighty fine.
Till some'ody shouted daddy!—Don't go down the mine!
—At the Rawtenstall Annual Fair.

* The Broken Jaw is the nickname of a notorious pub in Haslingdon now known as the Thorn.

In this version Bacup is a city, Rawtenstall a village, and Haslingdon a hamlet. There is an irony in this portrayal which suggests a relationship of hierarchy between these three towns, with Bacup in this instance placed at the top ahead of its rivals. Brad told me he swapped the names around, depending on where he was playing, although sometimes he left them the same when he played in Haslingdon and Rawtenstall—'to wind people up'. As we have seen, in the late 1980s there was a common perception in Bacup that Rawtenstall and Haslingdon were receiving preferential treatment, particularly from the local government, and growing, at the expense of Bacup. Bacup it was said had become the *poor cousin* of the three—a 'Cinderella town'.[8] For Brad to refer to it as a city is to recall its former glory, and to reinstate it above Rawtenstall and Haslingdon. With tongue in cheek, he subverts what is commonly perceived to be the contemporary hierarchy which has Bacup low down in the pecking order. He is also poking gentle fun at the rivalry existing between the towns. Recent immigrants also elaborate on idioms of city/village when they describe their reasons for settling in Bacup. When Bacup is identified as a village with the qualities associated with villages, it is either to underline its friendly or parochial ambience.

In English, 'city' and 'country' are culturally loaded idioms. They each embrace a cluster of qualities, different combinations of which have been pertinent in different periods of history (see Williams 1985).[9] They are conceptualized not only as separate but also as opposing entities and carry meaning over and above their definitions as particular kinds of places. Packed with inference, they are also aspects of each other and each gains its meaning in relation to the other. City and country bring to mind, then, much more than places 'on the ground': they suggest ways of life and types of social relationships. Part of their ability to do this is through connections they

[8] Like Cinderella, presumably Bacup gets left behind while her ugly sisters go to the ball.

[9] Raymond Williams writes of the kind of meanings that have been attached to 'city' and 'country' historically: '"Country" and "city" are very powerful words . . . On the actual settlements, which in the real history have been astonishingly varied, powerful feelings have gathered and have been generalised. On the country has gathered the idea of a natural way of life: of peace, innocence, and simple virtue. On the city has gathered the idea of an achieved centre: of learning, communication, light. Powerful hostile associations have also developed: on the city as a place of noise, worldliness and ambition; on the country as a place of backwardness, ignorance and limitation. A contrast between country and city, as fundamental ways of life, reaches back into classical times' (Williams 1985: 1).

evoke with culturally specific ideas of nature and culture.[10] But the village is not unambiguously associated with nature, nor the city with culture. Different permutations and blends of elements that constitute town and country, or city and village, are made up.

Bacup is neither a village nor a city.[11] It is what is commonly called a town, and a small one. It may be its status as a town—in betwixt and in between—to which Michael referred in his comments. But it is the symbolic purchase of the ambiguity itself which is of interest. My interest is not in locating Bacup, as a town, on a continuum between village and city. This would only distract us from looking at ways in which idioms of village and city are put to work, and not only in Bacup.

Stacksteads, Weir, Sharneyford, and Britannia all lie today within the Bacup electoral boundary. Each are also defined, from different Bacup perspectives, as separate villages in their own right. They are situated on the perimeters of Bacup and although I refer to them as satellite villages, I do not wish to impute to them a fixed status. My interest is in the way in which as *both* part of Bacup *and* separate 'villages' they are put to work by residents in a constant process of social differentiation.[12] The satellite villages are either connected or disconnected from Bacup: relatedness is both traced and curtailed. Places, like pasts and persons, both belong and do not belong.

Many elders recall that Stacksteads, Weir, Britannia, and Sharneyford were originally separate villages which grew up as settlements around particular mills. They remark on the loss of autonomy of these places since they were incorporated into Bacup. They talk in a similar way about Bacup, pointing out that it has lost its autonomy since being incorporated into the Borough of Rossendale. The social and economic changes which have occurred in Bacup over the past two centuries are imaged in, amongst other things, the shifting stature of the satellite villages. One woman who lives in Stacksteads told me it was now 'like the suburbs of Bacup'. Her comment embraces notions of upward mobility. Places no less than persons move. Today, for example, Weir is said to be 'posh' and its relative affluence is a focus of attention. Several young Bacup people expressed their ambition to move to Weir when they can afford it, while others pointed out that it was far 'too snobby' for their liking. People reminded me that Weir had not always 'been posh' (whether evaluated

[10] Strathern (1992*a*) has teased out, in the context of NRT, changes occurring in Western conceptualizations of nature. As technology intervenes in nature, then an idea that the activity of human beings (cultural practices) are grounded by a natural (given) world no longer holds the same place in the cultural imagination. In a post-industrial age, technology may be said to augment or assist nature, 'to give nature a helping hand', so that nature is perceived as requiring the activities of humans. As nature and culture are each the product of human activity so too is the country: what might have been a given now requires active preservation.

[11] Williams (1985) notes that by the beginning of the 16th cent. 'city' was commonly used to refer to a large town, in his own work he uses town and city interchangeably.

[12] See Rapport (1997: 653–72) for a discussion of 'the creative promise' of contradiction and in particular 'both/and'.

positively or negatively): like Sharneyford, I was told, it used to be called 'jam land'. They were given this nickname because villagers could only afford to eat jam butties[13]—an apocryphal observation portraying poverty, and furthermore a poverty more pronounced on the periphery in outlying villages.[14] The perception of these neighbourhoods both as separate villages and as part of Bacup provides, as we shall see in the next chapter, a means by which residents move conceptually in and out of Bacup.

For Edwin Ardener (1987: 49), '"remoteness" is specification . . . from an outside standpoint'. But from within Bacup there are many outside standpoints. Residents identify, and provide evidence of, those places nearby that they consider to be truly remote. Hence from Bacup, the satellite villages may be located on a periphery and those same qualities attributed to Bacup from the outside are now allocated to Weir, or Sharneyford, or Britannia. Listen to Mrs Jones talking about Glossop, in Derbyshire:

> I only lived there for eight months. I hated it—people—it's one of those places that if you've not lived there and your mother and father and grandmother and all those that belong to you, then you can't fit in. Mind you there's a place like that just up the road—Weir Terrace. Bacup's never been like that.

Weir Terrace is less than half a mile from where Mrs Jones lives. Recent incomers identify and enumerate the flip side of 'remoteness' when talking of what attracted them to the town initially. Now it is its remoteness that makes it charming. The locals of the Britannia pub identify the 'real locals' as other to them, and the youths in the theatre group are not *typical Bacup kids*. It is not, then, merely a definition imposed on Bacup from outside—a perception, as Ardener suggests, imposed from elsewhere—but is a conceptual resource equally available to residents of Bacup as it is to residents of neighbouring localities, or residents of Manchester, or, for that matter, social anthropologists. Like the polymeniscous gaze from the compound eye there are from within, as much as from without, myriad perspectives. And the English are adept at constantly formulating more or less inclusive and exclusive categorizations of their immediate social worlds.

What I try to convey in this and following chapters are the senses of distance, closeness, and remoteness mobilized in Bacup. There is an interplay between notions of mobility and fixity and one is transformed to the other depending on the hill on which one sits, and there are many hills in Bacup. The idea of remoteness is not only applied to Bacup, but also works inside, and can be brought very close to home. The people of Glossop or across the border in Yorkshire might be attributed with those qualities associated with remoteness but so too might neighbours. Relatedness is not axiomatic. Like family

[13] A butty is a sandwich.

[14] I was told on many an occasion, with mock sympathy, that Sharneyfordians have a further cross to bear, living, as they do, on the Yorkshire border.

members, perhaps once close but now cut off, fellow Bacup people, in the same neighbourhood, are not always 'like us'.

Informants and Information

Residents of Bacup with whom I worked, in telling me what they thought I ought to know first about Bacup and then about NRT, situated themselves in the town through selected and selective autobiographical detail. They contextualized what they wanted to say through narratives which revealed their origins, thus making explicit the authority from which they spoke. On many a first meeting, my co-conversationalists told me that they were either from Bacup or not from Bacup. Such a statement was often elaborated by detail of their own or their family's arrival in the town. In Chapter 1, I made the analogy between the anthropologist who situates her- or himself in a site of fieldwork through a narrative of arrival, with Bacup people who situate themselves in Bacup in order to establish the authority from which they speak. In this chapter, I draw on the narratives of six Bacup women, focusing on what they told me about their origins and arrival in the town. To call these women 'key informants', misrepresents, I think, the way in which their ideas emerge and are fashioned in interaction; it also sounds rude. The people whose ideas I present here did not exactly 'inform' me about the town, its residents, or NRT, but rather they explored these things with me (from different angles) and in this process put them together. If we take seriously the truism that anthropological information is generated in a discursive relationship between the anthropologist and her research subjects and what comes to be seen as 'information' is retrospectively construed as such, then we need a better word than informant and a more truthful one than collaborator to refer to those with whom we work.

The women whose autobiographical detail I borrow in this chapter, say something about where they come from—their origins. They ground their ideas and views about Bacup and its people in a narrative which says something about their arrival in the town.[15] In locating themselves in Bacup through their arrival, they create the context in which their subsequent views make sense. Here I highlight ways in which Bacup residents in 1987 and 1988 categorized themselves and each other through the links they made between Bacup and non-Bacup, persons, pasts, and places. In re-presenting what some women told me about their origins, I emphasize the point that none of us live categorical lives despite being categorized, and being adept at categorizing others.

[15] Denzin (1989) cites a study made by Horowitz (1969) of the autobiographies sociologists write: sociologists writing about themselves need, initially, to find a firm anchor for their life before they can begin writing about their sociological imagination. The anchors they often find are in the physical landscapes in which they grew up, or in what Denzin (1989) calls their 'family beginnings'.

Dwelling in Bacup

To be a Bacup person or not might seem an obvious starting-point from which to describe present-day inhabitants of Bacup. The ethnography of Britain reveals the way in which (in many places) residents identify themselves as local or from elsewhere; distinctions are made between those who belong and those who do not. In a Welsh village, for example, a distinction is made between 'Pentre people' and 'outsiders' (Frankenberg 1957), in the Yorkshire Dales between 'locals' and 'offcomers' (Rapport 1993), in the Shetland Islands between 'wir folk' and 'da folk sooth' (Cohen 1987), and in an Essex village between 'villagers' and 'newcomers' (Strathern 1981). Such differentiation is also made explicit in Bacup and is often couched in terms of *Bacup born and bred* and *incomer*. I refer to those who moved to the town before the 1970s as established immigrants and those who have moved since then as recent immigrants. The time-line is somewhat arbitrary but reflects indigenous differentiation between residents stereotyped as *commuters* or *yuppies*[16] and residents who, while not Bacupian, are *almost* or *more or less*. Recent immigrants speak about Bacup people as if they are homogeneous; as if they share certain characteristics by virtue of being local. Similarly, from Bacupian perspectives (*almost* and *proper*) all recent immigrants are incomers and are referred to as if they shared characteristics by virtue of not being from Bacup. While residents locate themselves differently in terms of their place of birth or length of residence, they nevertheless agree that a conspicuous and relevant distinction in Bacup is between Bacup and non-Bacup; what gets included in each, however, is not always self-evident. I refer to all present-day inhabitants of Bacup, regardless of their origins and ways in which they categorize themselves, as residents, my point is that they dwell in Bacup and my study is in Bacup.[17] All Bacup people at some point or other are incomers. I reserve the term 'Bacup people' for those who categorize themselves as such by virtue of being born in Bacup. My interest is in the ways in which residents perceive themselves and each other to be connected, or not, to Bacup.

Although the idiom *Bacup born and bred* appears at first glance to be self-evident and to refer to those born and brought up in Bacup, like *incomer* it is a chunky concept. It carries with it connotations of social class including labour, language, and houses. A single opposition between Bacup and non-Bacup or between, say, local and incomer, is inadequate for the descriptive task ahead. People connect themselves to each other and to Bacup through, for example, place of birth (Bacup or not Bacup) and disconnect themselves in terms of, for example, place of residence (Bacup or Weir). Distinctions are constantly made

[16] Yuppie (or yuppy) is an acronym of young urban (or upwardly mobile) professional (Collins, *Softback English Dictionary* 1993).

[17] In the often-quoted words of Clifford Geertz, anthropologists do not study villages, but *in* villages (1993 [1979]: 22).

and boundaries conceptualized which cut across and differentiate between people who otherwise, and for a different purpose, would include themselves in the same social category. Although being Bacup born and bred provides an umbrella of similarity, the birthplace of your grandparents, for example, may provide a point of departure; and although not being born in Bacup makes you axiomatically an incomer, whether you moved to the town fifteen or fifty years ago at times makes a big difference, while at other times it counts for little.

Bacup Born and Bred

The statement '[I'm] Bacup born and bred' embraces two significant aspects of English kinship. It juxtaposes what is perceived as an immutable place of birth with the effects of a variable upbringing: it is not enough to be born in Bacup, one also needs to be reared in Bacup. The experience of being *brought up* in the town is said to be influential: it moulds a particular kind of character. For example, poor working conditions, overcrowded houses, and a harsh climate are perceived to have moulded tough, stoical, and hard-working characters. 'Bacup born and bred' embraces and carries with it numerous connections: it is ripe with occupational and residential histories (factories, mines, quarries, and back-to-backs), language (Bacup dialect and Lancashire expressions), a toughness born of hardship (poverty), harsh environment (the weather and the bleakness of the moors), and uncompromising social relationships (marked by bluntness and honesty). The idiom evokes a working-class heritage: it ties *Bacup families* to the industrial development and demise of the region and to experiences of struggle in both economic and social spheres. One does not necessarily have to have been born in the town to have experienced such things, and indeed one may have been born in Bacup without ever having experienced them. Residents who readily claim Bacup born and bred status evoke a working-class background even if they currently sustain a middle-class position in terms of social and economic status. They are able to underline a working-class heritage by tracing the origins, occupations, and residential histories of their parents or their grandparents. The juxtaposition of 'being born' and 'being bred' allows always for some connection to be made. A claim to be Bacup born and bred invokes many associations and different combinations of them can be brought into sharper focus, bringing certain associations into relief and screening out others.

Within the category 'Bacup born and bred', further distinctions are made. Some residents are identified as belonging to a *real* or a *proper Bacup family*, often identified as big, and attached to a *real* or an *original Bacup name*, which include patronyms such as Ashworth, Hargreaves, Holt, Howarth, Heyworth, and Pilling. *Real* or *proper Bacup* is associated with certain places of origin, mostly rural counties of England, such as Cambridgeshire, Leicestershire, Norfolk, and Suffolk. Links made between particular patronyms and particular places of origin are also markers of ethnicity—in this case English. It is in the process of formulating particular kinds of Bacup identity that particular kinds of British ethnicity are formulated.

Mary Jones was the eldest of six children born between the turn of the century and the start of the First World War. Her mother's mother, Bella, first came to Bacup with her parents and six sisters. Mrs Jones thought Bella was the eldest child, she was not sure, but Bella must have been at the older end because she couldn't read or write. Bella's parents travelled from Reeth in Yorkshire in search of work when they could no longer feed their family by working on the land. They settled in Waterfoot, just outside Bacup, where Bella, who was by then in her early teens, worked alongside her mother in a cotton mill. Bella married John Holt, a fellow who came from Blackburn, and she moved to Bacup. Margaret, Mrs Jones' mother, was born in 1875, and at 19 years of age, she married Fred Howarth—'a Bacup lad'. One side of Fred's family came from Crawshawbooth, a nearby village, and the other side were from the Ribble Valley in Lancashire. Their daughter Mary was born in 1898 and, when she was 12 years old, she was apprenticed to a weaver in a cotton mill, 'to learn her a trade'. Mary Jones, née Howarth, recalled being employed as 'a tenter'.[18] She used to sing in the Baptist church choir, and loved playing whist. She met and married Percy Jones, a fellow from Northampton who had come to Bacup to work as an operative in one of the larger shoe factories. Percy never really settled in Bacup and he never grew to like it. Mrs Jones recalled the way in which he always criticized the quality of shoes manufactured in Bacup, always comparing them unfavourably with those made in his home town. For him, what he perceived as the cheap and poor quality shoes made in Bacup symbolized all that was inferior about the town and its people. Mrs Jones had two daughters whose education, she feared, was compromised because they had to move around quite a lot with her husband's work. They lived for a spell in Wigan and another in Glossop, and eventually settled back in Bacup in the same street in which she had lived as a child.

Newspaper reports from around the time Bella Holt was born reveal an interest in incomers who were then, as now, identified through their places of origin. An extract from the *Bacup Times* of 10 June 1876 shows how the idiom 'furriner' was used, as it is today, to describe incomers from other parts of Britain: 'There is quite a colony in Rossendale of what are termed "foreigners"—people from the Midland counties, in particular Cambridgeshire' (cited in Aspin 1983). Other places of origin named in family histories include Norfolk and Suffolk. Mrs Jones described the stigma attached to incomers from these counties of England: 'They were brought in by the trainloads to work in the mills [*pause*] they were called yellowbellies.' I asked Mrs Jones why they were called yellowbellies: 'Because they were foreigners—they worked for less. Some people say the Hoyle family ruined the town because they lowered

[18] The work she describes, indispensable to the efficiency of the mills, entailed tending (looking after) the looms by tying broken threads and changing empty bobbins. This relied heavily on the labour of children, who had small hands (Tom B. Thompson's 'nimble fingers'). Many elderly Bacup people recall being 'half-timers' when they were 12–14 years of age. As half-timers they worked in the mill during the morning and attended school in the afternoon.

the wages . . . bringing in these people.'[19] The Hoyle family, Mrs Jones informed me, were millowners. In another conversation she identified them as Catholic. According to Mrs Jones, *big* landowners were Catholic, the rest were local lads made good. A notion of local, and by extension *proper,* does not in Mrs Jones's formulation include Catholics, for her it is religious nonconformity that characterizes Bacup. She is, herself, Baptist.

For Barbara, her daughter, stigmatization of incomers such as the yellowbellies was a thing of the past: 'It's not like that now. When mother's generation die off nobody will remember where they came from—so they'll be Bacup people.'

For Barbara, a place of origin will no longer act as a distinguishing marker when the generation for whom it was relevant 'die off'. The place of origin will no longer be remembered; it will be un-known. The fact that people from Norfolk and Suffolk were called 'yellowbellies' will be forgotten and over time, distinctive features of dialect and clothing disappear. But there are always newcomers to occupy the conceptual space left by the yellowbellies. As one elderly Bacup man remarked: 'There used to be a lot of Irish that spoke Irish, but now their children's children are coming up they speak just like us . . . now they're Bacup people'.

A distinction between Irish families and Bacup families is still made, however, and in certain contexts is as relevant now as it was in the past. Although many Bacup people who trace their origins to Ireland have an equal claim on Bacup born and bred status to those who trace their origins to Cambridgeshire, they may not necessarily, or always, claim it. They may narrate, instead, connections to Ireland. And in doing this they make explicit their non-Bacup status. Although the man quoted above suggests that losing an Irish accent makes a person Bacupian (conversely an Irish accent is evidence that a person is not 'really' Bacupian) other aspects of Bacup identity, for example, being born there or having appropriate occupational or residential histories, can also be brought to the fore. And when they are they screen out connections (relevant elsewhere) to persons, places, and pasts in Ireland.

Patronyms such as Brody, Murphy, Donaghue, and Connolly came up again and again in my Bacup conversations. They are often said to belong to 'big Irish families'. A big family in contemporary English thinking is an ambiguous thing; it is both good and bad. 'Big', named families might be identified as Irish and Catholic, or as Bacupian and Baptist. But in both the ambiguity of 'the big family' is exploited: it is evaluated both positively and negatively—as

[19] Other residents identified Lincolnshire as the place where yellowbellies came from. Questions I asked about why they were called 'yellowbellies' more often than not elicited the response 'because they were from Lincolnshire', or as from Mrs Jones—'because they were furriners'. A Manchester graduate student told me a 90-year-old Lincolnshire acquaintance of his used to be called a yellowbelly. She told him it was because of their habit of rubbing their bellies with wheat in order to remove chaff from inside their clothes during harvesting.

mutually supportive or parochial. And from all Bacupian perspectives there is not always good reason to bring into relief Bacup born and bred status.

While Bacup people with both Irish and English origins equally claim Bacup born and bred status, they may also differentiate themselves by, amongst other things, places of origin and religion. But the model is, like all models, neater than reality. Intermarriage and a continuous process of in- and out-migration belie fixed categories of Irish and English Bacupian; of interest, however, is when and for what purposes such distinctions are brought to the fore. The idiom 'Bacup born and bred' contains its own possibilities of inclusion and exclusion which lie in the hybridity of a kinship that is Born *and* Bred.[20]

Laura Gray was born in 1967. She had always lived in the same neighbourhood of Bacup apart from a short period when she was first married and she and her husband lived on Mount Pleasant. Laura's mother was 16 when she first came to Bacup from Ireland. Laura still had family in Ireland, but hardly ever saw them, she also had family in north Manchester whom she visited frequently. Her father and her father's father were both born in Bacup, and according to Laura, were 'original Bacup people' with 'an old Bacup name'. Laura's mother and father divorced when Laura was in her early teens, and her father still lived in Bacup, while her mother remarried and now lived in the Midlands. According to Laura, her mother did not want to come back to live in Bacup, where in fact 'she never really felt at home', but with eight grandchildren she was connected and visited often. When Laura was 17 she married Alan—a Bacup lad—and they had two children. Several years later Laura's brother married Alan's sister and they also had two children. Laura's sister had four children and was settled with her husband in the same neighbourhood but, said Laura, with their own family responsibilities they did not see as much of each other as they used to.

While certain residents of Bacup define themselves emphatically as Bacup born and bred, others do so less emphatically and perhaps more selectively. The latter are often less ambiguously working class in terms of employment (unemployed or waged rather than salaried or self-employed) and residence (rented accommodation rather than owner-occupation). They tend to acknowledge readily the possibility for social mobility in extra-town relationships, and are more willing to perform an ongoing critique of Bacup. This in no way lessens their commitment to the town, or their wish to live and bring up their children there. It is not always relevant, however, to lay a strong claim to arenas in which one is unable to compete with equal effectiveness. Claims are

[20] I use hybridity here as a means of thinking about the relationship between being born and being bred which rely on each other for their separateness. It is not the case that one can be merely added to the other and that the two together make something different, but rather they both 'go together' and 'go apart'. For Kath Weston (1997: 168), hybridity compounds rather than mixes: her analogy is with 'a chemical reaction that transforms the whole into something different than its constituent parts'. My point in calling the type of kinship in which I am interested 'hybrid' is somewhat different—the significance of being born cannot be understood in isolation from the significance of being bred, but the potential to separate them is as available as the potential to join them.

therefore made on a status system wider than Bacup which includes access to modern consumer items and extra-town links.

Incomers

The incomers of yesteryear are the Bacup folk of today. Yet people who identify themselves as Bacup born and bred do not generally identify their ancestors as incomers (one has to be 'there' in order for others to come in); they do, however, remark on the origins of their ancestors (incomers, unlike kin, are unconnected). Elderly Bacup residents who moved to Bacup as children, usually because of the availability of work for their parents, are still incomers, albeit established and sometimes, in their words, 'almost Bacupian'. Two other waves of immigration were identified as significant. The first was evacuees during the Second World War, from cities such as Manchester, Liverpool, Newcastle, and London, who stayed. The second came in the 1950s and early 1960s predominantly, it is said, from Manchester and Scotland, due to the advertising of a surplus of local authority housing.

Rose Spencer first came to Bacup as a teenager in 1940, at the beginning of the war. She and her sister were evacuated from London. They were joined by their parents twelve months later. On the way to Bacup, her mother got chatting to a man on the train who warned her: 'Bacup is the last place God made and he never stopped to finish it.'[21] Rose's mother never settled in Bacup and, sadly, she died within twelve months of arriving. Rose's father returned to London but he also died not long afterwards. Rose explained that at that age (that is, the age of her parents when they moved to Bacup), it was difficult to make friends and to deal with such great change in your life. Bacup people, she explained, were very different from those her parents had been used to. Mrs Spencer described, for example, how horrified her mother had been when the milkman just walked straight into the back-kitchen, uninvited. Her mother stood up and shouted at him and told him to 'get out' and 'to knock next time'.

Rose married Donald Spencer—'a Bacup lad'—on Christmas Day 1943, and on Christmas Day, at quarter to midnight, four years later, their son was born. Rose's son and his family now lived in South Africa and she and her husband had already made one trip over there and plan to visit again next year. They also had a daughter who was married, lived in Bacup, and had an adopted daughter. According to Mrs Spencer, her husband belonged to an *original Bacup family*. She said her own family and other evacuees made up the first significant wave of incomers, before that there were only Bacup families in Bacup. 'Original Bacup people were all related, you know. Families such as the Spencers, Hargreaves and Whittackers and others go back centuries. The first influx of strangers were evacuees; but before that they were all Bacup people.'

With a few brief autobiographical details, Mrs Spencer made it clear she was *not* a Bacup person. She identified those who were and made explicit a

[21] A similar homily was presented by the president of the Nat who remarked: 'Bacup was last place God made an' he left tools behind, and they're still using them.'

distinction between her and them despite having lived in Bacup, at the time of our conversation, for over forty years. To be a member of an original Bacup family (like Mr Spencer), is somewhat double-edged in Mrs Spencer's account. They might be authentic and close, but they are also closed. She hinted that perhaps the evacuees demonstrated other (more sophisticated) ways of doing things: hence while the milkman may have been exhibiting informality and familiarity in his unannounced entrance, there is a place, suggested Mrs Spencer, for the manners and etiquette of being invited. There were other Bacup residents who had lived in Bacup as long as Mrs Spencer and who pointed, in our conversation, to their *almost Bacupian* status. They had brought up their children in Bacup and their children, in many cases, were born there. And they would, if they had not already done so, retire in Bacup. Their connections to the town, forged through time and traced via their children, attached them firmly.

Florence Nelson described herself as 'more or less Bacup'. She was born in Rochdale and moved to Bacup when she married a Bacup lad nearly forty years ago. All her children, she said, are Bacup born and bred; so she thought of herself as 'pretty much Bacup'. We played darts one evening in the Crimean and, after the game, stood talking at the bar. She told me Bacup was her home and she would retire here and, more than likely, she would die here. She did not contemplate living anywhere else. After all, she explained, 'this is where my roots are—it is where my children and their children were born'. She called to the landlord of the pub who was serving a customer on the other side of the bar and who, she told me, was an incomer like herself and had been in Bacup almost as long as she had: 'How long do you have to live here to become a Bacuper?' she asked him. He laughed: 'Well it shows *you're* not one—Bacuper!—it's a Bacupian!' We all, including Florence, laughed and she shrugged off this minor detail.

Mrs Nelson's attempt to enlist the landlord failed as he demonstrated his knowledge of the correct Bacup idiom. Never truly Bacupian, Mrs Nelson nevertheless considers herself to have a legitimate claim on the town and its resources based on forty years of residence and the experience of bringing up her children in the town. Her links with Bacup are mediated by her children who *are* Bacup born and bred and provide Mrs Nelson with roots in the town. Mrs Nelson is rooted to Bacup by her descendants. Although her idiom 'more or less Bacup' appears to refer predominantly to her length of residence in the town—forty years, she pointed out—it also embraces a similar range of ascriptions to those packed into 'Bacup born and bred'. To think of oneself as more or less Bacup is to claim those traits that belong to Bacup. Long-standing residents, such as Mrs Nelson, need not always identify themselves as 'almost Bacup' or 'Bacup more or less', they also have at their disposal the means of distancing themselves categorically from Bacup, its people, and its characteristics. To do this, they have only to make explicit an alternative set of connections to, for example, place of birth. When they do emphasize their almost Bacupian status, they evoke the resonances they perceive to exist between themselves and those who are Bacup born and bred. Should they create the context when such connections are not necessarily positively evaluated then they have the option to mobilize their place of birth which severs, albeit momentarily, connections traced via other mediators, such as houses, occupations, and dialects.

There are subtle differences, then, in the way in which incomers (who, according to sociological criteria, might be considered to belong to the same social category) speak of their connections to Bacup. They may identify closely with Bacup and the qualities it stands for, or distance themselves. Each requires making explicit certain connections and not others. While all incomers are able to draw on the conceptual resource of 'not belonging', they place emphasis on this at different times and again for different purposes. This mirrors the difference identified above between two categories of Bacup born and bred which I described in terms of different orientations to Bacup according to perceptions of equal access to the town's resources such as employment. Both examples show the way in which the perception of belonging to a social and economic class cut across (and disconnect) ideas about belonging to a place.

Olive Hughes is in her fifties. She moved to Bacup from Rochdale thirty years ago, and recalled that it was not a happy time. Her father-in-law was ill, and her mother-in-law unable to cope, and Olive was forced to move to Bacup with her husband and two young children in order to look after them. Subsequently, and ironically, her father-in-law recovered and he and his wife moved back to Rochdale. Olive and her family stayed on, initially because they could not afford to move. She used to hate Bacup, she told me, but things got better after a while, especially when both her mother and her sister moved from Rochdale. The three of them now live in adjacent houses. Olive considers herself to be well established in Bacup, her family forming 'a little community of its own' in a 'nice part of town'. Now she likes living in Bacup and gets on with most people. Although, she pointed out, 'Bacup folk can be funny, when they want to be.' They could be nosy and fickle, she suggested: 'One day they talk to you and the next they ignore you.' But having said that, she had many close friends here, felt at home, and was very unlikely to move away.

During the 1970s and 1980s there was a small but steady influx of households to Bacup from the conurbation. They left what many speak of as the cold, anonymous city to settle in 'the country' with what they perceived as its friendlier and more relaxed atmosphere. They commented on the beauty of the open spaces, the invigorating fresh air, and the community spirit with which the town is imbued. Bacup people also remarked on the beauty of the moors and they pointed, in passing, to the proximity of the hills as a positive feature of living in the area. While recent immigrants talk about Bacup as if it were itself 'the country', referring to it as a village and their move to Bacup as a move away from the rat race to a more laid-back environment, Bacup people position themselves on the outskirts of the country and speak about it as if it were readily and easily accessible. They may refer to Bacup as a village (particularly when differentiating it, and hence themselves, from the city and its connotations of unfriendliness and anonymity) but not, I think, as readily as recent immigrants for whom its villageness is explanation enough for their move to the town. I return to the symbolic import of 'the city' and 'the village', but the point to make here is that all Bacup residents have access to, and can put to work, such a conceptual resource. For all residents, villageness has attendant connotations of interrelatedness and mutual support; whether such interrelatedness is assessed in positive or negative ways does not alter the fact that meanings packed into villageness are shared. Some Bacup residents point to village-likeness of those places from where they came, such as Cowpe; or, in addressing a perceived threat to the integrity of Bacup from incomers, they may emphasize the village-like characteristics of Bacup over and above its industrial history; while more recent incomers point to Bacup's village-likeness as good reason for having moved there. In connecting those elements which make up villageness, the town's industrial heritage has not disappeared, it is merely screened out for the moment. A similar process takes place when emphasizing the town's industrial heritage rather than its other pasts.

Recent immigrants are sometimes referred to as commuters or yuppies. Like 'incomer' these terms obscure more than they reveal. Like 'Bacup born and bred' they are pregnant with connotations of social class. Although a common view from a Bacup perspective is that commuters or yuppies originate from, and then commute back, to Manchester (in company cars), many new residents have retired to Bacup, and others move from, and work in, surrounding towns such as Burnley, Rochdale, and Bury. Many women in incoming households secure part-time employment in Bacup, their children attend Bacup schools, and they join local organizations; and, while men may travel out of town to work, many do not travel to Manchester.

Carole Beckwith lived on the Orchards, a privately built housing estate comprising different-sized houses and bungalows built during the 1970s. Her husband, Keith, worked as an accountant in Radcliffe and Carole worked part-time in Bacup as a home help, and was employed in 1988 by the local authority. They had three children between the ages of 4 and 11. I met Carole first at a public meeting about the Poll Tax organized by the local branch of the Labour Party, and then several weeks later in the post office where, as a home help, she was collecting the pension of one of her clients. In the post office we chatted a while and I arranged to visit her, at home, on a particular evening. I arrived with a bottle of wine. Carole, her husband, and her two brothers were waiting for me. She had invited her brothers, one of whom had recently moved to Rawtenstall, while the other still lived in Manchester, so they could also, as they said, 'tell me about Bacup'. The children were in bed, put there early so as not to disturb us.

Carole and Keith began by placing themselves in Bacup, providing me with the autobiographical detail necessary for me to understand the authority from which they speak. They talked of their arrival in Bacup and the reasons for moving here. Their first home, they told me, was in a council house in Wythenshawe—an area of south Manchester where, said Carole, she was born and bred. Although Keith was born in Winchester in the south of England, his father was originally from Manchester, and his family moved back up north when Keith was a young child. Carole and Keith told me they discovered Bacup while visiting friends in Whitworth. Keith explained how he had never wanted his family to grow up in a city and Bacup presented an ideal environment in which to bring up kids. Property in Bacup was less expensive than in Manchester and if they moved to Bacup they could afford to buy a new house with a garden. They arrived in 1978, only a few weeks before the birth of their first child, and moved into a house on which the builders had only just finished working: 'It was a mess', recalls Carole, with feeling. But they soon felt at home and although now, as their children are growing, they would like a bigger house they would be happy to move just around the corner.

In using such terms as 'recent' and 'established' immigrant my aim is to convey a difference noted, for certain purposes, in Bacup itself. The distinction is not always relevant and all incomers share the possibility of excluding themselves and being excluded from the category of Bacup person. In both cases, more significant than length of residence are the attachments they trace, and are traced on their behalf, to Bacup. Established immigrants moved to the town in search of work or houses and they stayed; we do not meet, here at least, those who moved on. An assumption often made in Bacup is that recent immigrants perceive their sojourn in Bacup to be only temporary, and indeed many do move on in response to employment opportunities or, in the recent past, to exploit investment in property, but just as many appear to stay.[22] Many residents I refer to as recent immigrants are well established and will also trace their connections to the town through, amongst other things, their children who are growing up in Bacup, attending its schools.

Certain households are considered by Bacup residents to be distinctive in a particular kind of way. I refer to them here as fringe households, within Bacup they are said to belong to *Th'ippies*. While this term is commonly recognized, it is not used in self-definition, although those readily identified as such do make a distinction between themselves and what they call 'straights'.[23] They may refer to themselves as 'travellers' or 'freaks', or they may self-consciously reject all forms of classification as part of the fixing and classifying tendencies of the bourgeoisie, but they nevertheless recognize themselves as different. Ennew (1980: 117) describes a group of young people in the Western Isles in the mid-1970s as 'attempting to retreat from the 'pressures' of modern urban existence'. This pursuit resonates with ideas of members of fringe households

[22] Recent incomers, other than those who retire to the town, tend to be moving either into their first home or into the first home that they have owned. This contrasts with Elmdon, in Essex, in the 1960s where most incomers had established their households prior to a move to the village (Strathern 1981). The idioms 'incomer' and 'commuter' and variations on the themes are common to both Bacup and Elmdon. While embracing different patterns of residence and occupation they are nevertheless similar in the ways in which they are put to work in differentiating between categories of resident.

[23] I thank Sharon Macdonald (pers. comm.) for drawing attention to the gender parallels in these expressions: straight is placed in contrast with gay in matters of sexuality.

in Bacup in the late 1980s, but here membership is not confined to the young or to incomers. Adult offspring of either Bacup people or established immigrants are as likely as recent immigrants to belong to fringe households and to pursue what they perceive as alternative ways of living. They distinguish themselves from straight society in their rejection of what they perceive to be trappings and traps of modern urban life; theirs is also a selective rejection and, as in all expressions of Bacup identity described thus far, what is brought to the fore and what is screened out will relate to the reason for which rejection is relevant. Alison Irwin told me she was different from 'straights' because she placed a different value on material objects. She never used mail-order catalogues or credit to buy things for the house, nor did she believe in carrying out housework for its own sake. Alison was sceptical about the value of such effort in and of itself. Many fringe households, members of which may or may not identify themselves as 'freaks' are also attracted to what they perceive as the rural character of the area and, like other recent immigrants, by the availability of relatively inexpensive housing. Early fringe households were established on the edges of town in old farming property. One row of houses on an ancient bridle path, which is known by former residents as The Lane, and by other Bacup residents as Th'ippie Lane, now housed what both freaks and straights disparagingly refer to as yuppies. Members of other fringe households were in the process of renovating old, and what would otherwise be derelict, terraced houses in the town and a number of abandoned properties in a poor state of repair have benefited from their DIY skills and creative imagination. These Bacup residents placed a high value on the ability to travel and to change their place of residence frequently, and fringe households often contained individuals who were 'just passing through', or who had been just passing through and stayed. Extra-town links were valued and addresses exchanged with the promise and expectation of reciprocal hospitality.

The label 'hippie' might also be extended to individuals who would not consider themselves to be distinctive in this way. As symbolic resource it is used to differentiate; to include and exclude. It carries characteristics such as flamboyant dress and hairstyle, a liberal attitude to child care, the use of marijuana, and, for those who would identify themselves as different in this way, networks of comradeship across the British Isles. Whether they also described themselves as Bacup born and bred or almost Bacupian or said they were just passing through, they valued the possibility and freedom of mobility, whether they moved on or not. In contrast to recent immigrants I describe above, they rejected home-ownership and professional employment as straight and, as such, too constraining and unimaginative.

Judy Wilder was born in 1949. She was married with a child by the age of 17 and divorced by the age of 20. Judy was born in the Home Counties and moved to London when she got married. The bloke she married was an American GI who was quite wealthy, but the sedate life of a housewife and a mother soon, she said, lost its appeal and Judy found herself craving for 'a life'. She and her husband separated and Judy went to live and work in the city. Meanwhile her daughter was at boarding school and Judy took different jobs in other parts of the country and eventually in Spain, returning frequently to London to visit her daughter. Mark was from Liverpool and one of her circle of friends and acquaintances in London. She had a long-standing, albeit initially intermittent, relationship with Mark and one time went with him to visit his family. She was impressed with their kindness and the generosity with which they treated each other and she thought that when your family hasn't got much and unemployment is a familiar thing then you're more likely to slip your brother or your son a tenner and say 'get yourself a drink'. Her own family, she recalled, were quite different, expecting you to stand on your own two feet and much more critical of what you were doing.[24] A friend of Mark's on this visit to Liverpool told them of a house he had heard about in Weir. She remembered this friend saying: 'Shall we all go and live over there?' So they borrowed £4 for petrol, loaded up the truck and drove to Bacup. Judy got itchy feet almost immediately, and went to work in France picking grapes, and when she returned Mark left to work down south for a while. But by now Judy was 30 years old and she wanted another child. When he returned they moved together to the cottages up The Lane which were then almost derelict. The cottages needed a great deal of work to make them even habitable, but eventually they had running water and electricity and had like-minded and experienced travellers as neighbours. Meanwhile amidst the renovation and the installation of basic amenities, Judy fell pregnant. She gave birth to a son. Since then she had had two daughters and was at the moment doing up another derelict cottage in a different neighbourhood.

From the fringe, Bacup is perceived as a temporary base and the potential for travelling is valued positively. From this perspective, moving on is always presented as a possibility, despite the fact that many members of fringe households are settled in terms of their homes and the care of their children. Links with friends and like-minded people beyond Bacup boundaries are emphasized. More often than not maintaining a place on the fringe requires screening out connections (through birth and breeding, for example) to Bacup. 'Travelling' or 'freak' identities are forged in bringing together (connecting) elements perceived to be untypically Bacup.

Idioms such as 'straight' (implying bent), 'real' (implying unreal), and 'typical' (implying atypical), make explicit ever finer differentiations between categories of resident which cut across boundaries of Bacup and non-Bacup. Such idioms evoke connotations of social class which in turn cut across a gross distinction between middle and working class. Furthermore, they are evalu-

[24] I am reminded of an observation by Beatrice Webb's biographers about her impression of Bacup domestic life: 'She liked the kindliness of their home life. Unlike her own family circle, with its upper class habit of brutal frankness, these people were soothingly considerate, sparing each other's weaknesses and leaving unkind truths unspoken' (Muggeridge and Adam 1968: 105).

ated either positively or negatively depending on which set of connections is congealed and for what purpose. The notion of community has the capacity to bridge Bacup and non-Bacup persons, but like all powerful cultural symbols it is also deployed to do just the opposite—to make explicit the unrelatedness of persons and things.

'Community is Communication'

A group of youths had gathered in the youth club to tell me about Bacup. The participants were between 16 and 19 years of age and, all but one, the only young woman in the group, lived in Bacup. These young people met regularly at the senior youth club and, in 1988, formed the core membership of the Bacup youth theatre. It was the summer before two members, Joe and Dale, were to begin a course in theatre studies at the College of Further Education in Accrington. Joe was the son of Mary and Tom Shaw, both of whom he described as Bacup born and bred. Mrs Shaw was a welfare rights adviser and Mr Shaw an electrical engineer in a local shoe factory. Dale's parents were the landlords of a public house in the centre of town. Another member of the group, David, worked in a local shoe factory and attended college one day a week, where he was studying for a City and Guild qualification in industrial management. Judith lived in Waterfoot and was at school studying for exams. Joe, Dale, and David described themselves as Bacup lads. They made a distinction between themselves and what they called 'typical Bacup lads' and between themselves and 'proper Bacup people'. According to them, typical Bacup lads or kids are 'trendy' (what Pam Watson called 'the boy-next-door-look'[25]) and 'cause trouble'. Proper Bacup people are an older generation: honest, hard-working mill workers. Joe, Dale, and David, although born in Bacup, did not consider themselves to be proper or typical Bacup people. Apart from not wearing 'cloth caps and clogs', Joe remarked, they were unlikely to remain in Bacup. Their mobility, he suggested, excluded them from a category of proper Bacup. Another member of the group, Craig, told me that although he was not born in Bacup, he had lived here since childhood. He claimed his knowledge of Bacup through his length of residence, and more significantly through being brought up in Bacup. He was a trainee manager employed by a large chain of supermarkets. He told us his parents were middle class but, as a socialist, he was working class.

The youths perceived both proper and typical Bacup people to be attached (fixed) more firmly to the town than they. They agreed that as young people like themselves seek employment or educational opportunities outside Bacup and do not follow 'proper' Bacup occupations, such as factory work, real Bacup people would die out. They were, in the words of David, a 'dying breed'; and

[25] Clean-cut, with fashionable hairstyles, and clothes and trainers displaying designer labels.

according to Joe, 'they have no one to follow in their footsteps—they're dying out'. They mobilized idioms of kinship to portray vividly a class of people—Bacup manual workers—whom they perceived as not reproducing themselves.

We join a taped discussion at a point when Craig and Judith were describing 'real Valley people' or, as Dale put it, 'normal people'. According to Craig, a real Valley person was 'probably someone who has lived there all their life, worked in the slipper works and knows all the gossip about what's going on here and there'. Dale added that they had 'an average age of 60—they've come up through Bacup's wild and wonderful years—through all the goings on in the Valley'. I asked them what they meant by the Valley.[26]

CRAIG: I call the Valley, from Rawtenstall to Bacup.

JUDITH: Everybody misses off Haslingdon and Crawshawbooth which are probably the best parts of the Valley because they are little *communities*.

DAVID: But Crawshawbooth is in a different valley.

JUDITH: Its great. It's like a community. I love it—I was born there.

JEANETTE: What's a community?

DALE: A bunch of hippies on the road, all living together, going to Glastonbury, Stonehenge—if they don't get kicked off—being nice, cool, respecting each other.

DAVID: This is a community [*gesturing to those present*]. These are the only real people I see, because I couldn't name the person who lives next door to me.

DALE: In Bacup there's not just one community.

JUDITH: } There's not a community no more.
CRAIG: } There ain't a community any more.

JUDITH: There isn't *a* community in the Valley.

CRAIG: Well there is in a way, but there isn't. Because of public transport and that, people are just spreading out rather than staying in one village.

JUDITH: The streets are meant to be communities but they're not no more.

DAVID: It's people you know.

JOE: There is no community now, everyone is too worried about everyone else. Talking to my mother—you could [used to be able to] leave the door open and there would be people living downstairs and if anything happened everyone knew about it. Everyone joined in. If someone were lacking on food they'd lend them the food. It doesn't happen no more.

JUDITH: That's like our estate. It *does*.

DALE: It's like in our street no one ever talks to each other. Everyone's too worried about what everyone else says or what they're going to do. Keeping up with the Joneses. Everybody's got to be the same as everyone else—pisses me off.

JUDITH: Our estate's a community. Cowpe is a community.

JOE: Cowpe is.

JUDITH: Everybody knows everybody else's business—who you was with last night. What time you came in.

[26] I met twice with this same group of youths at the youth club and on each occasion they allowed me to record our discussion on tape. The excerpts presented here are transcribed from a recording made at one of the meetings. The brace around two names indicates an overlap between speakers. Emphasized words in speech are in italic.

JOE: I'd call that nosy.

JUDITH: A community is that, and also having a lot of old people and a lot of young people and the young people getting on with the old people—talking to them, doing favours for them, which is what I used to do when I was little and I used to love it and that's what I call community.

JOE: That's because Cowpe is smaller. If you look at Cowpe everyone is near enough the same—as in money status.

CRAIG: No there's a lot of people travel out of Cowpe, depends which end you're talking about. There's two ends to Cowpe. There's a posh end by the Buck.

JOE: If you go around the pub they've all got the same level of money.

CRAIG: No they haven't.

JOE: Well they're all on the same wavelength.

CRAIG: There are those who don't belong to Cowpe. The Cowpe community are those that go down to the Buck. Then there's the people who don't go down Cowpe—have their own little dos.[27] They have the Cowpe Dance—the barbecue.

. . .

DAVID: We moved into our house in Stacksteads twelve months ago and it took six months to start talking to the person next door. To acknowledge that I lived [there]—both sides.

JUDITH: I'd blame meself.

DAVID: They ignored me. Parts of Stacksteads *are* a community and parts not. A massive road runs right through the middle and that's it. Blackwood is a bit of a community.

JOE: Yeah, Blackwood's a bit of a community. Well it used to be before they knocked all the houses down.

JUDITH: I think a pub has got quite a lot to do with a community—a local pub.

CRAIG: Waterfoot used to have the Railway before they did it up. That used to be where all the pigeon fanciers used to go.

JOE: Pubs have got their own gangs. You've got the locals who go in all the time and they are a community to themselves although they don't live near each other.

JUDITH: Community is communication.

The conversation continued and the appearance of a consensus was reached. Bacup, it was agreed, used to be in a 'working-class valley', but now it was becoming a *dormitory town*, full of yuppies, and was losing its sense of community. From this perspective, all recent immigrants were yuppies—but fortunately they tended to settle at the other end of the valley. Dale told us that because the motorway did not run through Bacup it 'isn't as much a yuppie kingdom as Helmshore'. He elaborated, 'in Helmshore you're hard pressed to spot the normal' (by contrast with the yuppie?). I asked what a yuppie was. With little hesitation, Judith pointed at me. She said it was my hair-do, the way I dressed, and the colour of my hair that made me look like a yuppie. I must have looked quizzical, because on the tape I hear her patiently explaining: 'It's

[27] Plural of a 'do'—a party or an event.

the way you wear them [clothes], and the colours. You look like a young person with a lot of money—a yuppie near enough.' One of the young men added 'trendy', and there were no dissenters from this view. It led to disparaging comments about just how trendy it was to be a member of Greenpeace or CND[28] and, with a display of disdain, my co-conversationalists agreed that those who join such organizations were trendy and, they added, shallow and jumping on the bandwagon: I noted with relief that they seemed not to be including me in this category of trendy person.

It is clear that the trendy people who join Greenpeace, or the trendy people who wear burgundy, or the trendy people who wear Nike trainers and hang out in the town centre are not to be confused with each other. But nevertheless they share the trait of trendiness which, in whatever guise, packs a negative punch and constitutes an other; and, more to the point, an immoral other.

The conversation highlights many of the points this chapter makes. There is an admiration, expressed eloquently by these young people, for community and the values associated with it. It is, however, under threat. And the threat is posed by yuppies. Community is thought to be disappearing, although Judith makes a strong case for Cowpe still being a community. But there is a difference between Cowpe and Bacup, the latter having lost its sense of community. The fact that Cowpe is still a community reflects on Judith and her efforts, and in this she challenges the young men who need to make more of an effort at communication for, after all, it is this, not a pub, which makes community.

Community is not absolute, either present or absent and (like 'neighbouring', as we shall see in Ch. 6) there are degrees to it. Hence Blackwood, a neighbourhood of Stacksteads, is *a bit* of a community (not fully, but partly). Community is imputed to places which are thought to have changed the least: to those places which contain fewer strangers, in this example, with smaller numbers of recent immigrants. Community emerges from particular kinds of social relationships and need not necessarily correspond to the physicality of places on the ground. Thus members of the theatre group see themselves or hippies as good examples of community. A community is made up (in all senses of the phrase) of people who interact and communicate (but not, in this example, members of such trendy organizations as Greenpeace and CND). Community is both entity and social relationship. It is the forum for social relationships as well as emerging from them. Community is forged from the way in which people behave as well as from where they live. Ideally relationships of community entail reciprocation, mutual support, and respect. The same qualities attached to the family. Families and communities in common English usage are forged in similar kinds of ways: they are both things

[28] Campaign for Nuclear Disarmament.

and ways of doing things. They are both entities (born) and relationships (bred).

The young people quoted here perceive themselves to be more mobile than their predecessors whom they class as proper Bacup, and their peers whom they class as typical Bacup, both of which are connected to a future Bacup as well as its past. Criteria other than place of birth, or the ability to trace one's ancestors to the town, are drawn up to define a real or proper Bacup person. While connections can be traced to ascendants in the town, this is not necessarily sufficient criteria for proper Bacup status. One's ancestors may be perceived as given—as the English adage has it 'you can choose your friends, but not your family' (see also Schneider 1968 for American variants on this theme)—but how they behave is flexible, mutable, and intentional. For proper Bacup status, a criterion of being born in Bacup requires the addition of particular kinds of experience, such as working in mills, living in back-to-backs, and, in this example, having futures already circumscribed.

For both the theatre group and the locals of the Britannia pub, the real or proper Bacup person is male. He is marked by fixity, and carries with him, whether he wears them or not, symbols of working-class life such as cloth caps and clogs. He is attached to the industrial landscape and there he will remain, and none of the speakers aim to take his place.

The Tight-Knit Community

The idiom *tight-knit community* is invoked constantly in Bacup. It has both positive and negative connotations. In its positive guise, it portrays friendliness and mutual support stemming from interrelatedness. In its negative guise, the same interrelatedness is said to have resulted in a 'parochial' or 'cliquish' place. The tight-knit community contains either predominantly friendly or predominantly nosy inhabitants and, as a symbolic resource, may be evoked to either include or exclude the speaker from the community they are, at that moment, composing. From one perspective, the tight-knit community portrays relationships of mutual support, honesty, and friendliness said, perhaps, to be disappearing as more strangers appear. Here the tight-knit community is characterized by interconnectedness and interdependence not found in the anonymous and fragmented relationships of the city. Recent immigrants not only have access to the symbolic resource of the tight-knit community, but are also implicated in its maintenance. They associate themselves with what are considered proper Bacup characteristics (e.g. friendliness and neighbourliness). But we have seen how status can also accrue from dissociation; recent immigrants are also able to exploit their lack of connection to Bacup and its people. They can achieve this through putting the same idiom—the tight-knit community—to work in a particular way. Focusing on the fixity and lack of variety implied in the tight-knit community they now create and sustain a distance from it. Now recent immigrants bring to the fore their own mobility; mobility which now connotes movement on and up by contrast with fixity which implies stagnation.

From a number of different perspectives, as we have seen, the town is perceived to have changed immeasurably. The experience of shared hardship, where residents united in the face of adversity, is said to have moulded a particular Bacup character. The influx of recent immigrants has changed the town, for better or worse, depending again upon which hill one sits. Contemporary hardship, particularly in the face of unemployment, and growing up in Bacup also mould particular characters and influence certain alliances. I was often told that 'everybody *used* to know each other' and just as often told that '*everybody* knows each other'. Recent immigrants may perceive themselves to be more mobile than Bacup people and to bring to the town a vibrancy that was lacking. And Bacup people perceive recent immigrants to be merely temporary residents and their sojourn in the town fleeting, so that when they move on, as they inevitably will, their ties to Bacup will be severed. A commonly voiced complaint that came up again and again is that incomers 'give nothing back'; they do not to reciprocate in an appropriate manner. As one Bacup man put it: 'Approximately 2,000 people have come out of Manchester, but they haven't created income here. They are using our services—cheap services—but they haven't brought any actual work here.'

If incomers do not contribute adequately, how can they have a legitimate claim on those things perceived to belong to Bacup? One woman, in her mid-fifties and Bacup born and bred, described the people moving into the area in this way:

> It's people who don't work in the area. They come because the houses are cheap. The husband and wife both travel to work. They don't belong in the community, they don't play a part. It used to be that everybody went to Sunday School, bathed and clean and tidy. It was the only place of entertainment, the only social life [*pause*] leisure activity.

This woman expressed a common sentiment that recent immigrants exploit the town for their own benefit without playing a part in those activities which represent the unity and well-being of the place. They are not participating in the multiplex relationships perceived to characterize 'the community' which are necessary for its reproduction and endurance. If recent immigrants do not contribute adequately, then they have no legitimate claim on those things that belong to Bacup. Relatedness requires reciprocation, and belonging entails a claim on other things that belong. Those who lay claim to Bacup, either through length of residence or through being born and bred there, consider themselves to have a prior right to things that, like they, belong to Bacup.[29] Just as kinship entails a claim on persons (kin are perceived to belong to each other), so connection to Bacup implies a claim on the things that belong to it.

[29] For example its industry, its houses, and its hills.

The distinction between Bacup folk and incomers appears to have been as significant 100 years ago as it is today. The town then, as now, comprised those who were perceived to belong and incomers, and while the social characteristics which make up the protagonists have changed, the distinction remains. In the past two decades, middle-class incomers in search of 'the country' have replaced working-class incomers in search of work. Those who make up the most recent influx of immigrants have not for the most part moved to Bacup for reasons of employment, but to improve what they call the 'quality of life'. They either retire to the town or work outside Bacup. While most established immigrants (of 40 and over) competed for employment within the area, the main wage-earners of recent immigrant families tend not to compete for the same jobs and some return to the conurbation to work. Some women in recent incoming households, however, *do* work in Bacup; mostly in the domestic service industries, for example, in residential homes for the elderly, and often on a part-time basis.

The views presented by Bacup residents about each other, however they trace their origins, rely on caricature: yuppies, hippies, Bacup born and bred, and incomers are composite persons that do not necessarily represent the lives people live. In accounts given by recent immigrants, for example, they do not talk of their residence in Bacup as temporary, and may express a commitment to both playing a part in and preserving the community of which they are a part. They share with Bacup people ideas about what constitutes a real Bacup person—tough, friendly, hard-working, and living in, as well as creating, close-knit families which form a tight-knit community. They make explicit such a model as part of their rationale for moving to Bacup and as explanation for why it is such an attractive place to live. They also, however, draw on those very same qualities in disassociating themselves from Bacup: now the model is of a parochial and fixed community which has failed to move with the times. Certain characteristics are underlined which, on the one hand, affirm the idea of Bacup as tight-knit, friendly, and laid back and, on the other, affirm its parochial and cliquish nature. Evaluating the tight-knit community either positively or negatively, allows recent immigrants to include or exclude themselves within or outwith the bounds of Bacup.

This is not a prerogative of recent immigrants. These powerful idioms of exclusion and inclusion are cultural resources to which all Bacup residents have access. Thus established immigrants may describe satellite villages in ways which resonate with recent immigrant descriptions of Bacup as a whole. They identify 'remote' places also, but from this perspective remoteness may lie over the Yorkshire border, or on the outskirts of town. They mobilize the same idioms of fixity and mobility. As we have seen, the downside to the positively valued qualities of the tight-knit community—its friendliness and neighbourliness—is its cliquishness and nosiness. These are not, however, opposed to each other, but rather two sides of the same coin; an alternative of the same phenomenon—the tight-knit community. Recent immigrants in describing Bacup as insular or parochial disconnect themselves, and in its friendliness and mutual support they are reconnected.

Eva and George Anderson have retired to Bacup. They bought a new bungalow in Bacup and moved here in the summer of 1987. Before this they lived in Marple, Cheshire, for twenty-three years. Eva had been a manageress in a department store and George had worked as an electrical inspector for a large company. George took the opportunity of early retirement when it was offered and they were able to buy the bungalow outright partly from the profit they made from the sale of their house in Marple. George preferred Bacup to neighbouring towns and considered it to be 'the nicest part of the valley'. He thought that with its 'open spaces and hills, it has more potential' than other towns in the area. George described how Marple used to be a mill village but gradually it filled with 'strangers' and it 'lost its open spaces and it lost its community'. Mr and Mrs Anderson agreed that the changes occurring in Marple had precipitated their move, and they were not sorry to have left. Eva thought that, although Bacup needs 'cleaning up a bit', and the shops were not really adequate, people were 'very friendly'. They were both, they said, looking forward to becoming more involved in 'the community'.

What attracted Mr and Mrs Anderson to Bacup is that which they perceived to have been lost in Marple. They talked about changes that had occurred in Marple in the same way as Bacup people talked about changes in Bacup. The community that was once Marple had been infiltrated by strangers—people, that is, without prior social relationships in the town. If community (like family) is communication (in the words of Judith above) then it figures that the presence of strangers who do not communicate compromises the integrity of the community. Eva and George, however, live different lives and their intention and their desire is to interact with Bacup people. They intend in quotidian ways to be part of the community they have entered as strangers.

Talking of Wythenshawe, from where he and his family moved, Keith Beckwith explained how there the major local authority housing estate was built to accommodate military personnel demobilized after the Second World War. It was, he remarked, 'mostly skilled artisans, travel agents, firemen, policemen, and people like that' who lived in Wythenshawe during the 1950s and 1960s. It was called the Garden City because of its tree-lined streets and grass verges and, up until the 1970s, was 'a very pleasant place to live'. Throughout the 1970s unemployment increased. As the engineering industry collapsed, workers moved out to find employment elsewhere and, according to Keith, more 'labouring people' moved in. By the early 1970s the area was deteriorating and the changes taking place became tangible—'You could sense it; you could feel the violence,' Keith told me.

When they moved to Bacup, Keith was struck by the 'sense of community'; they 'got to know more people' in a very short time. This was due, he thought, to there being 'more community activity—a lot more community about the place'. Carole said that both local people *and* incomers were very friendly: 'the town engenders that'. Keith had no desire to return to what he called the rat-race of the city 'where dog eats dog'. With three children, they would like a bigger house but they would be happy 'to just move around the corner'. Carole pointed out that people smile at each other in Bacup, whereas, 'in Wythenshawe you feel daft smiling at people on the street'. 'Not only daft', added Keith, 'but you're in danger of getting injured.' In describing social change as they saw it, Carole and Keith were not merely presenting a chronological ordering of events—a selected social and economic history of Wythenshawe—but were locating themselves within those events and thereby formulating a moral present and their place in it.

Shrinking networks of friendship and kinship, decreasing numbers of significant social ties, a lack of connectedness and a diminished sense of belonging, are said to be features of modern urban life. Such traits of places, like of people, are known to be unhealthy: they generate violence. Residents who consider themselves Bacup born and bred describe Bacup in ways which resonate with Carole and Keith's description of Wythenshawe. They too draw on idioms of violence and trouble to chart social changes they perceive to have occurred. In so doing they also locate themselves in a present and in a place which is both moral and immoral.

The elements of their life together, presented by Keith and Carole, are selective. They emphasize only some and particular aspects of a rich and complex past. They make much of the former respectability and status of Wythenshawe, and tell of what made it initially desirable, and subsequently unattractive, as a place to live. Keith's categorization of residents draws on distinctions between skilled and unskilled labourers and between what he perceived to be the respectable and the unrespectable working classes. When unemployment hit Wythenshawe, it was those same 'skilled artisans, travel agents, police, and firemen', who had moved there after the war, who moved out: it was they, after all, who could. And they moved to places such as Bacup.[30] 'Commuter' is a symbolically packed social category. Associated with mobility, it evokes membership of the professional or entrepreneurial middle classes and of suburbia. A critical attribute of Elmdon commuters in the 1960s (Strathern 1981) was their orientation away from the village. This is also the

[30] Thinking about Keith and Carole's narrative, I am struck by some of the similarities between their housing history and that of my parents over a decade earlier. Throughout the first eleven years of my parents' marriage, their tenancies were insecure and by 1965, with six children and one semi-skilled labourer's wage, they had saved enough to place a deposit on a newly built house in Leigh (almost the same distance from Liverpool as Bacup is from Manchester). My father continued to work in Liverpool until he got a transfer to a depot nearer home. While he travelled to work, it would be misleading to talk of him as a commuter (to commute is to travel regularly, especially between suburban home and town office, see *Chambers Dictionary*, 1988). And this is again because of the meanings, particularly class connotations, packed into the 'commuter concept'.

way in which *commuters* are perceived from many Bacup perspectives. A common complaint, you will recall, is that they do not put anything back into the town. Yet for residents such as Carole and Keith Beckwith, work outside Bacup is but one orientation amongst many. They have no desire to live elsewhere and although they need a bigger house would be quite happy if it was round the corner. Their children were born in Bacup and attend local schools.[31] Carole works as a home help in the town, she participates in local campaigns, and in formal and informal organizations, and is critical of the town's services and local politicians. Carole and Keith's commitment to the town conspires against assumptions packed into the notion of 'commuter'. For analytical purposes, processes of becoming might be freeze-framed and called 'commuter' or 'Bacupian', but in fact neither are fixed and exclusive identities.[32] And both obscure more than they reveal.

In focusing on narratives of arrivals, I have shown how 'arrival stories' as genre not only situate persons and make explicit the authority from which they speak, but through them people also create the context in which their subsequent ideas make sense. I have wanted to highlight the kind of information about themselves that Bacup residents felt it necessary for me to have. I have also wanted to indicate some of the ways which they 'cut up' the social worlds within which they locate themselves. My interest in ensuing chapters is less in the way in which Bacup is made up of categories of resident, differentiated by such things as place of birth, length of residence, and type of housing tenure, and more on the range of perspectives people bring to bear on these similar substantive themes. People shift position according to questions they are formulating and addressing. Similarly, my interest in kinship is not so much in the terminology and structure of kinship and how they are related to, say, patterns of reciprocation, but more in the way in which different elements of kinship thinking, like being born and being bred, are brought into focus at different moments. In the autobiographical detail Bacup residents select to ground their ideas, they bring together (connect) disparate elements of their and their family's arrival in Bacup in a narrative which makes explicit relationships to neighbours and neighbourhoods, as well as to kin. The next chapter turns to the intentional activity of 'neighbouring' of which it is said there are greater or lesser degrees.

31 Carole corrected herself, 'Well, actually they were born in Bury hospital.' I am intrigued by the way in which my interlocutors in identifying birthplace moved between where they or their children were from and where they were actually born—usually a hospital, e.g. Rossendale, Rochdale, Bury, or Burnley. It is as if the moment of birth, as opposed to the social relationships birth entails, is brought to the fore. One or other, or both, are emphasized. Which one to draw attention to is partly dependent on the question they are addressing and what co-conversationalists know of each other and of the places and people to which they refer. I return to this point in Part 3 (and see Marilyn Greaves's comment and Ch. 5 n. 20).

32 A common stereotype, and one I hope to have shown is not borne out in the movement of labour, is that working-class lives are characterized by fixity, while mobility is a middle-class prerogative. The next chapter pays attention to the way in which social mobility is achieved in finely tuned house moves.

5

Houses and Homes

LOOKING across Bacup from one side of the valley to the other, one can see parallel rows of tiled roofs with chimneys. Some of the acclivitous streets, lined with terraced houses, are still cobblestoned but many have been 'landscaped'.[1] In 1987, in different neighbourhoods of Bacup, many shrubs and saplings had been planted and were struggling to establish themselves. During the post-Second World War 'slum-clearance' programmes, whole neighbourhoods (or sometimes only a street here or there) of back-to-back and terraced houses were demolished. Since then the tendency has been to build council and private houses in clusters rather than rows, to contain them within perimeter roads, and to call them estates. The largest council estate in Bacup was by the end of the 1980s mixed in terms of rented and owner-occupied dwellings.[2] It is named after the road linking what were originally three smaller estates built at different times, and I refer to it here as Mount Pleasant. There is another smaller council estate, the Meadows, on the opposite side of town. Both are backed by open land, neither contain high-rise dwellings, and the majority of houses have gardens to the back and front, which gives an appearance of spaciousness which is often missing from the council estates in northern English cities.

Local authority houses built in the 1930s and 1940s were mostly constructed from stone or red brick and on the whole it is these rather than the concrete and breeze-block dwellings of the 1960s which passed from local authority control to housing associations or to tenants who bought them under the government's right-to-buy campaigns. Consequently local housing authorities, not just in Bacup but across the country, administer some of the least prestigious and poorest quality dwellings. The encouragement given to council tenants to buy their houses went hand in hand with a diminishing political commitment to building more houses, and local authorities were actively discouraged from funding the construction of new houses for rent. The

[1] Which often means the streets have been resurfaced and modernized to accommodate cars as well as pedestrians.

[2] Throughout the 1980s, government-backed campaigns encouraged council tenants to buy their homes. Discounts and favourable mortgage rates were offered, and many council tenants across the country took the opportunity to buy council property. Mortgage holders were less protected against eviction, however, than council or housing association tenants and a wave of repossessions followed the tide of home-ownership. The repossession of homes by banks and building societies, government restrictions on the building of new council houses, and changes to the system of welfare benefits, particularly the restriction of benefits to 16–18 year olds, contributed towards a steady increase in the number of homeless persons in Britain throughout the 1980s.

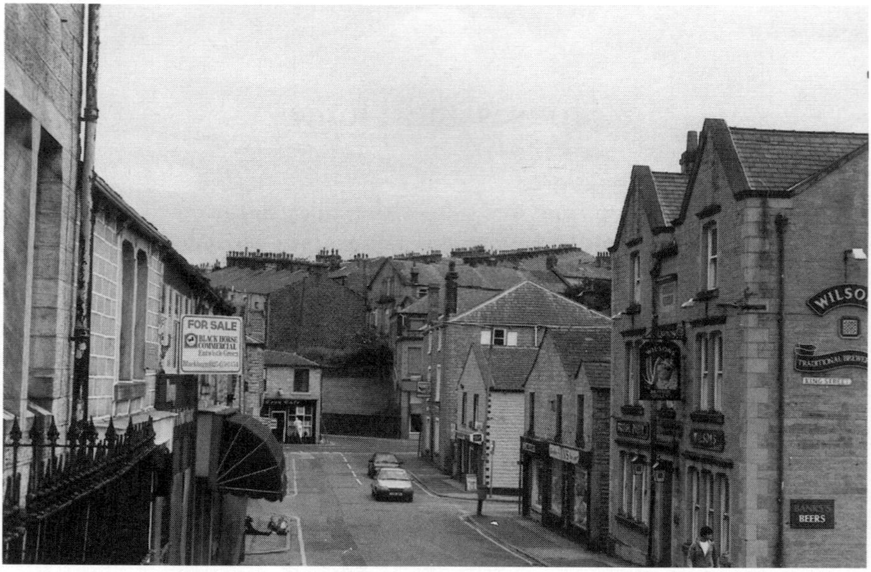

PLATE 9. Looking down Union Street to Cosy Café with rows of chimneys in background

last council housing development in Bacup was completed in 1975 and comprises a row of terraced houses—now called town houses—designed for the elderly.

It is said that in the midst of the slum-clearance programmes of the 1960s, there were many empty and derelict houses in Bacup. Stories are told of houses sold for cash in pubs, and I was told that, as late as 1975, 'you could pick up a little terraced' for less than £200. There does not appear to have been a shortage of inexpensive accommodation throughout the 1970s and early 1980s and in addition the rates (based on the value of property and payable to the local authority) were traditionally low in this region of England. Since then, following a rise in house prices and a decline in the private rented sector—both national trends but late to take effect in Bacup—the shortage of affordable housing for Bacup people setting up a new household is becoming an issue. In 1997–8 there were few privately rented properties, the stock of local authority rented accommodation was shrinking, and the cost of buying a house was rising. Houses are potent symbols of both social change and social differentiation and this chapter explores the prominence of houses on a Bacup landscape.

A Neighbourhood Office

The relationship between Bacup tenants (both actual and potential) and the local housing authority, based in Rawtenstall, is said to have deteriorated through the 1970s and 1980s. Complaints multiplied and many were about the difficulty in dealing with housing officers and the failure of the authority to repair and maintain the housing stock. Prior to my fieldwork in Bacup a series of initiatives to improve communication between the housing authority and Bacup residents, to carry out outstanding repairs and renovations, and to improve the environment of the council estates, had begun. A series of projects designed to improve the estates had been launched, and by the time I went to live in Bacup, Mount Pleasant had been designated an 'environmental improvement area', one of many estates across the country targeted as in need of special attention. Work on the estate continued throughout 1987 and 1988, under such schemes as the Priority Estates Project (PEP) and the Bacup Community Refurbishment Scheme. In an attempt to improve communication between the housing authority and its tenants, housing officers were moved to Bacup. A Neighbourhood Office was opened in the centre of town which allowed for rent to be paid and housing queries dealt with in Bacup rather than in Rawtenstall. When the centre opened, I heard its staff being assessed as though they were recent incomers.[3] Their arrival in town was watched with interest.

The Cosy Cafe is one of three cafés in the town centre and is next door to the new neighbourhood office. It is always busy and attracts a regular set of customers between midday and 2 p.m. and a more diverse clientele mid-morning and mid-afternoon. Market traders and workers from the nearby shoe factory eat their dinner in the café, while shoppers drop in for a cup of tea and perhaps a cigarette at other times. The speciality of the Cosy Cafe is their hot dinner, which comprises meat or fish (sometimes pie), potatoes, vegetables, gravy, and bread and butter followed by pudding (perhaps apple pie, or rhubarb crumble, or sponge pudding) with hot custard. For customers whose appetite or budget does not run to a full meal, half-meals are served for a little more than half the price. Consequently, as well as workers and shoppers, the café attracts some of the poorer of Bacup's residents, not only because it serves half-meals (which are cheap and substantial) but also because of the relaxed hospitality shown by the manageress (a self-designated title). Several regular customers are elderly, live alone, and are reliant solely on a minimal state pension, and the café provides inexpensive food and a warm place to sit for some who, in winter, can barely afford to heat their homes.

The window of the Cosy Cafe provides a clear view up Market Street towards the main Rawtenstall to Todmorden road. With the supermarket on the left and the entrance to the market on the right, Market Street is a busy through road, especially on market days (Wednesday mornings, Fridays, and Saturdays). One of my favourite places to sit, watch the passers-by, read, and bring fieldnotes up to date, was in the window of the Cosy Cafe. I often

[3] Most workers lived at the Rawtenstall end of the valley.

ate dinner there and often began, or was drawn into, conversation with the manageress and/or fellow diners. The window was also a favourite lookout for the manageress, Mrs O'Brien, who monitored the comings and goings of Market Street with or without comment. She often told me she knew 'everybody' in Bacup. The first time we spoke, she told me she was Irish. Her statement of fact, uttered with pride, seemed to me an exhortation, albeit implicit, for me not to mistake her for a Bacup person.

Sitting in the window one day, I listen as Mrs O'Brien gently teases one of her regular and elderly customers about the amount of sugar she (the customer) puts in her tea. She tells the woman, in a voice that can be heard only by some of us, that she will get fat (the woman is in fact extremely thin) and that if she carries on like this she'll bankrupt her (which is more to the point).[4] At that moment, a worker from the Neighbourhood Office passes the window carrying a bag of sugar and a bottle of milk. Catching sight of her, the manageress remarks loudly, in voice that can be heard by all of us: '*They* make their own tea.' In those few words she hints at a group of people who consider themselves above the likes of the Cosy Cafe. The manageress went on to relate 'exactly' how much it had cost (financially) to open the offices and asks, rhetorically but firmly: 'Was it worth it?' She continues, neither requiring nor necessarily expecting an answer: 'Do they actually put anything *back* into the town?' Unsaid, but clearly expressed, is a rebuke—workers in the Neighbourhood Office do not patronize the local café, and by extension local business generally, which belonging to Bacup entails. They brew their own tea and bring their own lunches. They not only withhold their custom but also maintain a distance; a distance readily interpreted by Mrs O'Brien as a deliberate means of maintaining social difference. From this vantage point, workers of the centre are not reciprocating in an appropriate manner: not only are they putting nothing back, but are also sending an implicit message that they consider themselves different (superior) to Bacup folk. The notion of appropriate reciprocation is something which emerged again and again in my conversations in Bacup and is a theme to which I return, but first a further look at back-to-backs.

Two areas of poor housing, which existed before the council development of Mount Pleasant, Plantation Back and Irish Back, were both densely populated neighbourhoods of back-to-back dwellings and described today as having housed poorer residents of the town. A knowledge of Irish Back, like Plantation Back, is put to use in the work of social differentiation. This is not confined to those who lived in, or even remember, the actual dwellings. Joanne Leary was in her early twenties, and a friend of Laura Gray. When I first met her, her son was 4 years old and he and Laura's son had just started school together.

[4] An example of the way in which social critique is couched in jest (see Ch. 6).

Joanne's mother is from Britannia and her father was born on Plantation Back. Joanne told me that Plantation Back 'used to be in the centre of town, but it was demolished before I was born'. She continued: 'All the Murphys, Learys, O'Briens—they were all born up there, it used to be the main street in Bacup . . . *all* the Irish used to live up there, as well as the local scruffs.' When her parents got married they moved to Broadclough and before Joanne started school they moved again to another terraced property in a different neighbourhood of Bacup; both these houses, Joanne told me, had since been demolished. Eventually her parents moved to a council house on Mount Pleasant and they and her younger siblings still lived there. Joanne lived in a terraced house near the town centre with her 'feller' and their son. They were buying the house and she told me they often talked about moving to a newer one, possibly on the Orchards: 'but we keep changing our minds'.

Joanne makes a distinction between 'the Irish' which includes her own family and 'the local scruffs'. From this vantage point, the feckless and irresponsible are not the Irish—they are '*the local* scruffs' who, from another angle, are original Bacup families.

A common residential pattern of an older generation of Bacup people was, on marriage, to rent accommodation from private landlords and sometimes from kin.[5] With the post-war state housing developments in Britain and then the 'slum-clearance' programmes of the 1960s, many tenants moved from privately rented to local authority houses and at the time compared the latter favourably with the back-to-backs in which they had lived as children. To evoke back-to-backs is not merely to imagine a type of housing now almost obsolete: their significance runs wider and deeper than their dominance on the landscape at the turn of the century. They carry with them knowledge of a particular kind of society including its histories and geographies as well as of particular families and the relationships between them. Named areas of the town, such as Plantation Back and Mount Pleasant, convey meaning above and beyond their significance as residential areas. It is generally agreed that overcrowded neighbourhoods such as Irish Back were not necessarily pleasant places to have lived. They were also, it is suggested, hotbeds of sedition. But sedition is not always a bad thing and sociality screens out discomfort. Whatever their characteristics, they are now an element in a shared history of hardship said to have formed a typical Bacup character whatever its origins. When Bacup people talk about the demolition of Plantation Back, they not only refer to the flattening

[5] When Bacup people talked to me about kin relations they invariably spoke of the expectation of mutual assistance without financial reward. Interestingly, several interviewees in a housing survey along with several informants during fieldwork told me they had rented accommodation from kin. The stipulation that one should not gain financially from kin does not appear to cover the jurisdiction of housing. For example, it is 'only right' that adult children 'pay their way' and contribute towards their board and lodging. The general prescription that money should not be exchanged for services within the family does not cover all eventualities. Finch (1989) pointed out, over a decade ago, that despite a strong emphasis on mutual assistance between kin, the way in which support is mobilized in daily lives cannot be predicted. In Bacup there is a dominant idea that kin *ought* to help each other, but so too ought neighbours and workmates.

of houses and the disappearance of neighbourhoods, but they also dwell on a shift in the quality of social relationships—a swerve in history. Mount Pleasant fills the conceptual vacuum left by such places as Plantation Back—partially.

When Plantation and Irish Back were demolished, many of their inhabitants were rehoused on Mount Pleasant and they recall that, after the dark and overcrowded tenements, the new council houses were light and spacious. Telling me about their residential history, many Bacup people remarked on how much more desirable the council houses were in comparison with the back-to-backs in which they had spent their childhood. They were modern, light, and airy, and had gardens and entrances to the back and front. But a transformation appears to have occurred in attitudes towards, and the value placed on, rented local authority housing.[6] From coveted and desirable residences when they were first built, their status has declined, and despite the vagaries of the housing market, the standing of local authority housing shrank along with its overall quality.[7]

Mount Pleasant, from some Bacup perspectives as well as from surrounding towns, is said to be a 'problem'. The name itself evokes a discourse of *trouble* and *troublemakers*, and many people claim an intimate knowledge of it without ever having been there. Barbara Jones told me that when she was a child she never knew anybody who lived on Irish Back, but she thinks Mount Pleasant is similar, at least it has a similar reputation. She has friends from the church who live on Mount Pleasant and they tell her of the stigma attached to having such an address. Not so long ago a friend of hers was refused hire purchase from a local electrical goods store because she lived on Mount Pleasant.

In a bid to ameliorate the stigma attached to Mount Pleasant, the local authority renamed the road after which it was called in the hope that the new name would spill over to the estate. This never happened, and the estate continues to be called by its original name which, in turn, continues to carry its infamy. A name, as an entity, might be changed, but what goes into a

[6] During the 1980s owning one's home increasingly symbolized achievement and respectability. A message, albeit implicit, sent by the government of the time was that self-respecting citizens should not be dependent on the state and renting houses from councils was tantamount to ignoring edicts of self-help and independence.

[7] A story told me by Judy Wilder provides a striking example of this shift in value. She described how her friend—'an alcoholic and who, at one time, was very wealthy'—had lived, as an owner occupier, in a succession of progressively less expensive houses. She had spent the profit from the sale of each house predominantly, said Judy, on alcohol. Her present accommodation was, according to Judy, at the 'bottom end' of the property market, and if she sold it in order to acquire cash, she would be forced to live in rented accommodation. Judy pointed to the severe implications of this in this telling comment: 'While she's got a house—she's eccentric. But if she ends up in a council house she'll be 'a dirty old drunk'". Herzfeld (1991:60), writing of Rethemnos in Crete, observes: 'The truly wealthy have the power to parade either eccentricity or simplicity: they can afford not to care' (See also MacLeod 1995 for similar views about low-cost housing from residents of housing projects in the United States.)

name—the package of social relationships for which it is but a shorthand—is not so amenable to transformation. The traces in the wake of a name, be it of places or people, remain.

The estate contains a number of properties that housing officials euphemistically call 'hard to let': houses or flats which stand empty for longer than average because tenants, if they have a choice, do not choose them. Some of the hard-to-let properties may be substandard in terms of repair (damp being a major problem) but a decision not to accept the offer of a council house is as likely to be made on the basis of its reputation as on the physical properties of the dwelling. It might be the reputation of the estate, or one particular area of it, or a specific street, or the block in which a flat is situated, which is taken into account. But once known, it is difficult for a reputation to be un-known. The bad name of estates and neighbourhoods is often laid on the doorstep of particular named families represented by specific patronyms. Knowledge of these families, their interconnectedness, and their connections to Bacup are brought to bear in local assessments of houses and housing areas. Links are constantly made which connect families, whether referred to as *big Irish families* or *big Bacup families*, to each other and to houses, which may be back-to-backs or council houses.

Suitable Material

The detached and semi-detached stone houses built around the middle of the nineteenth century for the merchant, professional, mill- and landowning classes remain dotted around the town. Some of the larger ones have been converted into residential homes for the elderly (one of a few burgeoning commercial enterprises in the region). They were often built overlooking rows of terraced houses which had been constructed rapidly and cheaply for incoming labouring families. There is a striking impression of a former architecture of surveillance. In the neighbourhood in which I lived, for example, the rows of terraced and back-to-back houses ran from where the factory stood, on the banks of the river Irwell, uphill to the house of the millowner. The factory workers were thus sandwiched between the mill and their employer—overseen at work and at home.[8]

During the 1970s there was a spate of private, speculative house-building which resulted in mostly detached and semi-detached houses placed in orderly

[8] For Michel Foucault (1979) the panopticon is the paradigmatic example of how technologies of power work to discipline bodies and control groups. The architecture of the panopticon not only allows for constant surveillance, but also for the constant impression of surveillance so that bodies discipline themselves (see also Rabinow 1984). While finding this paradigm analytically powerful, back-to-backs specifically and Bacup generally also suggest to me limits to disciplinary technologies: the reported behaviour (anything but disciplined) of working-class men in the town centre in the middle of the 19th cent. reflects an anxiety at the ineffectiveness of mechanisms of control (see Ch. 6); and today back-to-backs are deployed by their former inhabitants (for whom they are neither desirable nor prestigious dwellings) in formulating moral histories.

and ordered settings and enclosed within discernible boundaries. There appears to have been an attempt in the design and naming of these estates to capture a bucolic, or at least rural, calm. They are landscaped to make the most of geographical features such as streams and hills. Built with timber frames and precast breeze-block, they portray an image of fragile impermanence, placed as they are amidst the self-evident durability of local stone. One of the town planners (born in Manchester, trained in Liverpool, and living in Rawtenstall) was critical of the kind of materials used in the construction of new private houses. He argued that builders failed to take into consideration the altitude and the weather and consequently the houses they built required constant attention and continual repair. Speaking on behalf of the local authority—and clearly here on behalf of Bacup—he told me: 'We don't perceive the need for more housing—they have been building dormer bungalows out of unsuitable materials. We don't *need* more housing.' He also informed me that planning permission, which had been granted in the 1970s, was now being reconsidered by his department. The quality of the new houses was not the only reason for the change of heart, more significant to the town planner is the impact of such housing development on what he considers to be the *true* nature of the area.

> We are still seeing the results of large-scale planning permission that was given in the 1970s, for example, [one] for 180 homes—some of which have been built. But now the planning department wants to withdraw permission because they feel it is too large a development in an essentially rural area. It will have detrimental effects on the village and the community and put pressure on local schools et cetera.

If the 'essentially rural' nature of Bacup needs to be preserved, then the way to do this is to prescribe the type, and limit the number, of new dwellings. This is not an immediate preoccupation of many Bacup people with whom I spoke: the idea that Bacup is essentially rural is rarely mooted nor that the solution to degradation of the area is to prescribe and control the number and type of new houses. For them Bacup's preservation requires keeping its people (particularly its youth), and that requires employment. They draw upon an industrial rather than a rural past. They are not unconcerned about their vicinity (indeed they say a great deal about what they perceive to be a decline in the quality of local services, particularly since local government has been administered from Rawtenstall) but, in the context of housing, they focus their attention on the people moving into houses rather than the houses themselves. They talk of the kind of social relationships that incomers forge, or not, with local people. They put forward views on the characteristics of the kind of people they appreciate as neighbours, and dwell on the value of appropriate expressions of reciprocity and friendliness.

I met Mrs Sweeney at the weekly flea market.[9] She and two other women were working on a stall selling second-hand goods on behalf of a nearby hospice. I bought some hand-painted fruit dishes from Mrs Sweeney and she told me they were probably painted in Bacup as painting pottery used to be a common pastime of Bacup women. Our conversation continued and I explained what I was doing there, to which she responded that she was not herself *from* Bacup and queried whether, in that case, there was any point in me talking to her at all.[10] I assured her there was and she graciously invited me to her house and suggested I meet her husband. She explained she lived just north of the town centre, on the road to Weir, in a neighbourhood that was 'not *really* Bacup'. She also told me they had just built some new houses at the end of her road.[11]

I arrived on her doorstep a few days later, but she had forgotten I was coming and was, she told me, in the middle of having her hair done. She instructed me to return the following day. I did, and she greeted me warmly, made me tea, gave me biscuits and warned me: 'I don't know much about modern Bacup, because I don't have much to do with it.'

Mrs Sweeney was born in Cowpe, a village, she said, about four miles away, and she moved here (to Bacup and to this house) with her parents in 1939. 'I wouldn't call myself a Bacup person. I think I would put meself down as an Old Cowper. I wouldn't go back there now, though. It's altered.' She got married in 1947 to a 'Stockport lad' and he moved in with her and her parents. Her father died the following year, and she and her husband stayed on in the house with her mother. They took over the house when her mother died. She has a sister who lives in the same street, one son who does not live in Bacup, and a daughter who 'married an electrician up Cowpe'.

Mrs Sweeney thought there had been a great many changes in Bacup over the past few years. For example, a lot of new houses were being built, especially 'up Weir', although this was not surprising, she said, because 'it's so easy to get on the motorways to Manchester now and houses are a lot cheaper here than in Manchester'. Her own neighbourhood had not changed very much, 'except for the people', she told me. 'When we first came here it was very quiet. You had to wait for someone to die to get a house. I don't know the names of people who live here now. They're from the area, from Bacup mostly. The biggest part of them are local.' The new estate at the end of the road, she said, 'is alright'. It had 'tidied up' the area a bit and as long as 'decent people are coming in', she didn't mind what they built.

[9] The flea market was held on Fridays and was a vibrant affair with traders selling all manner of second-hand goods including clothes, domestic appliances, furniture, books, jewellery, and ornaments. There were usually two or three stalls fund-raising for local organizations such as the UWC, or local branches of charities such as National Society for the Prevention of Cruelty to Children (NSPCC).

[10] She evidently agreed with many other Bacup residents that expertise is a corollary of belonging.

[11] These were some of the same houses the town planner had been describing.

Mrs Sweeney's new neighbours were mostly from Bacup, but she didn't know many of them by name. Nor did she know, by name, the people who had moved into the new houses at the end of the street, but if they were 'decent people' they would 'keep the place tidy' and were unlikely to bother her. For the town planner, however, the preservation of Bacup required curtailing and monitoring development, especially in the construction of edifices and the appropriation of space. One of his concerns was the suitability of housing materials. For Mrs Sweeney, the preservation of Bacup depends on the day-to-day activities of decent folk, and decent folk, whatever their origins, were preferable as neighbours to indecent folk, wherever they came from. She was more interested in the material of neighbouring, than in housing materials.

As we have seen, one of the complaints often voiced in Bacup is that incomers neither worked nor socialized in the town and consequently were not 'putting anything back'. For the most part, the incomers referred to in these comments were recent immigrants and lived on the new private housing estates. Such comments are made just as readily by Bacup residents who consider themselves to be incomers—although they might qualify such a label with an 'almost Bacup' tag—as by those who are Bacup born and bred. A common complaint voiced by one woman is that incomers do not spend money in Bacup: they shop and 'go out'[12] out of town. With reference to housing, their motivations are questioned. In the words of one Bacup man: 'People are coming here because of cheap houses and rates, but they don't admit that's what it is'; they are exploiting, in other words, what does not rightfully belong to them. This man's accusation, however, leaves open the possibility that if incomers' motives for settling in Bacup were different (not merely for financial gain), or even if they were more honest about their motives, they could be accommodated with little risk to Bacup's integrity.

A Housing Survey

One privately built housing estate, the Orchards, has a tributary of the river Irwell running through it and, built in a hollow, it is hidden from the main road and from the view of passers-by. The houses on the estate are a mixture of designs and sizes. The contractor responsible for the majority of them built an additional row of two-bedroomed bungalows on the edge of the Orchards, which were completed and occupied by the summer of 1987. Four streets of older terraced houses, known locally as the Four Rows, lie in between the new bungalows and the council houses on the perimeter road of Mount Pleasant. I carried out a housing survey during the winter of 1987/8 in this area of town

[12] Meaning to go out of the house for entertainment: e.g. to pubs, clubs, restaurants, cinemas, and theatres. This observation on incomers momentarily screens out the fact that local people do the same.

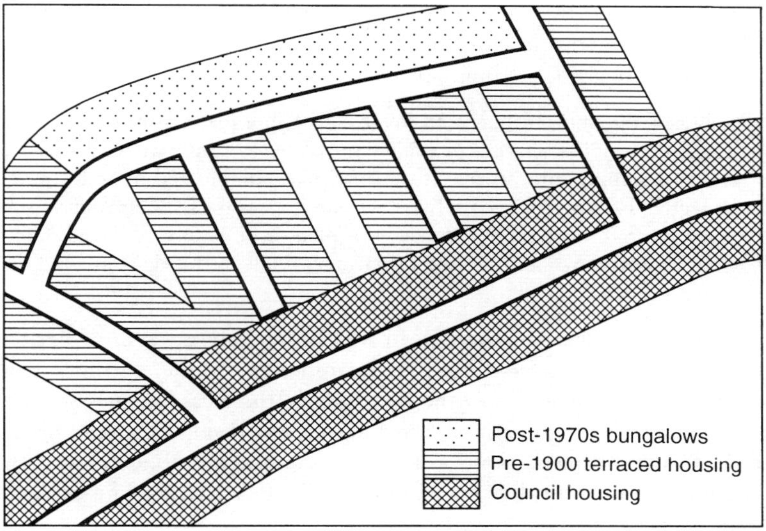

FIG. 5.1. Sketch of Housing Survey Area, showing different types of housing

(Fig. 5.1). To explain why I chose this area, I took my cue from a health visitor who, when I met her, had worked in Bacup for over twenty years. She told me she knew it 'like the back of [her] hand'. According to her there are three 'main types' of Bacup resident: 'There are the old Bacup folk who live in traditional terraced houses, the Irish Catholic community on the council estate, and the commuters who live in the new houses.'

Bethan Elliot similarly associated types of housing with types of resident. Bethan told me she was sent to Bacup by a London-based organization which places Christian volunteers in 'priority areas'. The volunteers are predominantly graduates who conduct a twelve-month period of service 'in the community' after university. Bethan was placed as a pastoral assistant in Bacup's Anglican parish church, evidently because Bacup is considered, from the perspective of this organization at least, to be 'in need' in matters of spirituality. This was a view also put forward by members of the Assemblies of God who had recently established a church in Bacup. It resonates with the way in which Bacup is identified as needy in other social domains, such as housing and housing estates.

Bethan told me her first impressions of Bacup were of a grey, drab, industrial mill-town. She thought it unattractive and unappealing. But following this initial impression she had come to like it a great deal, and to realize that 'visually, there's a strange kind of beauty about the place'. Moreover, any early negative impressions were always mitigated by the efforts Bacup people made to welcome her to the town and to make her feel at home. Her views on Bacup, she said, had changed dramatically as she had come to know it better and she could imagine, she said, settling here.

> As a member of the church there's an involvement in a place. I immediately know a large amount of people—sharing in their family life. I'm intimately involved in the town—always bumping into people. It's a small place dominated by industry. Everyone is connected. Bacup people have lived here for generations. Their sons and daughters live next door. They tend not to have travelled or be highly educated. Of course this is being broken down all the time by incomers. Given the right job and circumstances I could settle here.

Bethan went on to describe the way in which the congregation of her church is made up of a wide cross-section of Bacup people: there are the 'Manchester commuter types' who live in the new houses, the local 'business people like the millowners' and a majority of 'working-class—Bacup born and bred' who live in the terraced houses. She was not sure, she told me, about a few members of the congregation who live on Mount Pleasant: 'there are one or two from the estate who fit in somewhere different'.

A schema which links types of housing to categories of resident comes up frequently when residents talk about Bacup. The ever finer distinctions they make between each other is of a piece with the finely tuned distinctions they make between types of house, types of community (see next chapter for cities, towns, villages, and hamlets), and types of family.

In deciding to carry out a housing survey, I wanted to include the three types of housing that had emerged frequently thus far in my Bacup conversations. I identified an area containing houses built by the local authority (both rented and owner-occupied), post-1970 privately built houses, and nineteenth-century stone terraced houses. The area I chose was on the opposite side of town from where I lived, and was a neighbourhood with which I was, prior to the survey, unfamiliar.[13] Over the course of four months, I spoke with one or more residents of seventy-six houses (Table 5.1).[14] I used a brief interview schedule which included questions on the number of occupants in each house, their ages, occupations, length of residence, and previous place of residence. I also asked a general question about services. In some cases the initial survey questions led to lengthy conversations about Bacup, its inhabitants, and its particular kinds of services (often with reference to the past and change), and, in others, I was able to return and talk to respondents at greater length, in the

[13] One rationale being that it would broaden my horizons and help me get to know more people. The process of knocking on doors and introducing and explaining myself was lengthy and, initially, discomforting. I was a reluctant researcher during this phase of fieldwork: uninvited, I felt myself to be an unwelcome intrusion. For the most part, people responded with characteristic courtesy and willingness to help (me rather than research).

[14] Three houses in the area were empty. Residents of four houses did not want to talk to me and I was unable, after repeated attempts, to make contact with the residents of another four houses.

TABLE 5.1. *House type and tenure in the survey area*

House type	Tenure	No. in survey
Local authority	Rented	15
	Owner-occupied	7
Private terraced	Owner-occupied	32
Private post-1970	Owner-occupied	22
TOTAL		76

TABLE 5.2. *Length of residence in Bacup of adults in the survey area*

Type	Tenure	Bacup born and bred	>20 yrs in Bacup	<20 yrs in Bacup	Total
Local authority	Rented	11	4	—	15
	Owner-occupied	7	—	—	7
Terraced	Owner-occupied	26	4	2	32
Post-1970	Owner-occupied	7	1	14	22
TOTAL	51 (67%)	9 (12%)	16 (21%)	76 (100%)	

comfort of their home and with the luxury of time. In most cases communication in the survey interviews was brief and to the point.[15] The point to emphasize here is that, in talking about housing and services, respondents drew on idioms and images of kinship. They talked, for example, about being Bacup born and bred, or not, and of the origins and arrivals of themselves, their family, and their neighbours.

It was found that 81 per cent of the terraced, 82 per cent of the council dwellings (both rented and owner-occupied), and 32 per cent of the post-1970 houses contained one or more adults born in Bacup. This seems to bear out a general idea, prevalent in Bacup, that it is recent incomers who occupy newer privately built housing. However, the stereotype that recent incomers are mostly Manchester commuters (yuppies) is not borne out in the data. Tables 5.3 and 5.4 refer only to post-1970 houses. They indicate previous residence and present place of work of adult residents in twenty-two houses. Residents are not, as is commonly suggested, predominantly from Manchester or Cheshire; more than half moved to their present home either from another neighbourhood of Bacup or from a neighbouring town or village within a ten-mile radius of Bacup.

Unlike immigration into the Essex village of Elmdon in the 1960s (Strathern 1981), not all recent immigrants have established households prior to

[15] The survey is not meant to be representative of Bacup, but rather illustrative; providing examples rather than statistics. Without the signposts which came from fieldwork, from the conversations and discussions emerging from particular questions, I could have attached sparse meaning to survey information, and for my purposes the survey was more valuable in the discussion it generated and the relationships it enabled.

TABLE 5.3. *Previous place of residence of households in post-1970 houses (in miles from Bacup)*

Bacup	5–10	10–30*	>30	First home	Total
5	5	2	3	7	22

* Covers Greater Manchester.

TABLE 5.4. *Place of work of residents of post-1970 houses*

	Bacup	Ross	Manchester	Retired	Home	Other	n.k.
Male	1	5	6	5		3	2
Female	2	1	3	5	6	1	1

moving to Bacup. Apart from those who move to Bacup on retirement, there are many who are establishing a household for the first time. At the end of the 1980s, the cost of new houses in Bacup was significantly lower than in Greater Manchester or in those towns closer to the motorway links with the city. Of those who were setting up their first home, one person was from Bacup, seven from villages within a ten-mile radius of Bacup, and six from over ten miles away (which includes Manchester). Despite a common view that recent immigrants are predominantly from Manchester, and commute back there to work, there are as many people settling in Bacup who are from neighbouring towns and villages.

I first met Doreen Whittacker when I knocked on her door with a survey schedule in my hand. After answering my questions, she invited me to return and meet her husband, Arthur, who she said, coming from 'an original Bacup family', would be able to tell me much more about Bacup than she could. She also thought that given his background he would be very interested in my work. I returned, not once but several times, and on each occasion Mr and Mrs Whittacker welcomed me warmly. During my first visit we discovered mutual acquaintances from other Bacup forums. It turned out I had already met their son at a meeting at the Baptist church. We also discovered I knew Arthur Whittacker's business partner from the Nat, and Doreen Whittacker used to go to school with my neighbour, Barbara Jones. Making these connections was a pleasurable process, and along them credentials travelled.

The first time I met Mr Whittacker he treated the occasion with an authoritative formality: sitting me down in front of him, he asked me courteously what he could do for me. As a member of what Mr Whittacker also acknowledged to be an original Bacup family, he did not doubt his expertise and knew he was well qualified to provide me with information about Bacup. Mrs Whittacker colluded in her husband's status as '*original*' but as I got to know her better she made explicit the ambivalence of originality. She told me that she had once attempted to trace the family tree of the Whittackers: 'If you go back far enough', she said, 'there are lots of interrelationships.'

Mr Whittacker was born in the house next door to where he now lived. Mrs Whittacker was born in Sharneyford and her parents were from Ireland. After they got married, they lived in several different neighbourhoods of Bacup and in different types of accommodation, renting at times from family, and at others from private landlords and the local authority. Eventually when their children were still quite young they bought the house in which they still lived. In 1982, he was made redundant from the shoe factory in which he had worked for forty-one years. His father had worked in the same factory for fifty years. A year later he and two colleagues, who had also lost their jobs in the same wave of redundancies, opened a small shoe factory with their redundancy payments. Despite a rocky beginning, the company had so far survived. It relied on word of mouth for new orders and they had an advantage over larger competitors in being able to accept and supply small orders. Over the intervening years, they had carved out a specialist niche for themselves in the manufacture of satin or patent-leather dance shoes.

Dwelling on the changes he had witnessed in Bacup over the years, and drawing on his own and his father's occupational history, Mr Whittacker told me that, often, sons and daughters would work in the same mills as their parents, which meant that when one of the larger factories closed down and the workforce was made redundant, 'whole families' became unemployed. Families, he said, used to live close to one another in the same 'half dozen streets', and although a son might, on marriage, 'move to where his wife lived', he would nearly always, when he could, move back to where 'his family' lived. There was, he suggested, an expectation that daughters would move away from home, while sons would stay close to home.

Another woman I interviewed in the housing survey also told me sons tended not to move away from the area in which they were born and if they did, more often than not they would return. The suggestion that women were more mobile than men on marriage prompted me to look at information from the survey in a particular way. Of 134 adults in seventy-six households, seventy were women and sixty-four men. Thirty-seven (53%) of the women and forty (63%) of the men were born and/or raised in Bacup. Slightly more women than men came from neighbouring towns and villages but the numbers were too few to support a statement that marriage in Bacup is virilocal. Women do appear, however, to move further afield on marriage than men. But again, closeness and distance are relative concepts and the finer distinctions between what counts as near or far cannot be captured in a housing survey. These numbers are small and the point to make is that what might be asked of a survey such as this emerges from elsewhere. I noted in Chapter 1 that my second fieldwork in Bacup provided an analytical handle on the first. Likewise, information exchanged, say, in a conversation in the pub, provides a vantage point from which to regard information gained in a door to door survey and vice versa. Each contextualizes the other. In making connections we—in this case the anthropologist and Bacup people—create contexts.

TABLE 5.5. *Place of origin of adults in survey houses*

Type	Tenure	No.	Bacup born and bred	>10	>30	Other	n.k.
Local authority	Rented	37	27	2	2	3	1
Terraced	Owner-occupied	56	39	10	3	3	1
New	Owner-occupied	41	10	9	12	7	3

Bungalows

Different views as to the contribution of 'the new bungalows' emerged in answers to the survey questions. They were said, on the one hand, to have replaced an 'eyesore', and on the other to have replaced the garages and gardens of the old terraced houses. According to one respondent the area on which they now stand had been 'full of old pens', and to another it had been 'just full of rubbish and old sheds', but to yet another the new bungalows have meant that small plots of land for storage and on which residents of the terraced houses could grow flowers had disappeared. One respondent acknowledged the sheds *had* looked shabby, but explained this was understandable because it was hardly worth 'putting up new' when nobody knew for sure what was going to be happening to the land on which they stood. From this perspective, residents had understandably invested little in the way of time, money, and energy into the upkeep of sheds, garages, or pens in the event they would eventually be destroyed. From a different perspective, their poor state of repair was evidence that they were uncared for and this was legitimation enough for removing them.

The new dwellings and attendant landscaping were said, then, to have either improved the vicinity or augmented its decline. Whichever it was, it was said that the bungalows had created new problems, for example, cars were now parked on the newly built road creating a new hazard for pedestrians (particularly children), and in the next street where the cobblestones had been removed as part of the landscaping project, traffic travelled faster and children could now cycle or skateboard, posing a danger to themselves and pedestrians. Tied to conflicting opinions about the effects of the new housing and landscaping, was an ambivalence about the contribution and motivation of the builder, described by some as 'a local lad made good'. On the one hand, he had done a 'grand job'—tidying up the area and attracting incomers and wealth; in the words of one woman: 'He deserves a medal for what he's done for this area.' On the other hand, he was said to be motivated only by financial gain, and consequently to lack foresight and imagination. To illustrate this latter point, several interviewees told me there used to be underground mining in the place where the new bungalows were built. There was a risk therefore, they claimed, of subsidence. The suggestion, implicit in such an observation, is that anyone who knows Bacup would also know this. The 'local lad made good' is here assessed in the same way as the incomer we came across earlier—who was said to exploit Bacup (particularly its housing) without reciprocating. In each case, it is the motivation of those who gain financially from Bacup that is questioned. An analogy is made between the domains of kinship and community—both, in this context, are characterized by relations of mutual support, friendliness, and communication, and neither ought to be tainted by financial profit. Belonging to communities requires similar constraint as belonging to families. One woman remarked that 'the new bungalows' had 'ruined the community'. In her words: 'It used to be a right friendly neighbourhood this, but with all this [building] going on people are grumbling and complaining.' Her comment points not to the bungalows as, or as replacing, a physical blight on the landscape but as compromising, in complaint and criticism, the kind of relations which characterize community. The way in which interviewees explored the 'new bungalows', and the ambivalence the dwellings house, resonate with ways in which they explored other innovations in their immediate social worlds.

The example of the bungalows emerged in the process of carrying out a door-to-door survey. It is not, however, the research method which determines the kind of information generated, but rather the connections respondents are willing to make. Thinking about 'services' they dwelt on Bacup and its inhabitants; the kind of place it is and the kind of place it was. And in so doing they mobilized idioms of kinship.

Bettering Oneself

It is as an observer, a temporary resident, a guest, and a Christian (amongst other things) that Bethan Elliot (quoted above) views Bacup. The 'large amount' of people she knows are predominantly churchgoers and most are members of the Church of England. Like other claims to 'know everybody', her bodies are selective, and like claims to know about 'Bacup people' or 'incomers', the items she chooses as evidence, in this case of Bacupness, are selected. She remarked on the interrelatedness of Bacup people and what she perceived as their lack of mobility, both socially and spatially, placing a similar kind of value on mobility as other Bacup residents, suggesting analogies between mobility and progress. For her, it is newcomers like herself who provide impetus for change—who introduce new ideas from cosmopolitan worlds.

I met Mr Williams in the housing survey.

Mr Williams was born and bred in Bacup. He is now in his eighties, and lives in a two-bedroom terraced house very close to where he was brought up. He was born in a neighbourhood on the other side of town and his parents moved here to the Four Rows when he was 2 years old. When he first married he rented a back-to-back near the centre of town from a private landlord. When he was 30, and his daughters 5 and 7, his wife died. He remarried six years later and at this point moved to a house in the same street in which he was brought up, again renting from a private landlord. He went on to have two more children. He saved £100 and, in 1938, the Co-op gave him a mortgage for the other £100 and he bought his present house. This is 'a better area', he points out, 'there's more air and its breezier'. 'You can see, can't you', he asks me without expecting an answer, 'how I've kept bettering myself?'

To the untutored eye differences between the neighbourhoods in which Mr Williams has lived during his life are indiscernible and differences between the types of houses in which he has lived appear small. It might be suggested, from one perspective, that retiring in the next street from where one lived as child indicates little in the way of social mobility—such an observation might then be used to exemplify the fixity and lack of mobility often imputed to Bacup people. One of the town planners described it this way: 'Bacup people are the exact opposite to yuppies—they are not upwardly mobile. Although they call the place they don't want to move out.'[16]

But Mr Williams has been moving all his life. His reckoning begins from his first independent household, and with each progressive move, the quality of his accommodation and neighbourhood improved. Such mobility, for Mr Williams, is evidence of his self-sufficiency and his ability to look after his family appropriately. He has been bettering himself.

Mobility as a resource is as available to those who define themselves as Bacup born and bred as it is to those who consider their sojourn in Bacup to be temporary. Many people with whom I spoke acknowledged and applauded what they perceived as their children's mobility. Mr Sweeney pointed out that in *his* younger days he could not afford to buy and run a car, now he buys a new one (or at least replaces his old one) about every ten years. But it was different, he said, for his children—'they have bettered themselves': 'They go abroad every year. He [their son-in-law] was made redundant and then started his own business as an electrician. The order books are good. They are not short of anything. They have a good lifestyle—a lovely home—[they're] just having a garage built on and an extension.'

Mary Shaw is in her late forties, and describes herself as Bacup born and bred. She had been a welfare rights officer in Bacup for many years, was a key member of staff in the development of the Unemployed Workers Centre, and is a well-known and respected figure in Bacup. Her father was a quarryman and she was born on the Irish Back. She was one of five children and, in 1950, when she was 5 years old, her parents were offered the tenancy of a recently built council house in Stacksteads. It was a three-bedroom semi-detached house, with running hot water, 'sunshine windows', and kitchen units. Mary described the delight of them all on being able to move out of a privately rented, dark and dingy, 'one-up-one-down'. Their new house was, by comparison, spacious and light. It had its own bathroom and three bedrooms. Her parents were offered the house because a certain number were set aside for the families of

[16] To call is to criticize, i.e. call it names.

miners and quarry workers. The move, Mary recalled, coincided with the only period of time in her childhood that her mother did not have to work outside the home. Four years later they lost the house. Her father drank heavily and was unable to keep up with the rent payments and, when Mary was 9 years old, they moved out of their 'luxury' home back into a privately rented back-to-back. Without hot water and overcrowded again, they were all disappointed by the move, but it was particularly hurtful and difficult, Mary thought, for her mother. Two years later, although she passed her eleven-plus examination, Mary was unable to attend the Grammar School because her mother could not afford the school uniform. Mary was more saddened by the effect this had on her mother than by the fact that she never went to the Grammar School.

Comments from Mrs Shaw, Mr Williams, and Mr Sweeney on their and their children's housing histories reveal the relationship between moving house and 'bettering yourself', or not. Houses, fixed and immobile as they might be, symbolize social mobility. Moving house, in which people seem to have hardly moved at all, is yet packed with indigenous meaning and significance. This self-perceived mobility runs counter to the notion that Bacup comprises a fixed and static population. Houses symbolize much more subtle distinctions of class, than are available through gross categories of, say, housing tenure.

Mobile Local

There is a pub near the border between Britannia and Bacup, just over a mile north of the town centre. It is where the Coco-Nutters (a dance group) begin a marathon performance on Easter Saturday of each year (see Ch. 7). I had been meaning for weeks to visit the pub and to get the lie of the land before Easter. I wanted to meet and speak with the licensees about the Coco-Nutters and the forthcoming day—known locally as Nutters Day. Eventually I got around to walking up the hill. It was a cold and wet weekday afternoon, in March 1988. The man behind the bar, who I assumed was the landlord, was talking with three men sitting at the bar and the pub was otherwise empty.

The men were between 30 and 40 years of age; they listened as I introduced myself to the barman and as he introduced himself to me as Derek Morgan, the landlord. They carried on listening as I ordered a beer and sat at the bar a few stools away and as I haltingly explained to Mr Morgan my interest in the Coco-Nutters. The carried on listening as Mr Morgan told me he had only recently taken over the management of the pub in Britannia, and how he had a long history as a publican, mostly in Manchester. His voice carried the assumption that I knew (having come from Manchester) the implications of being a publican in the areas of the city he named. The customers resumed their conversation, and it turned to things they predicted a student of anthropology who wanted to find out about the Coco-Nutters would find relevant. Two of the men told me they were local, and it emerged that the other had recently settled, with his family, into a newly built private house on a nearby housing estate. He told me he commuted out of town to work and, again, in a way that suggested I probably knew what that meant. It became clear as the conversation progressed that they all thought of the pub as their local.

The men got around to the subject of pubs and trouble, and one of the Britannia men told me Bacup was 'a rough town', and the other that it was a 'hard place'. I asked them if they were from Bacup and one replied, for both of them: 'We're not Bacup—too much aggravation. We're born and bred around here.' They spoke of their origins in, and attachment to, Britannia. 'Britannia born and bred', said the other, thereby excluding both of them from Bacup. An argument then arose about who constituted the real locals, and the meaning of 'local' shifted between association with Bacup, Britannia, and the pub. This process, akin to shape-shifting, created, dissolved and reformed the contents of 'local', congealing different elements at different moments, allowing even the recent incomer, at one point in the conversation, to establish himself as a local (with reference to the pub). However, he was soon to exclude himself, albeit inadvertently, when he remarked to the other men, 'the only difference between me and you is that I'm more mobile'. This assessment was evidently problematic for the Britannia men, and one retorted that, as a long-distance lorry driver, he had travelled extensively and, if nothing else, was 'extremely mobile'. The other remarked that although he always came back to Rossendale, he had been 'everywhere' with the army. The incomer elaborated by noting his ability, if he chose, to move out of Bacup and live elsewhere. To the Britannia men, this was clear evidence he was *not*, indeed, a local and, in fact, did not even 'belong' to the pub. How could he be a local if he had neither prior nor future ties to Britannia, Bacup, or the pub? This was confirmed later in the conversation when he told them he came, from the south of England.

LOCAL: As business people, *you* come in, buy a house and when you sell it you make a killing. That's the difference—I'll be in a house until a die.

INCOMER: I see a house as an investment . . . I am quite happy to live in the same house for four years. The difference between locals and m'self is that I would live anywhere in the world as long as my lot was better.

ANTHROPOLOGIST: How do you mean, lot?

INCOMER: Standard of living.

LOCAL: It's not the standard of living but the quality of life that is important . . . Could you live down south?

INCOMER: I come from there.

LOCAL: *You're* not a local then.

Earlier in our conversation the incomer and locals had agreed that mobility was a good thing, now the Britannia men cut links between mobility and what they called 'the quality of life'. In bringing to mind 'the quality of life' they privileged it above the acquisition of money. A 'standard of living' was screened out in favour of an experience of living and there were more important things to life than material goods. But what are they? To bring to mind 'quality of life' is to trace connections to a different set of social actors. The incomer, while connected to money, is seen to be unconnected to a place (to a house or a town), and mobility curtails attachments to persons and pasts.[17]

Pushing the notion of local further, all the men, including the landlord, agreed that a particular corner of the pub is where the 'real locals' sat—a category from which they excluded themselves. The 'real local', in this context, embraces a number of defining qualities, none of which the men in the bar applied to themselves (except the fact that they are men). The 'real local', from this perspective, is male, elderly, and a former mill-worker, he has a broad dialect, may wear a cloth cap, and has not travelled far. The clustering of these characteristics connotes fixity—unchangingness and immobility. As the recent immigrant distanced himself from Bacup in terms of being more mobile, while at the same time locating himself firmly in Bacup in terms of being a local in the pub, so the Britannia men differentiated themselves from those they designated the real locals also in terms of mobility, while at the same time fixing themselves firmly, as locals, in Britannia and the pub.

Later in our conversation the incomer made a suggestion about what Bacup needs:

INCOMER: Bacup needs an influx of wealth. [There's a need to] persuade government to put money in villages and towns. It's the poor and people with lack of opportunities that cause trouble.

LOCAL: We don't want government in here; we want to keep it as a village.

The incomer associates Bacup with poverty and lack of opportunity, which in turn he connects to 'trouble'. In response, one of the locals associates 'the village' with autonomy and contrasts it, albeit implicitly, with the city, characterized by dependency particularly on bureaucratic and state intervention. I want to dwell for a moment on the notion that villagers are more self-reliant and resourceful than town or city dwellers.

I am reminded of the many conversations I had with Mr Charles Hardcastle. He was one of eight children, all of whom were Bacup born and bred. He told me frequently, and in different ways, that 'there are no poor today—not like there used to be'. In his opinion welfare benefits, particularly rent rebates, had eliminated poverty as it was. However, despite there being less poverty, he thought the quality of social relationships had deteriorated massively. He used to tell me that although Bacup had always been 'rough'—which he associated (as did the recent incomer cited above) with poverty, but (unlike the recent

[17] Furthermore, the Britannia men suggested it is exploitative to make money from Bacup houses when they do not belong to you: paying a mortgage, in this context, is not a sufficient criterion for ownership.

incomer) hinted that roughness in itself was no bad thing—the level of violence had increased. Mr Hardcastle and many of his compatriots suggested that autonomy and independence breed self-reliance.

The men in the Britannia pub suggested that city dwellers were more likely to rely on intervention from the state and from bureaucratic institutions than those who lived in villages. What is it about villages, then, that allows their members to get along fine without state intervention? What is it about the village that ensures its residents are cared for? We can only begin to address these questions if we go beyond seeing the village as a place (as entity). It is made up of social relationships, and what are perceived to be specific kinds of social relationships. Defining localities as villages or cities, or as urban or rural, draws on ideas about types of relationship. The village is characterized by a preponderance of mutually supportive (close) social ties—'everybody knows each other', while the city is characterized by a plethora of single-stranded, utilitarian, and anonymous relationships. Cities are stereotypically filled with cold, distant, and anonymous relationships, and villages with warm, close, and familiar ones. But while such stereotypes act to differentiate cities and villages as different kinds of place, they rely on their juxtaposition. Hence, the village connotes a locality where dense, multiplex relationships prevail, precisely because the city is cold and anonymous. Meanwhile, the city connotes a locality where simplex relationships dominate and where ties are transitory, precisely because the village has history, tradition, and depth in its ties. Bacup is both urban *and* rural: it is also neither. It is neither one nor the other, but both. It is a hybrid. Hence new residents are able to evoke the charm of a rural idyll, while seasoned residents dwell on its hard-working industrial nature. Both incomers and those who define themselves as Bacup born and bred draw on notions of town and country, and city and village, and they mobilize them not only to define Bacup, but also those places with which they are familiar. Such understandings and evaluations are familiar from the domain of kinship.

Recent and established immigrants agree that Bacup is friendly. Thinking of the past, Bacup people point out it is not as friendly as it used to be. However, when talking about the relationship between Bacup and nearby towns, all agree that it is more friendly than surrounding localities. Bernard Whittacker, whom I met at a meeting in the Baptist church, told me he commutes to work 'outside the Valley'. He is a teacher. When I visited him and his wife and young child at home, he told me his colleagues constantly 'call'[18] Bacup, asking him 'all the time' how on earth he can survive there. He tells them that Bacup people are 'the friendliest' he has ever met. He tells me the same, and reassures me that only a few 'rough 'uns' give Bacup a bad name. This is a theme which frequently comes up and one which I address in the next chapter.

[18] See n. 16.

Making Houses into Homes

Houses are not just entities; they are made through work into homes and the kind of home one creates is a reflection on the kind of person one might be. I met Mr Leary, Joanne's father, as a customer in his shop. After we carried out our transaction, I mentioned that I knew Joanne. He remembered he had heard something about me, and asked, 'but what *exactly* are you doing?' I did not get very far in trying to explain what I was doing before he intervened: 'There are different kinds of people in Bacup. Basically, there are ordinary folk and nutters.' He said I definitely ought to interview him, as he knew Bacup better than most. I agreed that this was a very good idea and we arranged a time and place. The next time we met he told me how he came to know Bacup so well. He also told me about houses.

When Donald Leary first got married he was buying a small terraced house from his wife's brother, and paying for it weekly as if it were rent. The council placed a compulsory purchase order on the property in order to widen the road and they were obliged to rehouse him and his family which was at the time 'growing by the year'. They moved into a council house on Mount Pleasant, and now they have been there seventeen years. Mr Leary is keen to buy the house from the council. There are, he argues, good financial reasons for doing so. First, after being a council tenant for twenty-three years he is eligible for a discount, which makes the house 'a bargain', and second as rents are increasing each year, a mortgage may eventually turn out to be less costly than paying rent. There is, however, a further reason for buying the property. In Mr Leary's words: 'A house is what—I'd consider—what somebody else owns and you're paying rent. But a home suggests something you own yourself—a nice comfortable little driveway, trees planted up and down, and its your own. . . . It gives you the heart to do repairs et cetera on it . . . You are independent, not restricted. The council can't say do this, do that, can't keep hens, et cetera.'

For Mr Leary, a home means autonomy—not being told what to do by landlords or neighbours. You can never really be at home in somebody else's house. A house might refer to an entity—to bricks and mortar—to the place in which a home is created, but homes require relations—relations between households as much as within. In the words of Barbara Jones: 'A house can be anybody's. It's the people that live in it that make it a home. It's not the things you have in it but how you treat people that come in to your home to make them feel welcome, and that sort of thing.' A home emerges from appropriate relations of hospitality. It is the way in which you behave towards those who enter your house that reflects your stature rather than the objects it contains. Effort needs to be put into homes and both material and non-material contents need to be organized. It is mostly women who are assessed in terms of their ability to create homes, and status is derived and allocated according to standards of housework and childcare (manifest, for example, in the ways in which children are dressed) but also in the management of social relationships. I was told, in a conversation with two Bacup women, that a neighbour of theirs had completely 'pulled the wool' over the eyes of social services after she had been accused of leaving her children alone at night. The two women were convinced that the children *were* being neglected (they were always 'playing out') but because the house was so clean and tidy ('and wouldn't you expect it to be if the children can't play in it') the social worker was fooled. She was lulled into a false sense of security, thinking the outward display of order reflected an ordered and orderly set of relations. Service providers in this example are gullible and credulous; not living in the neighbourhoods in which they work, they do not *know* Bacup, nor do they *know* Bacup families. They are criticized in terms of being unable to discern the subtle nuances which Bacup people are adept at seeing.

A contrast is often made between homes which, while not necessarily tidy, are friendly and welcoming, and those which are 'immaculate' but lack warmth and hospitality. One woman in her early fifties told me her brother-in-law (her husband's brother) admits to feeling envious of what he calls the 'homely atmosphere' of her house: he thinks her house is 'more of a home' and 'more lived in' than his own. His wife, she tells me, is 'prim and proper' and is obsessed with housework. But of course what is deemed an obsession in one context is a strength in another, and there are no end of possibilities for drawing on 'dirty houses' as evidence of unsociability and impropriety.

Ambiguity surrounds the notion of home: home is both the place where one lives and the place where one comes from. Just as child, in English kinship thinking, is both young person *and* offspring of parents, so a home is both an independent household and the place where one was raised. A home is both the dwelling where one lives presently and the place where the relationships from which one is made are located. Home is chunky: it is packed with the social relations by which it is constituted and is constitutive of. It is both the edifice that houses kinship and the arena in which it is formed. As the child is thought to contain the substance of its parents, so ties to home are not necessarily broken when one leaves it. Home can be where your parents live now, enfolding enduring kinship ties, or where you now live and call your own.

Neighbouring

The swimming baths in Bacup were opened in 1893 and built with a donation of £5,000 from Henry Maden MP, a local millowner and benefactor. In the spring of 1988, admission was free to the public during weekday lunch hours.[19] The same swimmers regularly used the pool at these times, and we swam sedately

[19] At the time of editing this, Bacup swimming baths have been closed down. There was a vociferous campaign against the closure and Bacup friends sent me newspaper clippings. One woman informed me that 'the council' wouldn't be allowed to 'just do what they want', and another that they could expect a fight.

from one end to another, counting the number of lengths under our breath, and occasionally stopping at the shallow end to exchange greetings and pleasantries. Such lunch-hour swimming sessions provided a marked contrast to the noise and activity in the same swimming pool on Saturday afternoons to which I occasionally accompanied my son. I got to know several of the women who swam and in the changing rooms, at the end of the lunchtime swimming sessions, they would ask me about the progress of my work. One day a young woman whom I had not met before joined us. I was introduced to her as somebody who was writing about Bacup. She was introduced to me as Jade. She told me she had just returned to live in the town after having lived on the Fylde coast for the previous ten years and, since she had been away, Bacup had 'changed enormously': 'It's deader now: never was a lively place but less so now.' Much to the discomfort of one of the regular swimmers, Jade told me that returning to Bacup had been 'like going back in time'. It was when she described Bacup people as 'hillbillies' that our mutual acquaintance reminded her gently but firmly that she 'shouldn't say things like that'. The conversation continued on a more cautious note and Jade, before she left, described what it had been like living 'on the Fylde': 'There's a lot of Rossendalians living [there], links from the old millowners [who] used to have estates and holiday homes out there. They're all still nosey but they've lost the sense of community, the sense of helping each other when needed. Really, they've got the worst of both worlds.'

For Jade, neighbourliness and friendliness are inherent in 'the sense of community'; without them the community does not exist and with them nosiness is no bad thing. The same fine line between friendliness and nosiness was drawn by a woman from Hertfordshire who was visiting her daughter in Bacup. Her daughter had just given birth to her fourth child and she was staying for a while to look after the house and the children. I met her out shopping one day and she was pleased to stop in the street and chat. Bacup is quite different, she told me, from where she lives in the south of England: 'People stop and talk to you here. There's a certain amount of nosiness—but it's different . . . there's a genuine interest.'

Bereft and disengaged from mutual support, nosiness is unappealing. A fine line is drawn between friendliness and nosiness, but where the line is drawn depends not on relative and measurable amounts of nosiness and friendliness, but on where the drawer places her- or himself.

We have seen how Mr Spencer and Mr Whittacker were not only born in Bacup, but are said to come from original Bacup families. Mr Spencer went straight from school, at 14 years of age, into his father's grocery business, where he worked until retiring at 65. He recalled that his father's uncle used to live above the shop, which reminded him that Bacup had changed immeasurably: 'People may have more money today but they are not as happy. Neighbours used to look after you and you never needed to lock your door.'

Mrs Spencer agreed with her husband that Bacup folk are neighbourly, but hinted at the downside of neighbourliness. Her family, particularly her mother (Ch. 4) thought it an insult for someone to walk into your house without being invited and were shocked when they moved to Bacup and people walked straight in to the back kitchen, without even knocking. She thought Bacup people were very friendly, but also very nosy. 'In the city', she pointed out, 'you do not interest yourself in somebody else's business.' One woman, who had also lived in Bacup for the best part of half a century, put it this way: 'Bacup people don't live and let live—they're always minding other people's business.' And a young man, an incoming spouse, tempered his enthusiasm for the town and its people: 'Ninety-nine per cent of people are fantastic, friendly [*pause*]—verging on the nosy'. Verging but not quite.

Kate Murray has two small children and, at the time I met her, was estranged from their father. Iris Hill had recently moved in with Kate and was contributing towards the bills. After explaining I would find Bacup people 'cautious' about talking to me because I was not from the area, Kate told me: 'It's a small, tight-knit community . . . everybody hears about everything, and they tell every bugger else in Bacup!' Iris agrees: 'There's lots of gossip', as well as a large number of 'narrow-minded people': 'Bacup is very cliquey: the unemployed stick together, the middle class stick together, and then there is some in the middle, like Kate, who like to bother with all walks of life.'[20]

Iris told me she was adopted when she was a baby. She did not appear, in her comments, to be including herself as a Bacup person. Moreover, although she pointed out that Kate was born and bred in Bacup, she also excluded her from typically Bacupian characteristics. Iris thought of Kate as a person who did not 'fit in' to a narrowly defined class, and was consequently not constrained by the confines of a particular clique. Later in our conversation, Iris switched to another way of looking at what is still the interrelatedness of Bacup people. What she loved about the place, she said, is 'the people', because '*everybody* is so close'.

Being interested in the business of neighbours is either a strength or a weakness. Neighbouring is expressed as an intentional activity, and one not only 'does neighbouring' but there are different degrees to it. One of my neighbours, a resident of seventeen years, told me: 'I'm not one for neighbouring myself. Can't be doing with sitting in people's houses all day. But if you go down Bacup you can always stop and have a chat with someone.' Many women

[20] In this context, to 'bother' with somebody is to be friendly with them. It can be used generally, as here, where it suggests that Kate can 'get on' with all kinds of people, or more specifically with reference to sexual relationships (usually adulterous): e.g. a young woman described how her mother had been very unhappy in her marriage and had 'started botherin'' with someone else. However, to have or to be in 'bother' usually means to be in trouble or to have problems; hence a young woman told me she was having 'a bit of bother' with her youngest child, and another with her boyfriend.

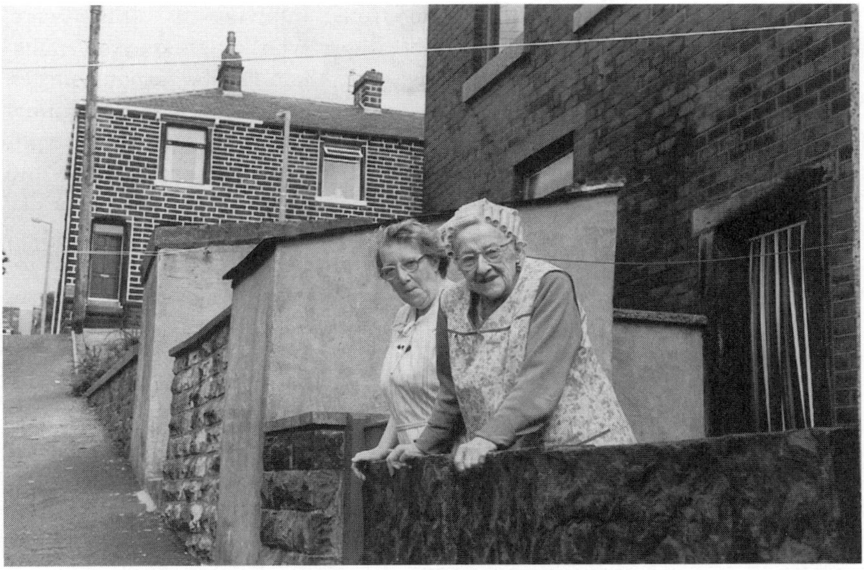

PLATE 10. Neighbours

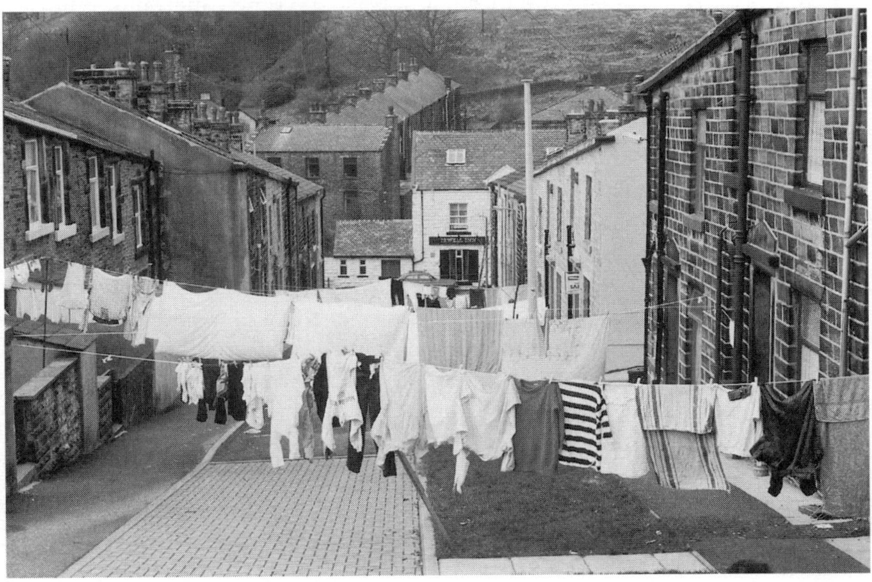

PLATE 11. Connecting neighbours: washing hanging across the street

told me they were not ones 'for neighbouring'; implying that others were. Neighbouring is morally loaded: there are those who 'neighbour too much' ('nosy') or who neighbour at the expense of their family responsibilities. Neighbouring is also a valued and valuable activity which entails sustaining more or less intimate social relationships. Mrs Sweeney was 'not one for neighbouring' herself, but observed that an older generation were better at it and the younger generation had lost the knack: '[I'm] not into neighbouring like mum's generation. Mother's generation they helped each other. The younger generation coming up today don't care less. Mother's generation would sit for a couple of hours; you'd see them at teatime coming out of each other's houses to get the tea ready. You don't see that today.'

It is not just that a balance has to be struck between not neighbouring enough and neighbouring too much, but rather that the concept of neighbouring is available as a symbolic resource and, as such, can be assessed differently according to the context in which it is rendered significant. Friendliness and nosiness are flip sides, as it were, of the same coin. Deployed for different purposes, they do not contradict one another even though they are contradictory. In conceptualizing categories of person who neighbour too much and others who neighbour too little, distance and closeness are achieved between the speaker (and people like us) and other Bacup residents (people not like us).

Lee Morris is in his late twenties. He was, at the time I met him, renovating a terraced house in the survey area. It emerged in our first meeting that I knew his cousin, Paula Seddon, and that I had also recently met and interviewed his mother who lived in the same street. He knew more about me than I about him. I asked Lee whether he thought there was a loyalty to particular neighbourhoods. He said, 'There are in these four rows, but its changing . . . The people who are now moving into the area do not speak to their neighbours—they're from Cheshire and Stockport and Bury—and they do not speak to each other like we do.' To illustrate what he meant, Lee described an incident from his childhood: from when he was a boy and living 'up the street' with his mother. He was playing the violin one evening in his bedroom. When he finished, the next-door neighbour poked her head around the door and informed him he had played a bit wrong and that if he brought the violin down she would show him how to play it properly. They ended up playing music together on the back street and neighbours came out to listen and, in the words of Lee, 'butties and brew were flying'.[21] Neighbouring, as a symbolic resource, is drawn upon to demarcate differences between types of Bacup person (as in my neighbour's example), between the past and the present (as in Mrs Sweeney's example), and also between Bacup and non-Bacup. In Lee's

[21] This is a wonderfully evocative expression, picturing a bevy of neighbours in adjacent houses hanging out of their back gates and making sandwiches and tea for each other.

narrative, neighbourliness (made manifest in the ability to intervene in neighbour's lives uninvited) with the reward of mutual aid and enjoyment in good company is a defining characteristic of Bacup.

Marilyn Greaves was born in Britannia—'Well Rossendale General, really'[22]—in the house next door to where she now lives. Mrs Greaves is in her fifties and has two married sons and four grandchildren. She says her husband is not a local lad and in fact he has little time for Bacup; if he had had his way, they would have moved to the 'family farm' outside the valley. Mr Greaves inherited the farm and has worked on it all his adult life. Mrs Greaves thinks her husband has never seen Bacup through the same eyes as she has: 'he only sees the bad tales'. She told me about the incomers who had, within the past five years, moved on to a new private housing estate near to where she lives.

> They're fitting in now. At first when they came—this is how I see them—like we've always been used to smiling and speaking to people, [but] they used to look at you like you was a bit funny, you know, speaking to strangers. But I think now they're fittin' in more, into our way of doing it. They come past here on their way to school—mostly Manchester people—now they'll smile and speak as they go past, whereas at first they used to look: 'what's she smiling at me for?' I seem to see a change in them.

For Mrs Greaves, the fact that recent immigrants have started to greet her and smile at her when they pass is a sign they are adapting to Bacup ways: 'they're becoming just like us'. Like Lee, she identifies friendliness and neighbourliness as true Bacup characteristics, and suggests that incomers, over time, will imbibe these traits.

Friendliness has no fixed form—it might entail the offer of a cup of tea, a kind word, or a joint. Friendliness can be made manifest in charity or conversation, but despite quite different forms of hospitality the value placed on reciprocity is shared. An image of the typically Bacupian character (friendly, mutually supportive, hospitable) is available and drawn upon by local and incomer alike. Neighbouring, as symbolic resource, is available to recent immigrants as it is to those who grew up in the town. And it is similarly used as a means of conceptualizing finely tuned differences between categories of person. One woman described herself as behaving in a more friendly manner than other incomers she knew. Other incomers, she pointed out, treat the town merely as a 'dormitory', whereas she actually 'lived' in Bacup.[23] Shades of incomerhood can be discerned in her commentary. She perceives herself, and not other incomers, as behaving in ways which resonate with Bacup. She differentiates herself from other incomers whom she accuses of ignoring the

[22] Again the ambiguity in birth (one is both born in a place and/or to kin) is exploited.

[23] The expression 'dormitory' (or dormitory town) is also intriguingly evocative. Dormitories suggest sleeping places and, juxtaposed with towns, they hint at the suspension of active, everyday, social relationships. A dormitory town comprises a population who only sleep in the town and fail to interact and, therefore, fail to create and sustain the kind of relations integral to community.

vernacular and neither forging nor sustaining Bacup relationships. In making this distinction, she formulates a category of incomer different to herself and in so doing composes herself as a 'proper' resident. While recent immigrants do not usually trace their ascendants to Bacup, or claim connection through being born there, they nevertheless place themselves in Bacup, and they make explicit their position in narratives which highlight, for example, the kind of relationships they forge (as neighbours and members of the community), or the permanency of their residence, or their commitment to the welfare of the town (exemplified in joining local organizations and joining in local campaigns against, for example, the closure of the swimming baths or the creation of a landfill site).

The social and economic changes which have occurred in Bacup throughout the twentieth century are portrayed through the survival or loss of certain Bacup qualities. Hence people are said not to neighbour like they used to, and doors can no longer be left unlocked. They are said to have lost their resourcefulness and their ability to cope in adversity and can no longer entertain themselves, but wait, passively, to be entertained. Recent immigrants say the same things about the places from which they came. They talk of Bacup as a safer, more neighbourly, and friendlier place than the cities and they admire what they perceive as the honest and hard-working character of its inhabitants. In turn, incomers may exhibit some, or all, of those same proper Bacup characteristics, in which case, knowledge of their origins is temporarily suspended. Lee, for example, made it clear that incomers could be assimilated into the community if they behaved in the same neighbourly manner as Bacup folk. He gave two examples as to how this might manifest itself: 'borrowing from each other' and 'leaving [the] back door open'. Such notions belie late twentieth-century experiences of urban life, but this is the point. Bacup is said to exert an influence—moulding the people who live in the place—and, while not born in the town, incomers can be socialized into its customs and expectations. Bacup grows persons. Neighbours do not come preformed and ready made, instead they are made into neighbours as much as they make themselves neighbourly. Neighbours present similar kinds of problem to those posed by the past and by kin. Who to select and who to leave out? How best to represent appropriate qualities of neighbouring? When is care interference, and concern nosiness? Neighbours can be too close (nosy) or too distant (uninterested); they can neighbour too much or too little—but however much they neighbour they are always good to think difference and similarity with.

6

The Same and Different

MANY residents of Bacup talk about it as an attractive and a desirable place to live. Recent immigrants come to retire or to bring up their children away from the city. They talk of the beauty of the moors and hint at a rural idyll. Such images are, however, belied by a landscape scarred and battered by successive generations of human activity. Surrounding the town, the land is dissected, seemingly haphazardly, by beautifully crafted drystone walls in varying degrees of disrepair. To the north, huge electricity pylons forge a straight and imposing pathway across hills with sides etched by quarries. It was local millstone grit that was used to build the town's dwellings, factories, and meeting places.[1] For me, there is something reassuring about this landscape; it is neither pretty nor cosy, but rugged and worn. It is peopled and used. Built, as it is, up the sides and on the floor of a valley, there is a view of hills from many Bacup houses. The combination of open moorland and a history of industry presents a contradiction put to work by residents.

Previous chapters have noted ways in which elements of the past are mobilized to exemplify the uniqueness of Bacup and to provide images of that which is distinctive about the place and its people. In the same way as the past is juxtaposed with the present, so place is juxtaposed with person, and analogies are constantly made across these different domains. Provinces of past, present, place, and persons are forever being connected up. This chapter also contains the past, and explores the way in which elements of it are selected in formulating a particular character said to be Bacupian. The notion of a Bacup character also has a wonderful ambiguity about it. It is both person and manner. Again there is a shift between entity and relationship, and each requires the other. I am interested in the way in which characteristics attributed to persons, both living and dead, tell us about present-day categorizations of immediate social worlds. In what follows, I try to preserve a sense of the way in which narratives about Bacup characters and characteristics emerge in conversation, and again I dwell on some of the autobiographical detail co-conversationalists select as relevant to the questions they ask and address.

[1] Out of sight, hidden in folds of the moorland, a landfill site has been initiated (and others predicted) to house, it is said, 'European' rubbish. A vocal and active group of residents is campaigning against the proposal.

A True Bacupian

> The character of the people is as marked as are the natural features of the Valley, pronounced, individual, blunt, sometimes even to rudeness. When once known, they are never forgotten, and are recognised the world over. Their dialect is peculiarly their own. They possess a two-edged wit and humour. It is said they love like angels and hate like devils. True as steel in their friendships, they are thrifty, but not mean, hard working and enterprising; quick to take advantage of any new thought and ready to pursue it to a successful conclusion. (Brearley n.d., cited in Bowden 1975: 88)

This description of a 'true Bacupian' was written by James Herbert Brearley (1874–1952) and is reproduced in *A Second Bacup Miscellany*. Brearley was a landowner and is reported to have built over 200 dwellings in Stacksteads and Bacup. He was one of the earliest Freemasons in the town, a founder-member of the Bacup Rotary club, Vice-President of the Golf Club and a member of the Nat. The quotation above is taken from an article he wrote entitled 'Random Reflections of a Bacup Historian', in which he briefly traces the history of the cotton industry in Bacup and the improvements made to the quality of life of its inhabitants by named individuals. He describes these people as the town's benefactors, 'pioneers who had vision'. It transpires they, also, are factory- and landowners, merchants, doctors, and politicians; what Nat members call 'the gentlemen of the town'. Writing of the development and growth of the Bacup Co-operative movement, Brearley notes it was 'started just over 100 years ago by working men who recognised the need for education to improve themselves' (Bowden 1975: 90). He goes on to pay a double-edged compliment to the success of its fourteen founder-members: 'Whether we agree with the principles of the movement or not, all honour must be given to these ordinary men who recognised the need for the improvement of the working class' (ibid.).

Brearley appears to be writing a history of the working classes in Bacup from a middle-class perspective, and it is not clear whether he claims or disowns the characteristics he describes as inherently Bacupian. In a different article published in *A Bacup Miscellany* (Bowden 1972), Brearley expresses the view that 'Bacupians' exhibit a 'suspicion of strangers' (whom they call 'foreigners') and are 'clannish even to stupidity'. Such a view of the clannishness of Bacup people finds its counterpart today in perspectives from outside Bacup which are equally found inside. They are also, as we have seen, part of the repertoire of those who define themselves as Bacup born and bred. Clannishness, like remoteness, can be brought very close to home and invoked to differentiate neighbouring streets as well as neighbouring towns.

Writing more recently, Benita Moore (1991: 4) describes her own interests and the people of Rossendale in the following way:

> I myself have lived at Rising Bridge on the outskirts of Rossendale for over twenty years, and have always been delighted with its beauty and Lancashire folklore. The

people of the Rossendale valley are a race unto themselves; hard-working, tough, parochial, zealously guarding their heritage and local traditions; yet I have never met with such kindness and humour.

Everywhere I went, people were always anxious to help and advise me, and their hospitality was truly Lancastrian.

Th'owd Characters

I called in to see my neighbour, Mrs Jones, one morning. Her daughter explained she was in bed 'feeling a bit under the weather'. She conveyed in those few words an assumption that, at 90 years of age, one was likely to have off days. Barbara was the younger of Mrs Jones's two daughters who were both born in Bacup during the depressed years of the 1930s.

Barbara's education was interrupted during her school years because her father often needed to move to different towns for work (a fact her mother now relates with a tinge of regret mingled with an edge of defiance—'that's just the way things were in them days'). The family settled back in Bacup when Barbara was a teenager, at which time she became increasingly involved with the Baptist church. Singing in the choir, teaching in the Sunday school, and actively fund-raising for overseas missionary endeavours meant Barbara had an active social life, despite her many household duties. Her first paid job was in Woolworth's as a sales assistant. She loved her work and through her conscientiousness and honesty eventually assumed a responsible position in running the store. Woolworth's was closed down suddenly in 1984. A decline in sales was the official reason given, although many Bacup people disbelieve this.[2] Barbara was made redundant and given only one week's notice after thirty years full employment. She had little prospect of finding another job and found unemployment very difficult to come to terms with. Now she wonders how she ever found time to work. Apart from looking after the house and her mother, she and her friend often take day-trips to places of interest in Lancashire, sometimes Yorkshire. She is an active member of the Ladies' Guild and the Baptist church. She no longer teaches in the Sunday school—a task she remembers as one of her most enjoyable undertakings—but is active in the Missionary Society and church fund-raising activities.

Barbara invited me in anyway and I took a look and made a comment on a massive, partly completed jigsaw on a card table in the front room. Jigsaws were one of Barbara's hobbies. Whenever I visited, I looked at the latest, which was usually more challenging than the last, and no matter how often or how long I looked I never seemed to find a piece that fitted into place. On this particular morning, Leonard Pickering, a lay preacher and minister of the Baptist church (and, I discovered, Mrs Hilary Hardcastle's younger brother) had also come to visit Mrs Jones. Much of his pastoral work, he told me, involved home

[2] The closure of Woolworth's is a significant event in the collective memory of Bacup. For many residents it marks the beginning of the deterioration of the town centre and, in particular, its shopping facilities.

visits to elderly parishioners, especially those who could no longer attend church.

Leonard was born in Bacup and had lived here all his life, apart from time spent in the army completing National Service.[3] When he returned to Bacup he worked in a shoe factory. His career in the church began, he thinks, when he used to counsel and listen to the problems of his colleagues in the factory. It was they who encouraged him to develop and use the skills he obviously had. When he joined the ministry he could have been posted to a church outside the area, and he considered himself very fortunate to have been granted the ministry in Bacup.

Our conversation, over tea and home-made cake, soon came around to Bacup's past. For my benefit, Barbara and Leonard compared memories of certain characters and events. Barbara spoke, again, of how 'whole families' came to Bacup in search of work because 'they couldn't make a living on the land'; they came from Lincolnshire (yellowbellies), Norfolk, and Cornwall, she told me. Leonard agreed and added that 'it was certainly a mixed up valley in them days'. They talked about the mills and millowners and Leonard is reminded of 'th'owd characters'

There was a lot of characters in those days. We've lost the characters now. [There's] bad characters today. Then, they were eccentric like Robert the Devil, Scotch Molly, and Alice from Wigan—she worked down the mines. We would call after them as kids but we'd respect them. Now, characters are more known for being hooligans; the old ones were eccentric, not bad. You used to see them down Bacup. Now everyone looks the same.

For Leonard, characterhood requires idiosyncrasy. He perceived there to be more of a uniformity in appearance today and when people are marked as characters it was because of their infamy—their bad deeds rather than their peculiarity. Barbara described how nicknames were given to people according to the things they did or the way they looked. Her mother's brother, for example, went to Paris and thereafter was called Paris Joe.[4] She agreed with Leonard that th'owd characters such as Ailse O'Fusser and Mad Ab were bizarre but not malicious. They were treated, and treated fellow townsfolk, with good manners.

They were called names but we still respected them. There was a fellow who used to walk up here and he'd be drunk as a mop and one time I saw him clinging to the bushes

[3] Throughout my fieldwork in Bacup, different members of the Baptist church remarked that Leonard was an excellent minister and he performed his pastoral duties with sensitivity and understanding. They often put this down to his knowledge of, and familiarity with, Bacup and its inhabitants; another example of a corollary between expertise and belonging.

[4] Ethnographers of Britain have focused on the use of nicknames both as markers of familiarity and as forms of abuse, jocular or otherwise. The old characters with such names as Ailse O'Fusser, Mad Ab, and Robert the Devil are familiar, and here nicknames act not only to individuate persons, but also to collectivize. 'Th'owd characters' represent a quirky, idiosyncratic Bacup and in telling of their exploits narrators provide evidence not only of knowing the place and its past, but also that they themselves are part of it.

all the way up the street, but if you walked past him he would touch his cap and say 'G'day to you ma'am'—polite—brought up like that, to be polite. Now, if you call people, it's in a nasty way like Phil the Thrill. It's not nice. You don't read things like that in a book.

The conversation continued and other characters were evoked. Characters such as Felix the Bobby[5] who gave the Pickering household a dog because they were getting their coal pinched. The dog has also become an established character. He was 'massive', Leonard told me, 'and would go into the baker's every day and pinch a 2lb loaf'. There is a suggestion in Leonard's comments that this behaviour would not be tolerated today, but of course it was unlikely to have been then. That, however, is not the point, as his clinching description of one man shows: 'There was a chap who used to keep live rats and for a drink would bite their heads off [*pause*], but he wouldn't beat up old ladies.'

The unsavoury and unsociable activities of this 'chap' have through time and telling been rendered safe. The significant thing is what he did not do—he did not 'beat up old ladies'—a quality that probably went unremarked when he was biting rats. Not all characters are suitable candidates for characterhood, and there are certain activities not considered as suitable items to be recorded and claimed as one's own history. For Leonard, biting heads off rats might not axiomatically exclude a person from characterhood, but violence towards the elderly would. And for Barbara sexual impropriety is not the basis of characterhood. The actions of Phil the Thrill (named thus because of his sexual proclivities) are not, for Barbara, suitable items for recording and identifying as 'belonging' to Bacup. Neither 'any old history' nor 'any old character' will do. A particular kind of history, like a particular kind of character—in these examples, peculiar but clean, polite and not violent (at least towards people)—best exemplifies Bacup.

Certain stories are repeated with humour and embellishment and, through their repetition over time, a pastiche of individuals and associated characteristics develops. The man with the rats, described above by Leonard Pickering, may be the same as the one mentioned in the following evocative description of a notorious felon (which belies the imputed harmlessness of all past characters), provided by a local historian.

His name was Robert Hame, but everyone knew him as Bury Bob, and he himself had forgotten his proper name. He had been guilty of every brutal crime in the calendar except murder. He was 34 years of age, he had been to prison 26 times, and had been dubbed a walking cutler's shop because of the number of pocket knives and penknives he had swallowed for wagers. He had also worried rats, wrecked public-house bars, mauled policemen. He was a terror. (Bowden 1982: 10)

[5] Bobby is English slang for a policeman. (Familiar form of Robert, from Sir Robert Peel, Home Secretary in 1828 when the Metropolitan Police Act was passed.)

This vignette has Bob from Bury swallowing knives and worrying rats. The story continues: in June 1882, Bob from Bury was converted to Christianity by a Methodist lay minister known as the Boy Preacher (himself a character in his own right). A pamphlet, 'Samuel Chadwick and Stacksteads', written by Kenneth Bowden, and sold on behalf of Stacksteads Methodist Church, begins:

> On a summery Saturday in the year of 1881, the 'boy preacher' of Burnley left his home in Junction Street and walked over the hill to begin a new chapter of his life in Bacup.
>
> His mother sent him on his way with the first kiss the lad could ever remember her giving him. He carried all his belongings in one tin box, and trudged the ten miles or so into Rossendale, finding his initial lodgings at the home of Mr and Mrs Thomas Disley and their young family at Fearns Bottom, Stacksteads, a cottage from which they later moved to Knott Hill House, opposite the entrance to Waterbarn Mill. (Ibid. 3)

The boy preacher's arrival in Bacup is described and he is anchored in Bacup in terms of houses, neighbourhoods, and a family before his work is explored.

Several photographs exist of a man known as Mad Ab.[6] One feature distinguishing Mad Ab as a character was his habit of clenching the lapel of his coat firmly in his teeth. He died in 1892. One explanation for his madness has it that on asking his 'lady friend' to marry him, he was turned down. This sad rejection caused a 'slight imbalance in his mental state'. Pam Watson told me how her teenage son and his friends use the expression 'Mad Ab' as a derogatory term of address or reference. She told me she had often heard the expression when she was a child, but always assumed it was a figure of speech, 'like mad as a Hatter'. It is only recently, she said, that she realized he had been a real person. Barbara and Leonard also told me about one of th'owd characters who used to sell oatcakes and always had a piece of rope between his teeth, but he was always, Barbara was quick to add, 'spotlessly clean'.

Ailse O'Fusser dressed like a labouring man and was imputed to have been as strong; she walked over the hills between Weir and Sharneyford transporting sacks of coal or lime. In her obituary in the *Rochdale Observer* she was described as a housewife, a description to which one local historian takes exception: 'although she has assumed larger than life proportions as a coal or lime carrier one thing she was *not* was a housewife' (Bowden 1982). Hence, while being a woman might not disqualify one from being an 'owd character', being a housewife does; characterhood requires nonconformity

[6] Photographs of Mad Ab can be found in *A Bacup Miscellany* (Bowden 1972) and *Bacup in Times Past* (BNHS 1987); an framed, enlarged copy of his photograph also hangs on the wall of a Bacup public house.

(within limits).[7] Leonard and Barbara ascribed similarly distinctive characteristics to a woman they called Alice from Wigan. Different names for the same person? Two different people? Does it matter? Over time, and through their repetition, contradictions emerge and questions such as these come to engage the attention of local historians whose interest is in sifting fact from fiction.

Characterhood draws on a pool of 'proper' characteristics which include strength, cleanliness, and respect. All in all, they are the same characteristics inherent in the perception of what constitutes 'decent and ordinary folk' from a contemporary Bacup perspective. Snatches of events, people, and places are handed down as established folklore and become the facts of history. Cohen writes of how Whalsay islanders continually express their knowledge of the past: of previous inhabitants, of how things were done and, importantly, how things were said. 'My subject has . . . been the pervasive presence of the past, its compulsiveness: it is the past as cultural resource rather than as ideological and rhetorical instrument, a resource which contributes to people's awareness of their difference and, thus, of the community boundary' (Cohen 1987: 133).

For Cohen, stories about the past 'act as an implicit statement about the community as a whole . . . suggesting its shared, quirky wistfulness and eccentricity' (ibid. 196). Th'owd characters of Bacup also act as a 'mnemonic of collectivity' (ibid. 195): familiarity with them and the ability to tell of their foibles, preferably with humour, express publicly an inclusive knowledge. And as in Whalsay, individuals are allocated idiosyncratic personae and stories recounted about their lives and their actions which act as a vehicle for the public presentation of intimate knowledge. But there is no *one* Bacup community. And stories about th'owd characters do more than create and maintain a boundary between Bacup and non-Bacup. Narratives which include th'owd characters are firmly grounded in the present and they image present-day social categories within Bacup as much as marking difference between Bacup and non-Bacup. Differentiation which has contemporary significance is brought to the fore, and the internal, present-day social divisions are of as much contemporary significance as is any awareness of 'the community as a whole'. Alongside the appearance and activities of th'owd characters, the linguistic skills of raconteurs are applied to humorous anecdotes which tell of contemporary events and living characters. Hence Phil the Thrill, or the Heinz 57 lot (see below), or named individuals, said to be *troublemakers* or *headbangers*, feature as large in Bacup conversations as do th'owd characters. Events assume no less a

[7] A story was told at a meeting of the Nat one week which provoked much laughter. It was about another character called Robert the Devil. Apparently he was extremely strong and for a living would carry loads on his back. One day he carried a heavy machine all the way up to Britannia. There was nobody at the place where it was to be delivered, so he carried it all the way back again.

mythical quality for having occurred last week as opposed to last century, and certain individuals assume no less a larger-than-life character for being alive rather then dead. Past characters are evoked to underscore the uniqueness of Bacup and to emphasize the distinctiveness of Bacup people: their strength, decency, and humour. At the same time, the quirkiness of th'owd characters sets them apart from their animators. Similar qualities are also attributed to contemporary characters, now with the possibility of subverting the value attached to them. So again speakers can also, if the occasion demands, dissociate themselves from such characters and characteristics.

A Troublesome Place

The expedience of moving to Bacup as a stranger and requiring assistance inevitably generated talk. One theme which repeatedly emerged in early conversations was the relationship between Bacup and trouble. The topic was broached in various ways but always came back to the notion that Bacup is 'bad news'. The electrician, who lived elsewhere in the Rossendale Valley, told me emphatically and with certainty: 'There's *always* trouble in Bacup.' And the carpet fitter, who *used* to live in the town but moved away several years ago, informed me, with feeling, that he would *never* live in Bacup again. In his words: 'It's a hole that wants blowing off the face of the earth,' and it had, he went on bitterly, caused him 'nothing but trouble'. An employee of the Gas Board who had never lived in Bacup, 'and never would', drew on the suspected gas leak he had come to investigate as evidence of the problematic nature of Bacup. In a voice of vindication, he suggested the leak (and by extension many other problems) was 'typical of Bacup!' Such observations were made by people who expected to have no further contact with me and they all suggested, in their own way, that I had made a terrible mistake in coming to live there.

Bacup residents themselves were more circumspect in their warnings and more selective in identifying and locating trouble, but they nevertheless pointed to it as a significant feature of the town. I was advised frequently to be careful with whom I got 'involved'. In the words of a neighbour: 'You'll like it here, as long as you mix with the right people. Just be careful who you get on with.' David Irving, a local builder who was working on the house, confided with an air of collusion: 'For its size, Bacup's a troublesome little town.' He continued, more loudly and with a different timbre to his voice: 'I doubt whether you'll last out the winter anyway,' given, he explained, just how much worse the weather is in Bacup (compared to places such as Manchester). David's work partner, Alan Gray, asked me repeatedly who had 'sent' me. The significance of the question, at the time, passed me by. Both he and David had settled on a mode of jocular banter early on in their interactions with me, and I thought he was merely teasing me about working for the Department of

Social Security or the Inland Revenue (just as I thought they were exaggerating the level of violence in the town). But, as in all good banter, barbed and pertinent social comments were smuggled in under the guise of flippancy. While I am convinced they realized quite soon that I had not been 'sent' by some state organization to collect incriminating information about the 'troublesome' Bacup folk, they carried on relentlessly with this line of questioning, and they did so partly to underline social differences they perceived to divide us. I was being placed, albeit temporarily, in the camp of 'the establishment'; a place which explained my interest in the affairs of Bacup and its people.

The present-day troubles of Bacup are said by some people to have stemmed from the open-door policy pursued by the local authority in the 1960s. Within Bacup today the source of trouble is, more often than not, located on Mount Pleasant. It is there that residents of other Bacup neighbourhoods and surrounding towns and villages, as well as housing, health, and social service workers locate *troublemakers*. In turn, residents of Mount Pleasant themselves identify specific areas, particular streets, or certain families as 'rough'. They draw on their knowledge of Mount Pleasant as residents and neighbours, or on their experience of growing up in the area, to make finer differentiations between neighbourhoods, streets, families, and types of person. They also, like recent incomers, point to areas outside Bacup as infinitely rougher than Mount Pleasant. Residents of Mount Pleasant qualify the association they make between the estate and trouble, and point out that it is only a minority of troublemakers who give the estate its bad name. In this they acknowledge that Mount Pleasant has a bad name, but in identifying the source of it they isolate trouble and divorce themselves from it. They are not responsible for the poor reputation of the estate, and furthermore the whole estate has been tarred by the same brush by those who obviously do not know it. Residents in other neighbourhoods of Bacup are often, however, far less discerning in their generalizations about the association of Mount Pleasant and trouble. They talk of Mount Pleasant and trouble in the same breath and either one triggers an association with the other. The analogy between Mount Pleasant as a whole and trouble generally is made from an outside (unconnected) perspective. Bacup residents who make the analogy trace their own connections to other neighbourhoods and to other types of houses. Both from inside and outside, Mount Pleasant can stand for Bacup: narrating links between Bacup and Mount Pleasant and by extension between Bacup and trouble, acts to exclude, and every act of exclusion is one of inclusion.

Punk Rockers

One afternoon, in the summer of 1988, I went to visit Laura Gray. Her friend, Joanne Leary, was there, and we drank white wine and Laura played us the latest Whitney Houston album. The music was loud, the windows were open and the children were at school. I asked them what Bacup was like today and Laura said she would tell me, but warned me to remind her when it was quarter past three as she had to go and pick up 'the kids' from school. I asked if I could go with her. She said 'of course you can' and we settled with two hours ahead of us.

Joanne and Laura began telling me about 'Bacup today' by remarking that 'the kids look older today' and consequently they get served in pubs at a younger age than they did. Apart from the fact her father 'would have killed her' if he had seen her in a pub drinking when under age, Joanne reckoned that she and her mates had a much better time just 'dossin'':[8] 'You can see the changes in the girls. They're not like we were [*pause*] they're more fashionable. I don't think they have half as good a time as we did though.'

Joanne was born in 1966 and Laura in 1967 and they started 'hanging around' together at the Meadows Secondary School. The only thing Joanne remembers liking at school was PE.[9] She and Laura were in the netball team together and Laura recalls their school had such a bad reputation they had to play all their games away because no school team in the league would come to the Meadows to play. They remembered how much fun they had between the ages of 13 and 16. 'There were rakes of us', Laura said, 'probably about twenty, sometimes more, and we'd all doss around on the Bonks.' The Bonks,[10] they explain, is the grassy bank sloping up from the main Rawtenstall to Todmorden Road, where Plantation Back used to stand. They used to send older youths for bottles of cider and went through a phase of sniffing butane gas. This phase was short-lived. A friend of theirs, a young lad, 13 years old, died. 'That used to be the local thing, didn't it—gas? Until he died and then, nobody, like . . .' Joanne trailed off sadly. A thoughtful silence, then she added bitterly: 'The shopkeepers who sold the gas knew what was going on.'

Laura continued: 'We didn't just drink though we used to play games like Greyhounds and Rabbits, Go and Find Them, and different chase games, and we'd sit there singing.' Laura and Joanne described how they would all sit on the Bonks singing country-and-western songs loudly. Laura explained the incongruous choice of music: 'Because me mum used to be into it, her dad is (pointing to Joanne), and Helen's dad is.' Helen, Joanne explained, is her cousin—'Helen's dad is my dad's brother.' 'So we'd sit there', Laura continues, 'dressed as punk rockers, singing country-and-westerns really loud.' I asked them what a punk rocker is. They looked at me with a trace of pity—a 'you've-never-lived' look.[11] Being punk, they told me, meant wearing a leather jacket, jeans, monkey boots, and loads of eye make-up. Lots of people thought they were rough—'we used to be right cheeky', admitted Joanne. Laura told of how they used to 'thumb it to Rawtenstall', have their photographs taken in the booths, and 'pull

[8] In Britain the legal age at which alcohol can be bought and consumed in a public house is 18.

[9] Physical Education.

[10] To bonk means to have sex (slang).

[11] Mrs Jones gave me the same look when I asked her what whist was. Although couched as a question, her response (when I told her I had never played whist) was a statement of fact: 'You've never lived, have you?'

people up in the street and say "I've lost me bus fare, can you lend me 20p?"' The only rivalry or conflict they remembered from that time was between 'the Bacup lot' and 'the Stacksteads lot'. 'We didn't used to like Stacky', explained Laura, 'but there was never any trouble'. 'Some kids would go home and watch Coronation Street and do their homework,' says Joanne, and although they would get oined[12] a little, they were generally left alone.

Not being exactly the same age meant they were not in the same class at school and were not always together. They also had different sets of friends. Laura used to hang about with 'the Weir lot' who, she says, 'have turned out to be hippies'. She has little in common with them now. She thinks they're scruffy, and 'there's really no need for it'. She names one lad who used to be 'right good looking and tidy' but has now, in her opinion, 'let himself go'. Joanne used to spend a lot of time up on the fields at the back of Mount Pleasant with her cousins, one of whom had a motorbike. Joanne and Laura's 'lot' are no longer punk rockers and most of them are now married and have children. Joanne said, 'they've all grown up now'. After some thought, she added: 'but we haven't changed *that* much, have we? We still like going out and having a drink . . . I haven't really settled. I still like to go out and enjoy myself.'

Joanne and Laura both left school at 16. Laura went to work in a shoe factory, and she hated it, but managed to 'stick it out' for twelve months. Joanne went on a Youth Training Scheme (YTS). During the twelve months of the scheme she had a variety of jobs but there was no 'proper' work available at the end of the training. Initially she was sent to look after children in a nursery which she describes, without enthusiasm and with a look of disdain, as 'all right'. The part of the scheme she enjoyed most, however, was working as a gardener in the public parks. As well as being outdoors all the time, this job meant she was able to travel around Rossendale. She also spent some time painting and decorating in 'old folk's homes' and did some bricklaying and plastering. The year they left school was also the year they both 'started courting'. They did not see much of each other then. They became pregnant round about the same time and both had sons who are also friends and who started the same school together on the same day. Laura had a second child, a daughter, just after she moved to her present house. Talking of the future, both Joanne and Laura wanted a different life from their own for their children. Laura did not want hers to grow up in the same way she did. She wanted to see them 'get out and get on'. Joanne, although she thinks the future might be bleak, did not necessarily want her son to leave Bacup but she hoped 'he'll have the sense to do something with his life'.

Joanne and Laura were punk rockers when they were younger. Punks were different from hippies, and different from those kids who watched Coronation Street and did their homework ('straight'). As well as there being a difference between punks, hippies, and homeworkers, the neighbourhood in which you lived also provided a means to differentiate between different categories of 'kid'. Hence, Joanne and Laura were axiomatically members of the 'Bacup lot' who were at odds with the 'Stacksteads lot' who sometimes hung around with

[12] Oined means worried. To oin somebody is to bother or to aggravate them.

the 'Weir lot' (here satellite villages are separate places on a par with Bacup). Laura used to be friends with the kids from Weir—'the Weir lot'—who turned into hippies. Joanne and Laura are no longer punks, nor are they hippies or, indeed, completely straight. They are married with children; they care for houses and families and would like to have paid work which fits in with their family obligations, but they do not perceive themselves, nor do they want to be perceived, as completely settled; as immobile or fixed. They still like going out and enjoying themselves and, in this sense, have hardly changed at all. So while now they might watch Coronation Street, and tackle housework and childcare with commitment and energy, they know these things do not represent, nor should they be represented as, the sum total of their social identities.

The Trouble with Talk

In order to tell me about Bacup today, Laura and Joanne situated themselves in the town. They presented what they perceived to be appropriate autobiographical detail of their growing up in Bacup to establish the authority from which they spoke and create the context within which their views were relevant. While Bacup had changed and the young did not have as much fun as they did when younger, they emphasized the fact that, despite outward appearances, which include homes, marriages, and children, they remain 'deep down' the same people. Their upbringing and childhood experiences had been formative and were constitutive of their present identities. Childhood experiences (being bred) had inculcated appropriate Bacup characteristics, including consistency, idiosyncrasy, resilience, and humour. I returned half-way through our conversation to my original question:

JEANETTE: What's Bacup like today?

JOANNE: It's a big hassle, to tell you the truth.

JEANETTE: In what way, Joanne?

JOANNE: It's the people; they get on me nerves half of them.

LAURA: It's not as . . . not as friendly.

JOANNE: Two-faced town.

LAURA: Can't do nowt, like everybody knows.

JEANETTE: Is this like—Bacup people?

LAURA: No this is the social [*pause*] the social side—the pub side.

JOANNE: Yeah but it's Bacup people as well, isn't it? You know what I mean? You've only got to do something and it's all round Bacup, over-exaggerated about fifteen times.

JEANETTE: Why do you think that is?

JOANNE: People like to tell tales. They like to *hear* about it as well, don't they?

LAURA: People like to see other people's [*pause*] you know, downfall. They like to see other people fall flat on their face, really, don't they? Nobody likes to see anybody get on.

JOANNE: They love trouble, don't they?

LAURA: Yeah they love trouble. They love it if there's been fighting at the weekend—it's something to talk about all week.

Trouble might fuel talk, but talk is equally as troublesome as fighting. Laura appears initially to be referring only to those Bacup people who go to pubs, but Joanne wants to extend it to a broader category of Bacup person. Joanne, whose cousins are known for being fighters, includes a wider constituency as problematic. From this perspective, Bacup people gossip, 'tell tales' and 'over-exaggerate' and this love of hearing about trouble is as much if not more troublesome than fighting. The Janus-faced nature of Bacup is displayed in the gossip of residents who are fickle—who smile and let on, but talk about you behind your back.

JOANNE: If you're nice, like, they don't like you, do they? Look at Jennie. Not so many people like her.

JEANETTE: Why?

JOANNE: She's just nice. Looks right well and that for her age. She's always going on holiday and that.

LAURA: She goes on the beer all day and that, and you can have a right good crack with her, yet people call her an old cow.

JOANNE: And she's not—she's far from one.

LAURA: She's not. She's right nice, looks right well for her age [*pause*] and other people of the same age—women of same age—call her.

Trouble is not only made manifest in fighting but also in envy. In the frame that Joanne and Laura present, Bacup people begrudge the good fortune of others. The experience of Jennie is evidence of this: criticism of her is provoked by jealousy. Jennie looks young for her age, she frequently goes on holiday, she enjoys herself, and these are cause enough for other women of the same age to be envious. They call her 'an old cow', Laura tells us, a derogatory label suggestive of sexual promiscuity. Laura and Joanne know she is not. They also know fighting might be confined to an 'insider lot' (pub-goers) but trouble is more widespread and caused by a wider category of protagonists (Bacup people) through their propensity to gossip and exaggerate minor incidents. For Joanne, Bacup is all right but 'it's the people' who get on her nerves. 'The people'—an idiom which emerges frequently as a means of differentiating oneself from others who from a different perspective might belong to the same social category. For example, 'it's the people' who are said to give the town a bad name, and 'it's the people' who do not support local things. In each case, a conceptual distance is created between the speaker and 'the people'. Describing Bacup as a 'two-faced town', Joanne dissociates herself from 'typical Bacup people' who from this perspective 'love trouble'.

Anna Brody, Laura's sister, lived on Mount Pleasant with her partner and three children. She called in on Laura one day while I was there. 'Still here?', she asked, not unfriendly, a slight irony in her voice (she meant Bacup, I think, not Laura's kitchen). She told me 'growing up in Bacup' prepared a person for life. It helped form, she said, an independent and resilient person. In her words, 'Bacup is full of anarchists. It's an education growing up in Bacup. If you can survive here then you can survive anywhere.' Anna, in her late twenties, made no explicit claim on the industrial past of Bacup, she did not talk about the mills, or back-to-backs, or th'owd characters, but she attached to Bacup and its people the same characteristics as those who did. A harsh environment, in terms of climate, industry, and poverty, was said to have moulded a particular Bacup character renowned for its strength and resilience, and so too for Anna. For her, it was the experience of growing up in Bacup, dealing with certain hostilities, and having to fend for oneself which developed particular Bacup traits, and these were characteristics she deemed an asset in a contemporary world which required skills of survival. These were also skills she knew herself to possess. With pride, she described Bacup people as 'anarchists'. She admired their propensity to eschew subservience—to fly in the face of the establishment. In the words of another interlocutor, Bacup people were 'far from soft—they know how to look after themselves'.

I noted the statement made by David Irving that I probably 'wouldn't last out the winter'. This theme was repeated, over the autumn, by other Bacup residents. There *are* physical factors influencing why Bacup should be blessed with more rain than surrounding towns, and a drop in temperature *is* noticeable when you arrive in Bacup from the lower plains of Manchester or Burnley, but it is also clear that these comments convey meaning over and above (and less than) the particularities of geography and climate. Doubt expressed about my constitution (as a city person) underscores the ruggedness of Bacup and its people. The weather is a hook on which to hang evidence of the distinctiveness and hardiness of the Bacup character.[13] It is not only that incomers (like myself) are 'softer' than Bacup folk, but also that we will not wish to persevere with harsh conditions; we will neither like Bacup enough, nor be sufficiently attached, to stick it out. The weather, of course, is a favourite topic of conversation of most residents, and recent immigrants also put the weather to work in distinguishing Bacup from the urban localities they left behind. Perhaps they remark on the beauty of the moors when covered in snow, and 'the community spirit' engendered when the town is snowed in. The weather is drawn upon selectively to affirm and legitimate their move to Bacup.

[13] Judith Ennew notes that Western Islanders say newcomers leave the islands because they cannot adapt to the climate: 'The locals blame the bad weather hinting at their own native superiority in being able to withstand the hardship' (Ennew 1980: 117). The weather, while said to be a favourite topic of conversation amongst the British, is of inordinate interest the world over. Apart from its direct influence on forms and means of subsistence, as a massively visual and tactile phenomenon it symbolizes all kinds of relationship, not only between persons and places, but also, of course, between persons and gods.

The Heinz 57 Lot

Laura and I went out one evening. She decided she would show me 'all the pubs in Bacup' and we managed to get through quite a few. We visited several pubs near the centre of town on each of the radial roads. Most are probably included in a local homily which has it that there used to be so many pubs in Bacup that if you threw a penny from the centre of town in any direction it would land on the doorstep of one. With an astute social eye, Laura described what she called 'the type of people' who drank in each of the pubs. The Crimean is where most of the 'ordinary folk' go, and this is where we were to end up for 'last orders'. 'Ordinary folk', from this perspective, are 'the lads' who play football (such as her husband) and their wives and girlfriends. Mostly between 18 and 30 years of age, they like to sit in the back room where the juke-box plays, and play pool in the games room. Elderly regulars (locals) and visitors usually sit in the lounge, and although single people might call in at the Crimean for a drink it tends not to attract the trouble-makers. Laura said the lads who drank in the Crimean had been nicknamed the 'Heinz 57 lot'. This nickname stemmed from a 'spot of trouble' a few months before. One of them had been obliged to go and fight a young man at the Victoria (another town-centre pub). The lad in question turned up at the Victoria with several of his Crimean drinking friends. This provoked the remark from one of 'the Victoria lot' that it was 'the Heinz 57 variety' who had come to fight. The comment suggested that not only are 'the Crimean lot' a motley crew, but also, despite their bravado, they could only come and fight in numbers.

Laura took me to the Kings Head, and then the Albert. We went on to the Garden, which had recently been refurbished, and was where, she explained, 'the trendies' drank. Trendies dress up in fashionable clothes, they are a younger crowd, 'they like teeny bopper music and they can't hold their drink'. We went on to the Victoria which Laura explained is 'full of headbangers'. This is the last place in Bacup were people barred from other licensed premises can still get served, and it is renowned for 'trouble'. Several people told me how a succession of licensees had been harassed by troublemakers and each, in turn, had been forced to leave. The result was that the pub was closed for periods of time in between landlords. During my stay in Bacup, it also suffered more than any other pub from periodic bouts of window smashing which occurred after closing time (usually in the early hours of Saturday morning). One young man told me that the window smashing sprees were usually an act of revenge against licensees who had refused to serve certain individuals. On our tour, Laura described the Victoria as 'the worst' and 'roughest' pub in Bacup. This was a view also expressed by Peter Miller who regularly drank in the Crimean. He told me he had stopped going to the Victoria after he had seen one of 'the headbangers' in there with a baseball bat under his coat. The names of Bacup public houses, like the names of 'real' Bacup people or of neighbourhoods, are far from inert. They carry with them persons, and evoke particular collectivities with their own kinds of identities and social relationships.[14] Laura and I ended up, that night, in Horace's.

Horace's is a nightclub (some call it a discotheque—but, by the late 1980s, the term 'discotheque' was losing its chicness). It is licensed and serves alcohol until 2 a.m. In 1988 the entrance charge was £5 and most people agreed this was expensive. Nevertheless, after 11 p.m. it attracted a large and lively crowd and was a popular venue for some regular pub-goers especially on Friday and Saturday nights. On the two occasions I visited Horace's it was crowded. The music was loud and conversations were conducted mouth to ear. Regular dancers came prepared: dressed lightly in white they coped with the heat and achieved the best effect from the ultra-violet lighting. Newcomers and visitors (like myself) are often spotted (in all senses of the word) because they wear unsuitable clothes: too many and too dark, so as well as looking uncomfortably warm, under the ultra-violet light they appear to be speckled, unattractively, with dust or dandruff. I had been warned by several friends and acquaintances not to go to Horace's because it was 'rough'. One young man, who lived in Waterfoot, advised me *never* to go to Horace's. There was, he warned, a 'clique of Bacup lads, always causing trouble'. He suggested I go, instead, to a club in Waterfoot which he said was 'not as rough and cheaper'. He had never been to Horace's himself, he told me, and had no intention of going there.

When I first visited the club, it had not long been taken over by new licensees. I had been told the new owners were from Manchester, that they had made few changes and invested little in the enterprise. One young woman described how she had been banned from the club for fighting. She related the incident to me in gory and victorious detail and claimed she was 'not really bothered' (about being banned) as there had been 'nothing but trouble' in the club since the new people had taken over. In her opinion they were to blame because, coming from Manchester, they neither knew nor recognized 'the troublemakers' and consequently were 'letting in all the nutcases'. For her the troublemakers had been admitted and there was inevitably trouble, and then the wrong people had been banned; which all went to show the new owners could not and did not recognize the real troublemakers. To know Bacup is to recognize its troublemakers, and knowing its troublemakers is half the battle, because if you *know* the troublemakers, you can pre-empt trouble.

Pubs and drinking in pubs are forums which image differentiation between types of Bacup resident: pubs display attachment. One woman made a distinction between three categories of Bacup resident: those who, like herself,

[14] Such as the town-centre public house nicknamed the 'Little Vatican'.

'go out in Bacup'; those who stay at home; and those who 'go out' outside Bacup. She added, 'you don't see a lot of people who've got more money because they don't drink in Bacup'. 'The posh don't drink', another young woman told me. These statements and the view that the new owners of Horace's have invested little in the business, are used as further examples of the way in which recent incomers exploit the town for their own gain without reciprocating in an appropriate manner. Such views disconnect recent immigrants and give voice to the idea that they choose not to participate in the day-to-day life of Bacup and therefore do not know the town (through experience). If they knew the town they would be better connected. Yet their presence in Bacup pubs and clubs can also be used as further evidence that they exploit those things which do not belong to them. Recent incomers cannot win: they are too distant if they do not go out in Bacup, and too close if they do. But winning or losing is not the point: they are useful to measure connection and disconnection by. Pubs, like houses, not only belong to those who belong to Bacup, but also provide a visible space where belonging or not is made manifest.

Laura tells me she does not know a lot of people who 'do *not* go out'. In other words, her friends and acquaintances, those with whom she connects herself, are those who go out to the pub and who enjoy similar forums of sociability. These are the same people between whom conflict arises and antipathy is sustained. Going out in Bacup, then, is a means by which symbolic boundaries between categories of person within Bacup are marked. It can act as a broad statement of social class (yuppies spend their money elsewhere) so that notions of, for example, self-help and household management, which are deployed for other purposes of differentiation, are eclipsed. Thus Joanne made explicit a distinction between those, like herself, who managed to find work and those who 'are lazy and just collect their giros'. Cross-cutting this distinction are other distinctions between people who go out and people who stay home, or who go out in Bacup and who go out elsewhere. Laura also pointed to women who have high standards of household management—whose homes are 'spotless' and their children 'always dressed well'—but who may be 'buggers' when they have had 'a drink'.

Somehow people had more fun in the past, they entertained themselves, they were more tolerant and less malicious. Similar views emerged from Bacup residents who appeared to have quite different ideas about appropriate forms of sociability. Like Joanna and Laura, Nat members compared how they occupied themselves when they were younger—'we were never bored'—with what they perceive as present-day passive and solitary pastimes. For Nat members, the television, videos, and being plugged in to Walkmans symbolize such passivity. For Joanne and Laura, getting served in pubs at an early age means that young people no longer *make* their own entertainment. Both members of the Nat and Joanne and Laura complained that forms of sociability are becoming more individualistic and insular. While the content of what is deemed appropriate sociability differs greatly between the two, the way in which it is assessed is similar. Residents who recall the Bacup cinema, which is now the Bingo Hall, point out there is nowhere now to watch a film. In the same vein, there is nowhere to dance or listen to live music since the dance-halls closed down. Videos at home cannot replace going to the cinema, and Walkmans are no substitute for singing country-and-western songs out loud on the Bonks. It is the loss of social forums (where watching films and singing songs can be done communally) that these remarks address. Nevertheless meetings of the Nat and the Women's Guild are well attended, and on Friday and Saturday nights Bacup pubs and clubs are full. Groups and informal organizations meet on different nights of the week in, for example, the Conservative Club, the Baptist church, the Leisure Centre, or the Working Men's Club. It would seem that narratives about the lack of 'things to do' and diminishing forums of sociability address questions of appropriateness rather than scarcity.

The Trouble with Kids

At the youth club one week, I got talking to three young women between the ages of 14 and 16. One was making a screenprint of her pop hero, Duran Duran, with a view to making a cushion for her bedroom. Our conversation rested on their question of why I had come to Bacup 'in the first place'. One of the girls told me 'there are two types of people in Bacup—those who cause trouble and ordinary people'. Another said 'the lads' (Bacup lads) did not like them going out with boys from outside Bacup: 'they chase strangers out of town'. It is these lads who 'cause trouble' and they do so, it seems, in the name of Bacup—shoring its defences and repelling outside incursions—and the girls have to meet their out-of-town boyfriends out of town.

Later the same evening, Philip Glass, one of the youth workers, told me the troublemakers are the lads who look 'dead trendy'. He explained they were the ones you would least expect if you were judging by appearances. Philip wanted me to know that appearances could deceive. A 'trendy look' here included trainers (certain makes only), jeans and jackets (sporting particular designer labels), short hair, and generally appearing 'clean and tidy'—what Pam Watson called 'the-boy-next-door-look'. Pam, who worked in the youth club part-time, told me her own teenage sons refused to join the club because of the Bacup lot. This 'Bacup lot' sport a trendy look, are between 14 and 16 years old and hang around together on street corners.

I was frequently told that one of the big problems in Bacup is that 'there's not enough for the kids'. Ideas put forward about youth and their potential for disruption resonate with ways in which other troublemakers are identified, and 'self-help' emerges again in narratives about appropriate youthful behaviour. One recent incomer, with two teenage sons, disputes the commonly expressed view that there is not enough for 'the kids to do'. She claims there is 'plenty to do in Bacup if you just look for it'. She lists, amongst other things, the dry-ski slope in Rawtenstall, horse-riding, and Scout, Cub, Girl Guide, or Brownie camps. She suggests that rather than a dearth of activities being the problem, it is the lack of initiative of kids and their parents.[15] Of course, for children living with unemployed or low-waged parents, the cost of skiing, horse-riding, or Scout camp is prohibitive, and it might be argued that this kind of self-help is a costly exercise. The point to make, however, is that the idea of helping oneself rather than passively waiting to be entertained is as dominant a theme when people talk about 'kids' as when they talk about 'locals', or the makers of trouble. In previous chapters I have described similar ideas put forward by Nat members, by the clientele of public houses, by those who define themselves as Bacup born and bred, almost Bacupian, and incomer.[16]

In the summer of 1988, Laura Gray and Joanne Leary told me the unemployment situation in Bacup was getting better, but a lot of people were still on 'schemes' as opposed to 'proper jobs'.[17] 'Of course', Joanne said, 'there's always the few lazy things who just like to get their giro[18] and go and get pissed on it'. Joanne identifies a category of Bacup person who does not conform to standards of self-help. She and Laura dissociate themselves from those they mark out as the feckless few. From a different perspective, the distinction is screened out: thus when talking about the availability of decent, affordable housing they connect themselves up with those who elsewhere they exclude as profligate. Now those excluded as 'not helping themselves' from one perspective, are 'in the same boat' from another. When immutable economic classes are brought into focus, they screen out mutable behaviour. Recent immigrants, who might for another purpose exemplify virtues of self-help and social mobility, are identified as yuppies.

A conceptual opposition which constantly emerges in Bacup, then, is between the respectable and the feckless. Social categories of the deserving and undeserving poor have historically been a feature of service provision in Britain since the Middle Ages. While membership of each category may shift according to the social preoccupations of the era, it is nevertheless a powerful cultural idiom tied to an inflated value placed on the ability of individuals to help themselves. Adults are meant to be responsible, through their own efforts, for

[15] I am reminded of a commonly voiced complaint (not confined to Bacup) that local people suffer more than others from apathy.

[16] Furthermore, the centrality of ideas about self-help and the positive values placed on it, are not peculiar to Bacup. They are clearly part of broader thinking which is also not confined to 'the English' (see for example Macdonald 1997).

[17] Not long after this conversation, both Joanne and Laura started work in different shoe factories. The intention of both women was to earmark their wages for something specific: Laura's for the deposit on a house (which she and her husband intended eventually to buy) and Joanne's to pay for a holiday in the United States.

[18] Unemployment benefit or income support (now job-seekers allowance) is usually paid by post office cheque—a giro.

their own welfare, and they encourage their children in their independence and autonomy. Peter Howarth (n.d.: 4) in his study of leisure and educational services in Bacup between 1850 and 1880 is puzzled by the ever-present dichotomy in Bacup between 'the godly' and 'the ungodly'; the respectable and the feckless.

> One major problem, which is never quite surmountable, when looking at Bacup a hundred years ago, is the difficulty of reconciling the two images of the town which are constantly thrown together. The first exemplified by the large number of churches and chapels, the early establishment of a Mechanics institute . . . the town's early development of co-operation . . . all combine to present an image of a town characterised by thrift, godliness and a total dedication to the belief of the perfectibility of man. The second, evidenced in . . . newspaper accounts of gambling, drunkenness and hooliganism.

This dichotomy is only a problem, however, if we attempt to attach the two images of the town to two discrete classes of person with fixed and opposing social characteristics. It becomes less of a problem, although no less of a problematic, if we regard the categorizations salient to contemporary residents, which appear to be remarkably similar to those presented 100 years ago, as facets of each other. The troublemakers, whether they be personified as the poor, as residents of council estates, as the rough element, or as members of specific patronym sets, are said to give Bacup a bad name. By attaching trouble to a specific category of person it is placed; it is never not evaluated. Moreover, incomers are not the poor, real Bacup people do not constitute the rough element, and to have an unmarked patronym means you do not belong to the families being named. Trouble is always located, and always elsewhere.

I had not asked about trouble or troublemakers, but participants in the youth club set their own agenda and took both the opportunity and the trouble to tell me what they thought I should know. The lads who cause trouble were said to intimidate other youths, fight frequently, and be involved in petty criminal activities. They are also said to be interrelated, and to come from big families. Philip thinks Bacup has a much worse reputation than it warrants. He does believe, however, that 'Bacup kids *are* different'. He explains: 'they seem slower to develop, naïve in some senses, and slow to embark on relationships with the opposite sex'. His view echoes a stereotype of Bacup as a parochial and insular place with a somehow fixed population that is somewhat behind the times. Youth cannot win: they are either too precocious (urbane and old before their time) or too childlike (unsophisticated and more immature than their years warrant). They gather on the street and are said to 'doss around'.[19] It is

[19] To doss is slang meaning to sleep, esp. in a doss-house (cheap lodging-house) (*Concise Oxford Dictionary* 1988). Here it is used to mean to hang around, or to do nothing (in late-1990 Mancunian slang, 'to lounge').

assumed they need to be kept occupied lest they cause trouble, hence there is never 'enough for the kids to do'. Adolescents are thought to be a disruptive category of resident (not only, of course, in Bacup, and not only in the late 1980s). While we might acknowledge that adolescents, as a socially sanctioned age set, behave in ways appropriate to adolescence, 'the kids' carry with them more than their behaviour. As Bacup is seen to be declining economically and socially, youth symbolize a contemporary malaise. Place and person are juxtaposed—Bacup is suffering (ignored and marginalized) and youth have nowhere to go and nothing to do. The survival of Bacup depends on it being able to contain its young people (to guarantee its future). But in the same way as it is perceived to be unsuccessful in keeping its factories, or its houses, or its autonomy, it is also unsuccessful at containing its youth.

OfRoughness

Bacup is said to be rough. Incidents of fighting and belligerence are cited, families associated with trouble are named, and views on troublemakers constantly put forward. The idea of Bacup as a hard place is not without status. From different Bacup perspectives, stature lies in resilience and resourcefulness. Such characteristics are made manifest in the ability to fight (to stick up for oneself) and in industriousness. These two qualities are not mutually exclusive. Both to fight and to work in an appropriate manner requires fortitude, and each of these activities reveals positively valued qualities of autonomy and self-help.

A man who had moved from Manchester ('away from the rat race') informed me that several years ago (before his arrival in Bacup) there had been a report in a national newspaper suggesting that, per head of population, Bacup had the highest crime rate in the country. He told me this in a local pub and went on to say, lowering his voice and making sure we were out of earshot of anybody else, there was no comparison between levels of violence in Bacup and levels of violence in particular areas of Manchester.[20] He believed Bacup's reputation to have been 'blown out of all proportion'. The same report was cited by a number of Bacup people as evidence that Bacup is 'not as bad as it used to be'. People who were teenagers ten years before, and embroiled in contests for stature and recognition played out on the streets, argued that Bacup was much worse then. For them, the troublemakers have, for the most part, married and settled down.

I was often told Mount Pleasant *used* to be much rougher than it is now, and I was just as often told 'it is getting worse'. John Doyle, in his late thirties, told me he was born and bred on Mount Pleasant and he and his wife had recently

[20] The fact that my co-conversationalist took care not to make this opinion public, suggests he also recognized the prestige inherent in toughness, and to opine that Bacup is not as tough as it is made out to be is to impugn the courage of its people, particularly its men.

bought a terraced house in a different neighbourhood of town. He thought Mount Pleasant was 'levelling off now—it was much rougher ten years ago'.[21] 'When I was a child it was a model estate—people came from miles around just to look at it . . . In them days everybody helped each other.' For John, the majority of Bacup people are 'sound' and there is 'just a handful of idiots'. But he knows the idiots and greets them when he sees them. They have their good points, he tells me, but sometimes it 'does them good to get a good hiding'. According to John, it is not those who are known to him, however idiotically he thinks they may behave at times, who give the estate a bad name, but 'druggies and squatters'. This category of troublemaker was identified by some residents of Mount Pleasant who suggested that empty or hard-to-let properties are squatted by drug users. From here, it is the druggies or squatters who are beyond the pale. Perceived to have no prior ties to the area, they are the new incomers, and are identified as the real troublemakers. In turn, those categorized in this way point to the prejudiced and parochial nature of Bacup people, and to troublemakers on the estate who are violent and out of control, and who give them a hard time. The point to make is that trouble is always located and always located elsewhere.

Recent immigrants do not usually compete for status within Bacup; they have no past in the town to live with. They compare Bacup with the urban areas they knew and left behind and, for them, it is not a dangerous place. Alan Gray remarked towards the end of my first fieldwork that, not having been 'involved', I could never 'really know' Bacup. It was trouble to which he referred. I, like all recent incomers, share the experience of not being involved. Our social relationships in the town have no history of conflict; no experience of violence to 'blow out of all proportion'. The man, on the other hand, with a broken nose from a baseball bat attack, or the man who told me that over the years his father has had his ear bitten off and his brother has been stabbed, might well perceive that, if anything, the level of violence in the town is underestimated and is, in fact, worse than records could possibly indicate or I could possibly know.

Similarly the experience of Black and Asian residents, or homosexual men, belie a view of Bacup as idyllic and filled with mutually supportive inhabitants.[22] On several occasions during fieldwork, I was asked (sometimes disin-

[21] The town planner, quoted in the last chapter, told me that 'ten years ago' the estate became so bad, and communication between residents and the council so poor, that a major renovation programme was devised. I was also told it was 'ten years ago' when the name of the major road through the estate, from which it derives its name, was changed in an attempt to relieve the stigma attached to it.

[22] In 1987/8, lesbians in Bacup had a much more visible and open profile than gay men. Socializing as a group, women were open and assertive about their homosexuality with little apparent harassment, even if the focus of overt gossip (but, I would suggest, they were the focus of no more gossip than other residents of Bacup deemed to be troublesome in different ways). I think it would have been impossible for gay men during this period to have visibly asserted themselves in a similar way. Incidents related about harassment and prejudice against homosexuality always focused on men not women.

genuously) why I thought there were no Black people in the town. I was told they would inevitably be harassed and ultimately driven out. Examples of this having occurred were given and incidents recounted, again with disdain (Bacup as a parochial, backward place) or pride (Bacup as a hard place). Such accounts act within Bacup to identify a backward and unenlightened category of resident—again, 'there are just a few "dickheads" who give Bacup a bad name'. Whether it is Bacup people as a whole, or certain families, or particular neighbourhoods, or just one or two 'dickheads' that are identified as racist, sexist, or homophobic, their interrelatedness is identified as a cause of their parochialism. The same perception of interrelatedness is also evaluated positively and underwrites a self-satisfaction in the ability of Bacup to repel outsiders/strangers.[23]

Such examples are deployed as further evidence of the way in which 'Bacup people' are either 'troublesome' or 'tough'. The same examples are drawn upon to highlight both the parochial, homophobic, and racist tendencies of Bacup people (negative) *and* their down-to-earth, no-nonsense attitude to life (positive). Both are caricatures which tell us as much about the way in which Bacupness is construed as they do about the workings of racism and homophobia.

Bacup people acknowledge that Bacup has a bad reputation as far as surrounding towns are concerned. According to one young woman: 'Rawtenstall people' think Bacup should be walled off at the Glen (a narrow gorge which lies just beyond the boundary of Bacup, between Stacksteads and Waterfoot, and through which the main road passes). She also said Bacup seems to be blamed for everything, but that if you study the newspapers then you see there is more trouble at the other end of the Valley than at the Bacup end. I took another look at the local newspapers as she suggested. I had been collecting the free newspaper delivered every Tuesday to 22,500 households in Rawtenstall, Bacup, and Haslingdon, and what the editor called its sister paper sold in newsagents on Fridays and with a circulation, in June 1988, of 16,350. The news offices and reporters are based in Rawtenstall, and I went to talk to the editor in his office. He told me he was born in Bacup and now lived at 'the other end of the valley'. He emphasized that he retained an affection for Bacup and a concern about its problems. He described his role as serving the town. In this context, he had initiated a dialogue with the local police over the best way in which to deal with violence and intimidation in Bacup, and with the local Member of Parliament over the way in which official unemployment figures failed to represent a true picture of unemployment. Over a two-month period during fieldwork, there were two front-page stories which directly mentioned Bacup in terms of violence: the first was a report about a Bacup pub which was forced to shut down due to a 'barrage of violence and intimidation' against the landlord, and the second reported that

[23] I was told repeatedly about a man living on Mount Pleasant who had been persistently harassed because he was homosexual.

'hooligans and drunks' had forced the bus company to withdraw the last bus to Bacup through Waterfoot on a Friday night. There were many more reports about the financial troubles of Bacup, and the trouble caused by the closure of its factories and it shops.

Sparring Partners

An exchange of sparring partners and spouses seems to have traditionally linked Bacup to Burnley, Rawtenstall, and Rochdale (see Ch. Five). Today immigration to Bacup from these towns, although small in numbers, continues, and the image of a small town surrounded by larger and more powerful places remains. There is a need, it is said, for Bacup to defend itself, and trouble, like all symbols of community, has its upside.

Joe Prescott had moved from Rochdale three years earlier, after a divorce. He lived alone in one of the bungalows in the survey area. He was in his mid-forties and thought that Bacup had improved immensely since he was a lad. When he was younger, he recalled, Bacup had a reputation as a 'place to fight', and young men would travel in gangs from Rochdale to Bacup in order to have 'a good scrap'. These kind of incursions were described by a Bacup man in this way:

> Bacup is surrounded by big towns. It had a lot to live up to for many years—just like England had a lot to live up to with America—Bacup boys are very proud people. They don't like outsiders coming in. They will fight if they have to . . . They used to come in from Nelson and Colne to fight—gone back with their tail between their legs. Some very big families, not [necessarily] hard people, tended to stick together.

A friend of his added: 'Rochdale gangs used to come and fight because Bacup lads were so hard'. The success of Bacup fighters was due to their 'hardness' and hence they were a challenge to lads from neighbouring towns. But their success was also due to their interconnectedness. Of interest, here, is the way in which an idiom of kinship is mobilized in order to portray the kind of solidarity that was needed to overcome more powerful adversaries. Bacup fighters were having to defend their reputation against bigger and mightier foes, and the interconnectedness within and between big Bacup families was put to good effect. Solidarity between those already related resulted in a strength which made up for what they may have lacked individually in terms of hardness.

Men, talking about how they used to fight but don't anymore, say that Bacup has improved enormously; they say it is nowhere near as rough as it used to be. Yet, addressing a different question, they told me it was 'getting worse'; a sentiment echoed by many other Bacup residents. Two things epitomize the perceived deterioration: the first relates to the *way* in which fights are fought, and the second to the protagonists. Fighting is said to be conducted 'nowadays' in an inappropriate manner (weapons and unfair tactics are used) and between inappropriate protagonists (between Bacup lads or family members). In 1988, hostilities between groups of young men were described in terms of place—antipathy between, for example, Rawtenstall and Bacup—and in terms of *feuding families* to whom I shall return.

The awards ceremony of the amateur football league, in which a number of Bacup teams compete, is held at the Leisure Centre at the end of the football season.[24] Players are allowed one guest and, in 1988, they mostly invited a male relative or friend. After the ceremony, groups of men continue their celebrations at a nightclub in a nearby town. On the evening of the annual dinner dance, I was with the wife of one of the football players. She said she hoped the men ended up in Waterfoot rather than Burnley. If they got to Waterfoot, she explained, there would be no trouble, whereas if they went to Burnley, especially in such large numbers, they would inevitably get into a fight. Waterfoot is closer to Bacup than Burnley, much smaller than both, and within the Rossendale Valley. Burnley is perceived as a separate place, a locality with no axiomatic ties to Bacup. Bacup lads are able to drink in Waterfoot with impunity as there are inevitable friendships and alliances between the two—they are interconnected. Burnley, by contrast, has its own alliances and foes; it is big enough to gain strength from its own connections and has no need to forge or sustain links with Bacup. Consequently, Bacup lads, in gangs, are likely to be perceived as an incursion and repelled. The same logic is reversed when applied to Waterfoot lads in Bacup. Listen to Joanne and Laura describing the young men who fight:

JOANNE: Waterfoot lads won't drink up Bacup at all. Bacup lads don't like anybody else in, do they?

JEANETTE: Is that that macho thing you were talking about?

LAURA: I don't think it's because they think 'oh they're going to take all the women'. I think it's just they don't . . .

JOANNE: They don't like them in the pubs. But yet *they* can go down there. Waterfoot lads just go out for a good time. Whereas these, up here, they just like to go out and have a fight at the end of the night.

LAURA: It's not a good night for them if there's no scrapping.

JOANNE: Rawtenstall's quite a bad town as well, isn't it?

LAURA: All the lads from Bacup could go to Waterfoot and they could go down and they could cause hassle in the pubs and they wouldn't really get much hassle back would they? But if they went to Rawtenstall and did it, there would be a fight, more than there would in Waterfoot.

JOANNE: But then they've been down there [Rawtenstall] and sorted half of them lot out, haven't they? They're a hard bunch up here, really. They're a crazy lot—I think they're the craziest about.

LAURA: But I don't think that's *all* the lads.

[24] Teams are generally attached to pubs, clubs, or factories.

JOANNE: Oh no—just a bunch. But I'll give this for them, if there were, like [*pause*] a fight down Rawtenstall, just a normal lad, like, they'd back him up, wouldn't they? They'd be there to back him up.

LAURA: If it's just an ordinary lad, like, that's not really a fighter.

JOANNE: They'd help him out, wouldn't they? Even though [*pause*] they're not a bad lot really. They'd certainly help you out of trouble. They're not the kind to sit back and let it all happen, are they? They'd certainly stick by you. That would be anybody in Bacup that, wouldn't it?

Laura and Joanne begin by creating a conceptual distance between themselves and Bacup lads by focusing on men's territorial proclivities: they point out that Bacup lads will not *allow* Waterfoot lads to drink in Bacup. That same belligerence, however, may be put to good use, so that the same lads will defend a non-fighter, from Bacup or otherwise, against Rawtenstall lads. They will champion, in other words, the less powerful. In this they share part of the Bacup character which is identified by Nat members, amongst others: namely, a keenness to observe justice and fair play. Aggression is both positively and negatively valued and in its positive guise it means defending the underdog and coming to the assistance of those in need. Hence, although particular patronyms are associated with trouble, and members of such patronyms' sets are defined as troublemakers, their activities may also be interpreted as appropriate and proper Bacup behaviour. Consequently, the good side of men and women, excluded elsewhere as 'headbangers', is emphasized through mobilizing a different set of connections. Now their willingness to come to the aid of the defenceless, or to contribute financially to collective action in times of trauma is brought to the fore. In mobilizing idioms of trouble, people locate it; in identifying the 'real' troublemakers they dissociate themselves from the category. However, troublemakers are not always making trouble; they also participate in community affairs, are generous and mutually supportive. As Joanne Leary put it:

> half these what talk about you, you know what I mean—the bad lot—when anybody dies they're there, aren't they? At the funeral, collecting and stuff like that. They're right good, you know, that way. That's one thing I've always said for the Murphys and the Doyles—if anybody's died they're always the first ones to go round with a collection and flowers and that. They're all a good lot in their own ways, they'll help you out if they have to. I suppose like everybody. Everybody has their good side and their bad side.

Changing Forms of Hostility

Newspaper reports from 100 years ago describe rowdy scenes as a regular occurrence in Bacup town centre. It is reported that large groups of young men gathered and jeered at passers-by, making offensive remarks, swearing, and generally making a nuisance of themselves. The *Bacup Times* of Saturday, 27

October 1887, carried an item which described an obstruction at Bull's Head Bridge at 3.30 p.m. the previous Sunday.[25] Between 200 and 300 people are reported to have assembled and the 'highway was completely blocked'. On being asked to move on, the crowd began to 'hoot and jeer at the sergeant'. The Chairman of the Council, in response to a question about the incident, is reported to have said: 'This loitering on the streets was a great nuisance to the public generally and the authorities were determined to put a stop to it . . . [People] pay rates so that the streets can be kept orderly and decent and not be obstructed in this way' (*Bacup Times*, 27 Oct. 1887).

A booklet published by the Natural History Society to mark its centennial celebration presents similar quotes from around the same time. They are published under the heading: 'A glimpse of Bacup over 100 years ago'. Examples include:

> That horrid bridge, Bulls Head, with its assemblage of young cads, middle-aged rakes and old loons, on Sunday afternoons, is enough to make one blush for his manhood.
>
> The language to, and looks at, respectable passers-by, male and female is unendurable.
>
> Scenes of riot and disorder occur at Broadclough on almost every Sunday. They come reeling out of the Inn at Higher Broadclough. They range in age from 25 to 35. They are unwashed, and clad in their dirty weekday dress, with clogs and caps.[26]

The original authors of these statements were obviously commenting on a category of Bacup resident distinct from themselves: 'young cads, middle aged rakes and old loons' and those with 'unwashed' bodies dressed in 'clogs and caps'. Nat members, in presenting these particular snippets, are interested in a comparison between today and yesterday, but they are also writing a history about, and on behalf of, a working-class Bacup. To select such items is to formulate an anarchic history which, on the one hand celebrates an absence of subservience and, on the other, shows up the fecklessness of the labouring classes. Nat members have themselves risen above such squalor and roughness and, like the original authors, through these examples distance themselves from the behaviour they report. In selecting what from another perspective might be considered the least attractive aspects of Bacup's past they celebrate a history of trouble, anarchy, fortitude, and resilience.

A prominent way in which residents of Bacup in late 1987 and 1988 measured social change was through crime and violence. People often remarked that you could no longer leave your back door unlocked, [27] and many residents

[25] The river Irwell runs underground through Bacup. Before it was covered over and hidden from sight, it was crossed by the Bull's Head Bridge (named after a nearby hotel) in the centre of town.

[26] From BNHS (1978).

[27] They were the same people who talked about living in houses without back doors (back-to-backs), which underlines my point that such statements are as much matters of differentiation as matters of fact.

expressed concern that 'the streets' were unsafe, particularly at night.[28] Recent immigrants said the same thing about the urban localities they left behind. From this perspective, Bacup was safe, and was not as bad as 'the city'. A view of the tranquil character of Bacup rests uneasily, but not impossibly, alongside a view of Bacup as rough and getting rougher. Residents of Mount Pleasant may have argued that the estate was not as bad as it used to be, but they pointed out that the forms available for resolving or playing out conflict had changed for the worst—they had become more violent. One man explained, in the past, a fight would take place between 'two lads', while 'today they don't have the guts to face man to man', so they recruit the help of their brothers and uncles. It becomes a family affair and a matter of honour and pride. 'Families' cannot 'be seen to be losing'.

A significant difference in meaning was attached to inter- and intra-town conflict. In fights between Rochdale and Bacup lads, for example, a positive value was placed on the ability of the 'Bacup lot' not only to defend themselves, but to 'sort out' (humiliate) their opponents. The same people who described with pride the ability of the Bacup lot to defend themselves against gangs from nearby towns, looked askance at fighting within the town. They deplored what they perceived to be an increase in gang hostility and contrasted it with what they perceived as a more acceptable means of resolving conflict 'man to man'. Both men and women described changes in the nature of violence and argued it had become more cowardly. They pointed out that weapons (such as baseball bats) were increasingly used, and fights were increasingly taking place between unequal numbers of opponents. Unevenly matched fights, or attacks on an individual by a group, were regarded as unfair and cowardly, but were said to be on the increase.

According to James Whittacker, there were fights between men from Bacup and men from neighbouring towns in the past, 'but there weren't the unruly mobs or the violence in them days'. 'Any rowdiness', he continued, 'used to come from Todmorden.' Fighting was not a new phenomenon, then, nor indeed was rowdiness and unruly behaviour. But while Bacup men may have fought in the past, they were not, in Mr Whittacker's word, rowdy. And while there may have been unruly mobs and rowdiness, they were not to be found in Bacup. Here we see again the way in which the past is mobilized to render visible contemporary social differentiation. Mr Whittacker identified a class of Bacup person without scruples or integrity made evident in the ways in which they conduct themselves in their fights. One woman, in her early fifties, told me that although there had always been a few 'rough families', fighting never used to be a 'serious matter': 'There might be a fight with somebody from Rochdale but you didn't get involved. It was more a skirmish—a fun thing

[28] And not confined to Bacup: a strong perception of the late 20th cent. is that we live in more violent times.

then—not real animosity. Now it's a hate thing. Today it's not clean fighting. They go in with the boot in.'

A common idea that fighting is qualitatively different today from how it was in the past also addresses what is perceived to be a more violent and more fragmented society generally. One with less cohesion and less mutual support between members. It also addresses differentiation within Bacup, which in an economic framework, and/or from an outside perspective, is hardly discernible. A distinct category of 'troublemaker' is defined by whom they fight (their foes), whom they fight with (their allies), and the ways in which they fight (their techniques). Who they are, however, depends on the perspective from which they are viewed: either 'typical Bacup lads' or 'just a minority' they nevertheless give Bacup a 'bad name'.

'Kick One and They All Limp'

Recent immigrants might identify Mount Pleasant as a 'rough estate', but generally thought Bacup less troublesome than the urban localities from which they 'escaped'. Bacup people who had been privy to ongoing hostilities argued it was 'getting better', while others, particularly older residents, pointed out it was 'getting worse'. All tended to agree that Bacup has a bad reputation due to a 'rough element'—a minority who gave the town a bad name. This minority were 'headbangers', 'hoodlums', 'hooligans', 'tosspots', 'dickheads', or 'clowns'. They were different. One man told me that trouble is caused by 'nutcases, 20-, 21-, and 22- year-olds, all sound lads when they haven't had a drink'. The same few patronyms came up again and again in the context of trouble.

Trouble was perceived to be passed down from generation to generation, usually from fathers to sons, and those who fought together were connected by kinship. The offspring of siblings (cousins) were said to form alliances, usually under the umbrella of a particular patronym. In the words of Laura and Joanne:

JOANNE: They're all fighters in this town like. They're not a soft lot [*pause*] are they? Far from it.

LAURA: Oh no. Bacup's known as a fighting town.

JOANNE: They'll certainly stick up for themselves.

JEANETTE: But who? Is it people coming from the outside that they're fighting?

JOANNE: No it's inside lot, isn't it? They all live here.

JEANETTE: What's it about?

LAURA: It's just carrying on from generation to generation. The fathers fought the fathers an' . . .

JOANNE: I think a lot of it is because they have big families and then they have big families. It's just like a macho kind of thing, isn't it?

Trouble is imputed to named families. These families are always said to be big, and those linked to particular patronyms are closely connected. It is assumed you have a vested interest in those who share your patronym. The more people who share that patronym the more likely they are to defend themselves as a group, to participate in one another's conflicts. The interconnectedness of these families is imaged in expressions such as 'kick one an' they all limp', or 'kick one an' a bruise comes up on t'other', or 'push one an' they all lean'. These are wonderfully evocative and portray vividly the idea that individuals are connected, so much so that, like a ripple, a shove on one body passes through an adjoining body and from there to another, and so on. Or so much so, that to injure (bruise) one body (with a kick) is to injure all connected bodies equally and in the same place. Such images portray the impossibility and perhaps the futility of trying to separate out individuals. The effect of a hurt may just as readily manifest itself on one part of the collective body as on another.[29] These expressions, you will recall, were also used to describe Bacup people as a whole: recent immigrants and residents of neighbouring towns said, for example, that Bacup was characterized by big families who intermarry ('everybody is related to everybody else'), and 'kick one and they all limp'. Furthermore those defined as real Bacup families with English surnames such as Whittacker, Hargreaves, Howarth, and so on, were also said to be big and to intermarry. The troublemakers were also said to belong to big families, this time with names that had their origins in Ireland, such as Murphy and Doyle, and these families were also said to intermarry. The image of the tight-knit family is juxtaposed with that of the fixed and interrelated community, and the tight-knit community with the fixed and interrelated family. Neither the community or the family so described is unambiguously good or unambiguously bad. They are both.

While trouble is linked to particular patronyms, residents without personal experience of conflict rarely knew, nor could they identify, individuals who comprised a particular named family. Bernard Whittacker told me it was only recently he had even heard of one of the surnames currently associated with trouble. He described how 'there have always been family names that struck fear into people'; when he was a child, he recalled, it was 'the Brodys' and 'the Donahues' who, he said, were cousins. 'The Brodys' comprised two or three brothers as did 'the Donahues', and together they formed a gang and, according to Bernard, recruited other cousins.[30] The leaders of the gang, at that time,

[29] 'There is no better image of the logic of socialization, which treats the body as a "memory jogger", than those complexes of gestures, postures and words—simple interjections or favourite clichés—which only have to be slipped into, like a theatrical costume, to awaken, by the evocative power of bodily mimesis, a universe of ready-made feelings and experiences. The elementary actions of bodily gymnastics, especially the specifically sexual, biologically pre-constructed aspect of it, charged with social meaning and values, function as the most basic of metaphors, capable of evoking a whole relationship to the world' (Bourdieu 1992 [1984]: 474).

[30] Cousin is used generically here to cover in English kinship thinking relations on 'both sides'—that is both mother's *and* father's siblings' children (e.g. MBD and FBD). It also covers first (e.g. MBS) and second (e.g. MFBS) cousins. How close or distant different kinds of cousin are perceived to be is variable (and see Strathern 1981: 146).

were the Donahues who, Bernard recalled, looked alike. Now, he said, they had grown older, settled down, had children of their own and were not heard of any more.

I was often told that trouble in Bacup was due to feuding families, and it was also pointed out, on more than one occasion, that these families were, in fact, cousins. In making explicit the fact of their relatedness, a further layer of opprobrium is added to their fighting in the first place. In the example of 'the Donahues' and 'the Brodys' an alliance was formed between sibling sets who were related to one another (in this example as cross-cousins). Troublemakers are conceptualized as a discrete group of kin who, in turn, can be divided further into more exclusive groups of kin. As well as forming natural allies they can also form natural enemies. Hence cousins (like the Donahues and the Brodys) might join forces but the potential is also there for them to fight each other. The concept of a feuding family is ambiguous: it can embrace two unrelated families or two branches of the same family. Patronyms act both to include and to exclude: to imagine exclusive and inclusive categories of kin. There was one patronym that frequently emerged in many of the conversations I had which meandered (inexorably) towards trouble. I was told the name belonged to a 'big' and 'tight-knit family', but for residents who knew individual members of this family, or for members of the family themselves, finer distinctions were made. For example, the *real* troublemakers, those who gave the family a bad name, were identified. If you can 'kick one and they all limp', you can also 'tar them all with the same brush'. The idea of their interconnectedness can be put to work both to castigate and to defend them.

The solidarity assumed and predicted between sibling sets is expected as much of women as it is of men. Mavis O'Connor was a sewing machinist in a local shoe factory. Despite low wages,[31] and periods of short time,[32] she professed to enjoy her work and in particular 'the crack'.[33] However, she was going through a difficult patch, and told me about difficulties she was having with certain colleagues. Two of her co-workers were sisters. She referred to them by their patronym, expecting me to have heard the name, and therefore that she would be able to leave a certain amount of detail implicit. It turned out that each of the sisters was in fact married and had a different surname, but Mavis could say more with fewer words by invoking their patronym. The sisters were backed in the dispute between them and Mavis by the floor manager who, Mavis told me, had married into the family, and by their cousins

[31] In 1988 the average take-home pay for a 40-hour week, as a machinist in a shoe factory, was £76. I discovered this when I met a colleague of Mavis while out shopping one afternoon, she had just left work and was angry. She showed me her pay-slip and told me they had just been awarded a cost-of-living pay increase—it amounted, she said, with disgust, to less than £2 extra per week.

[32] Periods of part-time work due to a fall in the number of orders.

[33] Fun, gossip, ambience (social relationships and events with, in this context, colleagues): to have a crack (Scottish Gaelic and Irish).

who also worked in the same factory, but in a different section.[34] Mavis spoke of how they closed ranks. In her words 'you kick one and you kick them all'; it was impossible, she said, to have an argument with only *one* member of 'that family'. Eventually hostilities subsided and, in becoming friends with one, Mavis said, she automatically became friends with the rest.

Ursula Murphy pointed out that her son and partner were assumed to be 'Murphys' although they were not. She thought the name was 'hated in Bacup' and was 'known all over the Valley'. She worried for her son who, despite not being called Murphy, would probably 'get a bad time' because people would '*think* he's a Murphy, even though he's not'. She described his father as 'right quiet' but he 'gets oined as well, because people think he's a Murphy'. When she applied for jobs, she never gave her real name and anyway, even if she changed it, she said, she would still 'be classed as a Murphy'. She told me her family had been forced to defend themselves because of the response elicited by their name: 'They don't have to do anything—they're hated straight away. Half of my family are straight. They've never been done for burglary.' She listed the acts of violence and harassment committed against members of her family and added, 'they're always fighting because they *have* to. They're not idiots—they're not just gonna lie down and take it.' In this context, Ursula is referring to her father's brother and his children—those who share her patronym—as her family. Ursula was known as 'a Murphy' and she believed from a Bacup perspective she would always remain so whether she changed her name or not. She valued, however, the ability to defend oneself against abuse. Only idiots, she suggested, suffer in silence.

Just as Bacup needs to defend itself against surrounding towns, or Bacup people against outsiders, so families also have to defend themselves: not to defend oneself—to sit back passively and wait to be beaten—is foolish.

If certain patronyms were identified with trouble and certain families said to be feuding, how did trouble and feuds manifest themselves? Josh Clark was in his early twenties and although he was born in Bacup he had lived in Burnley, a neighbouring town, for eighteen years. He was, he said, the only member of his family to have returned to Bacup and his mother, who still lived in Burnley, wished he had not. His wife, he told me, belonged to one of 'the families who are feuding'. He described her family as big and able to look after itself. The latest incident in the ongoing hostilities occurred four days before his wedding when his wife's brother, who was due to be best man at the ceremony, was ambushed and beaten by two men. Witnesses to the attack, according to Josh,

[34] At the time, Mavis was on piece-work, which is paid for by completed unit, that is, by piece or quantity. On a production line the speed at which one person can work is dependent on the supply of materials to them. In this case shoe uppers were being cut out and had to be supplied to the machinist at the same rate (or faster) than the rate at which they could be sewn. There is the potential for either co-operation or conflict along the chain of operatives.

refused to testify because of fear of reprisals. He also argued that the police knew who was responsible but were also scared. Josh said he knew those who carried out the attack, and although it was a 'small family—they think they own the town'. According to Josh, they had lived in Bacup all their lives and were 'all Ireland, and all Catholic'. Later in our conversation he conceded it was really only one man and his sons who were 'the real troublemakers'; the man's other brother, he told me, had settled and calmed down as he had grown older. Talking of the conflict between them and his wife's 'family', Josh said: 'Even though it is me family I'm not involved. We've [he and his wife] got a lot of friends in town—we're protected. This is my town and I'm not being intimidated. If it's not sorted out legally—then our lads will do something.'

Josh thought that although there was 'trouble everywhere you go, it is more noticeable [in Bacup] because it's always the same people'. He also thought Bacup was improving all the time and he resented the bad name it had acquired. Although he would have preferred to live somewhere else—'for the sake of the kids when they come'—his wife was 'basically tied to Bacup'; her parents, grandmother, and brothers and sisters, he said, all lived within five minutes. Kinship tied his wife to the town and although he personally could handle intimidation he wished his children would not have to face the same experience.

Josh has a claim on Bacup, he belongs, and will not be intimidated in his own place. He is both involved and not involved in the conflict; it is both his family and not his family. Josh connects himself to his wife's family. He makes explicit his connections to her relatives ('our lads'). On the other hand the same affinal tie can be used to imagine exclusion. It is mobilized to make explicit the *distinction* between Josh and his wife's family. Affinal ties provide a means of inclusion and exclusion—of solidarity *and* differentiation.

Cousins, particularly cross-cousins, are an ambiguous category of kin, and interestingly it is they who emerge as major protagonists when the subject of feuding families (itself ambiguous) is raised. Cousins feature frequently in ideas about Bacup as a troublesome place. A notion that 'cousins marry cousins' is also commonly evoked as a further example of the parochial nature of Bacup. Couched in terms of 'intermarriage' it has both positive and negative connotations: as well as parochialism (exclusivity) it also exemplifies mutual support (inclusivity). I have focused on the way in which trouble is associated with 'big families', members of which are perceived to form formidable foes when they join forces, or who fight bitterly amongst themselves. Both cousins in conflict and cousins who marry are problematic, they are perceived to be both too close to be hostile and too close to reproduce, despite the fact they are allowed and do both.[35] To suggest 'cousins marry cousins' or 'families feud' is to tweak at

[35] To put it crudely, cousins ought neither fight nor fuck.

idealized images of appropriate forms of sociality. Cousins are both kin and potential marriage partners, and families are both havens of protection and forums of antipathy, and such ambiguity is also why natives of neighbouring towns are legitimate sparring partners and spouses.

I recall a conversation I had towards the beginning of fieldwork not long after I had moved to Bacup. One Sunday I went with a friend and my son on a fungus hunt, organized and guided by the warden of a country park just outside Whitworth. Ten adults and six children, mostly from Rochdale, turned up for the event. Only my son and myself had come that day from Bacup. With the help of our guide, we tracked and identified a variety of mushrooms and toadstools. We collected in plastic bags those we were told were edible, except for ones that looked too unlike food to be edible, and we were suitably wary of, and impressed by, the rare 'deadly poisonous' specimen we were shown. One man in the group, in his mid-thirties, told me he had recently moved from Manchester to Whitworth, and I told him we had recently moved to Bacup. We swapped removal stories and he proceeded, like many people I met in those days, to inform me about Bacup, despite never having been there. 'A funny place', he said, 'lots of intermarriage, you know? Cousins marrying cousins.' He spoke authoritatively about the town and its people, and admitted not only to never having been there but also to having no intention of going. I was constantly surprised at how many acquaintances, friends, and colleagues (sociologists and social anthropologists included) proffered a view of Bacup when they discovered I was working there. Many commentators before, during, and after my fieldwork in the town, hinted at its 'troublesome' nature or the proclivity of its people for 'intermarriage' (often couched in terms of cousins marrying cousins). Many readers will, no doubt, be reminded of places, maybe villages perceived to be remote, or council estates perceived to be rough, that are described in similar terms: perhaps also in terms of 'intermarriage' or with reference to 'interbreeding'. Such descriptions are not confined to Bacup: fishing villages in Cornwall, rural communities in the Appalachian mountains, council estates in Greater Manchester, the smaller of the Canary Islands are all amongst many of the places I have heard described thus. Such idioms are mobilized as much from within Bacup as from without. They are part of a common currency of ideas which it is tempting to think of as Euro-American except we know little ethnographically about similarity and difference across European and North American contexts.[36] None the less, similar descriptions are mobilized to differentiate between categories of person in places other than Bacup and are part of cultural repertoires other than English. While the persons and places to whom these idioms are applied may not be comparable

[36] I am also warned about the exclusiveness of the American in Euro-American which often refers to North American (Verena Stolcke, pers. comm.). Strathern (1996) uses it fruitfully and explicitly to refer to a 'largely middle-class North American/Northern European discourse of public and professional life'.

the process of differentiation (of inclusion and exclusion) which construes them is (see also Strathern 1991).

I never explicitly set out to discover whether cousins marry cousins in Bacup, and I only ever came across one example (during a pilot interview for the housing survey). It could be argued that a dearth of cases suggests the practice is stigmatized and therefore kept quiet, or that it is a myth. Either way, we miss the point if we dwell on the scarcity of actual examples, or make too much of the fact that the one example I did record was of a couple who were not themselves from Bacup. The interesting question is why the idea of marriage between cousins should emerge as significant at all (there are no legal or religious restrictions on the practice), and, furthermore, what is being conveyed when certain places are identified as places where 'cousins marry cousins'. A common view of Bacup, from the outside looking in, is that its population is densely interrelated: it comprises an interconnected and fixed community—one marked by dense networks of kinship. Interconnectedness, as we have seen, has both positive and negative connotations depending on the angle from which it is viewed, or indeed from the hill on which one sits.

From outside Bacup (a perspective also found inside), Bacup people are described in terms which suggest the interconnectedness of their intimate relationships. Implicit in statements such as 'cousins marry cousins' is a comparison with all the places Bacup is not. The formulation of interrelatedness in this way has Bacup people as inward-looking and residents of, say, the city as outward-looking. It is a strategy of differentiation, distinguishing the speaker as a different kind of person; at the least, more mobile. But as we have seen such ideas of interrelatedness are as much part of a Bacup repertoire as they are of other places in Britain. And cousins are at the cusp of interrelatedness: they are both 'too close' and 'too distant'.

7

Common Knowledge

CHANGES on the physical face of Bacup are marked. Its rapid growth as an industrial centre, when houses, factories, churches, businesses, public houses, and transport systems 'appeared overnight', gave way to a contraction when, one after the other, factories closed down followed by other small businesses and the railway station. One unused and slightly crooked factory chimney remains standing, and gives little intimation of what, 100 years ago, was a vista dominated by factory chimneys. Residents who appropriate Bacup's industrial history as their own talk of changes that have occurred as part of a general deterioration in 'the quality of life'. The present is thought of as qualitatively poorer than the past (see also Cohen 1987; Macdonald 1997). In bringing the past forward to comment on the present, the poor and arduous living conditions of earlier times, which are elsewhere and for a different purpose foregrounded, are for now screened out. It is not that they are forgotten, it is just that, in this context, they are irrelevant. Instead the image of Bacup as a thriving, densely populated place, at the centre of activity and industry, is put to work.

One woman recalled that Burnley Road would be so full of people on a Saturday night that 'you had to jostle to get a place on the pavement'. Another recalled the clatter of clogs on cobblestones which made a huge 'racket' when factory whistles went and workers were let out for the day. And you will recall the adage that if you stood in the centre of town and threw a stone (or perhaps a penny) in *any* direction, it would land on the doorstep of a public house.

A decline in industry and population is perceived to have gone hand in hand with diminishing autonomy. Residents remembered that in the harsh(er) winters of the past snow would be cleared quickly by an efficient Bacup Borough Council and an excellent water supply was maintained by Bacup's own Water Board. Snow clearance and the quality of water have come to stand for general deterioration in council services; a deterioration dated to when Bacup was subsumed under the Borough of Rossendale and ceased to administer itself. A common complaint today is that Bacup 'gets left out': it has become, in the words of one man, 'a Cinderella town'.[1] And just as individuals and families need to be able to defend themselves, so too does Bacup. Rivalry between Bacup and neighbouring towns is framed, amongst other things, in

[1] But Cinderella—left at home to clean the hearth while her stepsisters go to the party—wins out in the end.

the uneven spread of local authority resources: Rawtenstall gets preferential treatment and Bacup is ignored, and local authority services are not as efficient or as thorough as when Bacup administered itself. Residents remarked that new industrial or commercial enterprise tended to concentrate at the western end of the valley (which is, of course, a bad thing if you want a job in Bacup and a good thing if your aim is to retire to 'the country').

Yet Bacup, like many Lancashire small towns, is a hive of social activity. On any given night, numerous groups of residents meet. The Nat has a full house for its Saturday evening lectures, and on Thursday when its members meet, drink tea, and do business, members of the Bacup Women's Guild meet in The A, B & D Centre (Aged, Blind, and Deaf). On Wednesday evenings, at least half the public houses in Bacup will be hosting a match of the Ladies' Darts League.[2] The Soroptomists, Rotarians and Freemasons, and the Camera Club meet regularly, and the Bingo Hall attracts a crowd most evenings. There is a local branch of the Red Cross, and more than one pack of Brownies, Girl Guides, Scouts, and Cubs, as well as two youth clubs and a youth theatre. The Rossendale Players rehearse in Bacup's theatre which was bequeathed to the town and maintained through voluntary contribution and labour. Sometimes they stage their performances at the Leisure Centre, more often than not to a full house and almost always to vociferous local praise. Each church congregation (including, Church of England, Catholic, Methodist, Baptist, and Assemblies of God) has its own series of meetings, fund-raising, and social events. Public houses are especially busy on Friday and Saturday evenings when groups of young women and separate groups of young men, striking in winter for their renunciation of outdoor clothes, walk from one to another and perhaps meet up at the end of the night in Horace's. Bacup amateur football teams, affiliated to places of work, public houses or working men's clubs, attract local men to the pitch and bar on Saturday afternoons, at least during the football season, and during the cricket season the local cricket team attracts paying supporters to their well-kept ground, while the Cricket Club is open to members all year round. The Working Men's Club and the Conservative Club have their own clientele, while members of the keep-fit class, Labour Party, Greenpeace, and the local Conservation Society, to name but a few, each have their favourite place in which to continue discussion after, and perhaps in between, their formal meetings (Fig. 7.3). The Britannia Coco-Nut Dancers of Bacup meet once a week in Stacksteads to practice their dance, teach their apprentices, discuss business, and perhaps have a drink together. It is they who are the focus of the first part of the chapter.

[2] I played occasionally on the team that was attached first to the Blossoms and then to The Crimean (they moved because they perceived a lack of support from the licensees of the Blossoms, who were said neither to look after the trophies nor provide supper on match nights); had I been a better darts player, I might have been encouraged to play more often. As it was, I was generously tolerated occasionally.

THE ROSSENDALE PLAYERS

present

SEE HOW THEY RUN

a farce by
PHILIP KING

Produced by
ELIZABETH LLOYD

at
THE LEISURE HALL, BACUP

WEDNESDAY, SEPTEMBER 7th
to
SATURDAY, SEPTEMBER 10th
1988

at 7-30 p.m.

PROGRAMME 20p

FORTY YEARS ON

The Players do not often repeat themselves but the present play is an exception.

SEE HOW THEY RUN was first presented by the Society in 1948 and was described by the Rossendale Free Press as "the funniest thing seen on a local stage for years". The two local newspapers devoted between them over two thousand words to reporting the production. An extra performance was arranged for the Saturday afternoon to satisfy public demand, making eight performances in all. Admission was 2/6d real money (12½p).

The cast included JACK DAVEY and EDITH FILDES as the Toops, HILDA THOMPSON as Miss Skillon and DOROTHY HISLOP as the maid. OWEN RYDER played Clive Winton and HAROLD HELLIWELL was the Rev. Arthur Humphrey. The cast was completed by DONALD McCLAY, JOHN STANSFIELD and H. C. CAISTOR. DONALD McCLAY also produced the play.

Under the heading "Woolly Vest", the Bacup Times reported that "one of the leading characters needs a woolly one-piece. He has not one himself and feels that the present cold spell will not encourage a fortunate possessor to loan an ankle-length garment of such comforting warmth". The Greenfield Players of Darwen apparently solved that problem.

Summing up, the Bacup Times reporter said "On looking I noticed smiles everywhere, with roars of laughter continually filling the auditorium". Let's hope that Philip King's farce has the same effect forty years on!

FIG. 7.1. Rossendale Players present 'See How they Run', September 1988

CHURCH DIARY FOR FEBRUARY.

Tues.	2nd.	Men's Fellowship - 7.30 p.m.
Sun.	7th.	Morning Worship - 10.30 a.m. Communion Service - 3.00 p.m. Olive House Service - 6.00 p.m.
Mon.	8th.	Social Committee Annual General Meeting.
Tues.	9th.	Ladies' Fellowship - 2.30 p.m.
Sun.	14th.	Family & Parade Service - 10.30 a.m. Afternoon Worship - 3.00 p.m.
Tues.	16th.	Tuesday Club - 7.30 p.m.
Sat.	20th.	Tuesday Club Coffee Morning 10 a.m. - noon.
Sun.	21st.	Morning Worship - 10.30 a.m. Service of Healing in Worship - 3.00 p.m. NEWSLETTER NOTES DUE.
Tues.	23rd.	'Man Alive' at the Astoria, Rawtenstall.
Wed.	24th.	Annual Church Meeting - 7.30 p.m.
Sun.	28th.	Morning Worship - 10.30 a.m. Afternoon " - 3.00 p.m.

LOOKING AHEAD.

Friday March 4th. Womens World Day of Prayer - 2.30 p.m.

March 12th./13th. "AUSTRIAN WEEK-END" with Pastor Porkorny.

Friday March 18th. Scripture Examination 7.00 p.m.

Saturday March 19th. Beetle Drive.

FIG. 7.2. Trinity Baptist Church programme for February 1988

THE CLASSES

All the classes we have on offer, at the Centre, are free to the Unemployed and their partners. Fee-paying students are made equally welcome.

Most of the classes are run in conjunction with Accrington and Rossendale College of further education. Some of our classes are run on a Skill sharing basis, this means that the time and expertise of the Tutors are given freely so that the classes are given free of charge to all. This term the Skill sharing classes are - Typing, French and German.

The classes are run in a very informal, friendly atmosphere. There is no set curriculum so if you miss a class due to sickness, bad weather or any of lifes ups and downs, you will be allowed to carry on at your own time and speed.

If you have a young child, they will be well taken care of in our supervised creche.

For more information concerning the classes or any other function at the Centre. Why not call in and see us for a chat? The kettles always on.

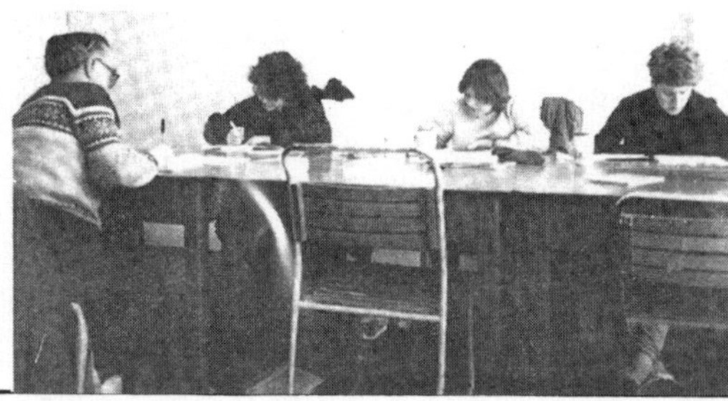

The Timetable for the Classes

MONDAY	ART FOR ALL	1.00 - 3.00pm.
	*FRENCH	1.30 - 3.30pm.
TUESDAY	HAIR AND BEAUTY	10.00 - 12.00am.
	*TYPING	1.30 - 3.00pm.
WEDNESDAY	BASIC MATHS	9.30 - 11.30am.
	BASIC ENGLISH	1.00 - 3.00pm.
	*GERMAN	7.00 - 9.00pm.
THURSDAY	FABRIC PAINTING & HOME FASHION	1.00 - 3.00pm.
FRIDAY	BUDGET DRESSMAKING	1.30 - 3.30pm.

*Denotes Skill Sharing Class

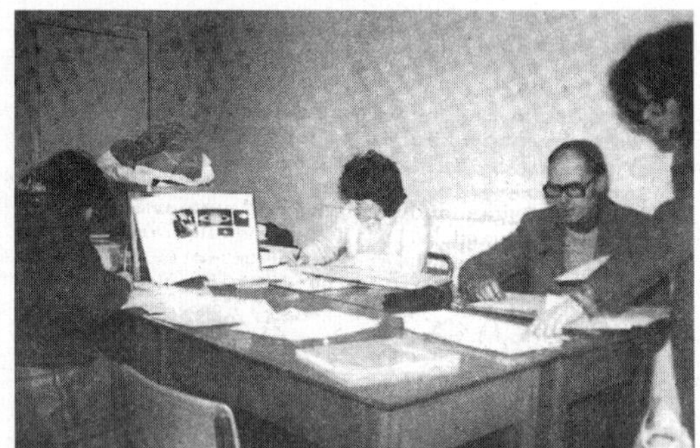

FIG. 7.3. Timetable for classes at UWC, 1987–8

The Britannia Coco-Nut Dancers of Bacup

Appeals to an idyllic past, or evidence of Anglo-Saxon battles, or a harsh climate and rugged environment, all feed in to the idea of Bacup as idiosyncratic and unique. Th'owd characters such as Alice from Wigan, Robert the Devil, and Mad Ab embody qualities perceived to be inherent in the Bacup character. Their bizarre and idiosyncratic appearance and behaviour convey a distinctiveness and eccentricity which set them apart. They stand for Bacup and person and place are interchangeable; telling of their exploits reveals the uniqueness and idiosyncrasy of Bacup and the expertise of the narrator. In addition to the old characters, there are new characters also claimed as truly or typically Bacupian. Chapters 5 and 6 dwelt on ways in which certain family names are associated with original or typical Bacup people, and the different evaluations made of such stature. I want to extend a similar claim to the Britannia Coco-Nut Dancers of Bacup, known locally as the Nutters.[3] They also provide a powerful symbol of the distinctive and idiosyncratic nature of the town. They are considered to be typically and uniquely Bacupian, and are therefore invoked in both inclusive and exclusive ways. Symbolic boundaries, conceptually separating and thereby creating categories of person are not fixed and nor do they bound empty space.[4] They collectivize and, at the same time, locate those collectivities inside or outside moral communities. The idiosyncratic and unique character of the Coco-Nutters may be evoked as an asset or as a failing, but either way the power to do so rests on the notion that they are typically Bacup; that they are, in other words, exclusively attached and inextricably connected. As such, they personify Bacup and provide, on the one hand, an image for inclusion (positively embracing all that is typically Bacupian), and on the other, an image for exclusion (rejecting all that is typically Bacupian). The Coco-Nutters serve to conceptualize inclusive and exclusive boundaries not only between Bacup and non-Bacup but between categories of person within Bacup.

The explicit analogy I wish to make between the Nutters (of the present) and th'owd characters (of the past) is not one made in Bacup itself. My reasons for linking the two lie not only in the singular appearance and inimitable activities of both, but also because they are both made to stand for Bacup: either all that is good or all that is bad, depending on the angle from which they are viewed[5] and the reason for animating them. Furthermore, the Nutters are evidence of an unbroken continuity with the past and their public appearances symbolize the survival of a unique and resilient Bacup in the face of social and economic change. Patty Cooper, an incoming spouse from Haslingdon,

[3] For a detailed description of the dances, readers are referred to Buckland (1986).

[4] I am grateful to Ursula Sharma (pers. comm.) for prodding me not to forget that symbolic boundaries have contents.

[5] Or the hill on which one sits (Le Guin).

observed, 'History is very important in Bacup. Where else has a museum like Bacup? and look at the Coco-Nutters. Without the Coco-Nutters, Bacup would lose its pride.'

Patty often commented on the distinctiveness of Bacup and often implied that my choice of fieldwork site was both wise and obvious. She thought Bacup a fascinating and intriguing place and particularly good for my purposes as a student of social anthropology. She assumed, despite my explanations to the contrary, that my interest was in real Bacup people and not people, such as herself, who came from elsewhere. She reminded me often that she was not herself 'from Bacup' and consequently her knowledge of the town was limited. But, at the same time, she also believed herself to be well placed to tell me about Bacup, particularly as she married into a real Bacup family. In her comment about the Coco-Nutters, she explicitly associated their survival with the survival of Bacup. Just as people need pride, so do places.

The Coco-Nutters are a group of men who, with blackened faces, colourful costumes, and ornate clogs, dance a series of complex choreographed dances at least once a year in the streets of Bacup. The dance troupe comprises eight dancers and a 'whipper-in' or 'whiffler'. Once a year, on Easter Saturday (known locally as Nutters' Day) they dance on the streets in a circuit which symbolizes the perimeters of Bacup. The day begins at about 9 a.m. in a public house on the southern boundary of Bacup in Britannia and ends early evening

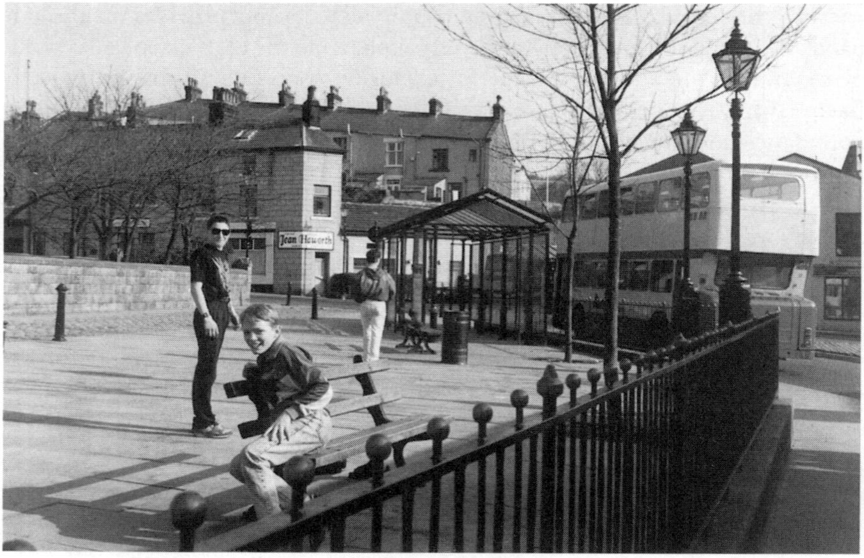

PLATE 12. Town square paved with Yorkshire stone

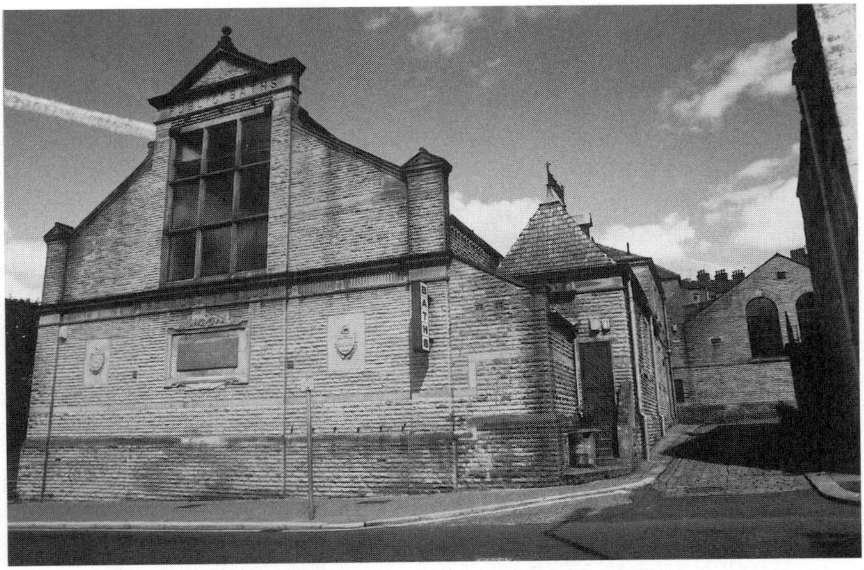

PLATE 13. Swimming baths

on the western edge in Stacksteads. Dancers are preceded by the Stacksteads Silver Band and flanked by supporters and friends shaking collection boxes and urging spectators to make an offering.

The Coco-Nutters perform two types of dance—Nut Dances and Garland Dances. The Nut Dances feature the rhythmic sound of nuts (hard wooden discs) being brought into contact with each other and one of the Nut Dances allows dancers to progress, at speed, along the route. The dances are well suited to the hilly terrain of Bacup and what were once predominantly cobblestoned streets. The sound of iron-soled clogs on the cobblestones would have augmented the rhythmic and loud ringing of the nuts as they were brought into contact with each other. The Garland Dances are performed in quadrille formation, at prearranged sites along the route. These dances revolve around garlands which are hoops of cane decorated with red, white, and blue ribbon and crepe paper. Buckland (1986: 142) describes their repertoire thus:

> This corpus consists of five garland dance figures, performed in quadrille formation and known by number, one to five; a coconut dance executed again in quadrille formation; a road dance consisting of stationary figures interspersed with a running polka step, which is danced by two files of four dancers staggered on each side of the road; and the 'Nut dance' performed in a linear stationary formation by all eight dancers.

The dancers blacken their faces with face paint (they used to use lamp black). They wear white cotton hats to which red, white, and blue pom-poms are attached, and black sweaters crossed diagonally with a band of red, white, and blue. There are 'male' and 'female' dancers. The 'ladies' have a blue rather than red ribbon on their hats, and their bands cross the left shoulder rather than the right.[6] All the dancers wear short white skirts circled with hoops of red and worn over black, knee-length breeches. Knee-high white stockings cover the lower part of their legs and on their feet are highly polished wooden and leather clogs. The clogs have leather uppers, with intricate patterns beautifully etched into the leather, and they are the focus of much attention and admiration. The wooden soles are trimmed with 'irons' and a full day of dancing on Easter Saturday will, it is predicted, completely wear out one pair of irons.

Several derivations of the name of the dance troupe are given; all associate the name Coco-Nutters with the hard wooden discs (the nuts) attached to the wrists, knees, and waists of the dancers. The nuts are generally made from maple and are about four inches in diameter.[7] A loud, ringing sound is created as the wrist nuts are brought repetitively and elegantly, with a circular movement of the arm, into contact with each other and with the knee and waist nuts.

On Easter Saturday the dancers pay a visit to most public houses along the route, as well as to working men's clubs, residential homes for the elderly, particular neighbourhoods, and the fire station. Spectators line the route, some follow the dancers all or part of the way, and a crowd gathers at each Garland Dance venue. Performances in, or outside, pubs and clubs are usually rounded off with dancers, the band, and followers having a drink (usually beer) and some venues lay out sandwiches for the participants. Mr Dearden, a Coco-Nutter for thirty years, a highly accomplished dancer, and often delegated as the group's spokesperson, told me that although the Nutters had a reputation for being hard drinkers, it was not true. The rumour, he said, stemmed historically from the fact that troupes of dancers always met in backrooms of pubs in order to change and black up. Some stories of origin, however, include the fact that dancers were predominantly poorly paid millhands and money they collected from dancing on the streets went to pay for beer.

Origins: From Moorish Pirates to Cornish Coal Miners

The Coco-Nut Dancers have compiled a brief history of their activities which they copy and distribute to interested parties, and which includes ideas about the origin of the dances. It comprises a bricolage of items, some pertaining to economic class and others to religion, which portray an exotic and extraordinary past. The blackened faces and unusual costumes have been attributed,

[6] One of the dancers told me he learnt as 'a lady' when he joined the Coco-Nutters in 1958. He explained that in the Garland Dances, 'the gents' part is twice as easy—the ladies have to do all the work'.

[7] Nuts were originally made from the tops of bobbins (Froome 1953).

say the Coco-Nutters, to Moorish pirates which, together with the nuts, has led to speculation that the dances originated in the South Sea islands. Closer to home, the dances are said to have arrived in Bacup with immigrant miners from Cornwall, and more specifically with two Cornish miners who settled in Whitworth and taught the dances to local men. In this story, the nuts were inspired by the discs worn by miners to protect their hands and knees whilst crawling underground. Further evidence for this story of origin lies in the choreography of at least one of the dances. Each dancer, in turn and in line, cups his hand behind his ear as if listening out for the preceding sound which is passed along the line. This sequence is said to mimic the way in which miners communicated underground, relying on sound rather than sight.

Other origin stories include items about pagan rituals performed to ensure fertility of the land and the well-being of the community. The whipper-in or whiffler, who precedes the eight dancers in line formation, carries a whip. In one exegesis his role is to drive away evil spirits from the dancers and, by extension, from Bacup (today he also controls traffic and spectators). Dancers disguise themselves from those same evil spirits (and it is said from colleagues and neighbours) by blackening their faces. It has been suggested by different commentators that in tracing the boundaries of Bacup and in chasing away evil spirits the Coco-Nut dancers traditionally played a crucial part in spring agricultural festivals, ensuring fertility and abundant harvests.

Stuart Watson, an incoming spouse from Rochdale, related the pagan ritual exegesis, and likened the Nutters to 'modern-day ghost busters'. He was one of the few residents of Bacup who, when I asked about the meaning of the dances, appeared even vaguely interested in the question. It was Stuart who described my role as 'a folklorist—binding the community together [by] collecting people's stories'. Generally Bacup people appear not to be interested in attaching meaning to the Coco-Nutters and their activities. They neither tell stories of origin, nor provide explanations for the event. They do, however, locate themselves in a history which includes them. Thus, several residents described how as children they accompanied the dancers every Easter Saturday; they talked of the festivities associated with the day and the crowds which gathered to celebrate the event. Elderly residents recall that there used to be an array of dance troupes each associated with a particular neighbourhood and usually a specific mill. Implicit in many of these comments is a comparison between what used to be a thriving and busy mill town and a present-day economically depressed community marked by unemployment and out-migration.

In their own history, the Coco-Nutters have appropriated and retextualized some of the many stories crafted about them. Certain myths of origin have been inspired by the romanticism of middle-class *aficionados* of folk-dance, who in their self-ascribed task of preserving what they call tradition and antiquity, have been interested in presenting an image of an idyllic rural peasantry whose traditions and rituals were in danger of being irretrievably lost. But the Coco-Nutters themselves acknowledge the uncertainty surrounding the stories of origin. For them a search for a *true* etymology is best left to others; what appears to be more significant to the Coco-Nutters themselves is their role in the present. They conclude their own history by emphasizing their present-day impact: 'whatever the history one thing is certain, wherever the "Nutters" go their appearance and the name of Bacup remain vivid in the memory of the people, because nowhere in Great Britain is there a traditional team quite like us. In a word we are unique.'

The synthesis of stories of origin presented by the Coco-Nutters in their own potted history has been partly inspired by the concerns of those who have taken it upon themselves to write the history of the dances on their behalf. It is also inspired by commonly held views which conflate the Coco-Nutters with Bacup. Their idiosyncratic and unique past mirrors an idiosyncratic and unique Bacup, both past and present. The perception of uniqueness is valued positively—as an asset—but at the same time its value can be subverted and, from another perspective, the same uniqueness used to set both the Coco-Nutters and Bacup apart.

Nutters' Day 1988

The dancers, the band, and their supporters meet on Easter Saturday morning on the northern Bacup boundary. In 1988, a crowd of twenty or so spectators had gathered to see them set off. The dancers emerged at 9 a.m. to a cheer and they performed the first Garland Dance of the day. Then they danced downhill, in a line, from Britannia towards Bacup, stopping briefly for a Garland Dance outside the next public house along the way. They then took a detour, away from the main road, to Olive Mount, a residential home for elderly people. They danced outside the entrance and staff of the home helped less mobile residents to doors or windows so they could see the dances and hear the music. The dancers, band, supporters, and accompanying spectators (whom I shall call followers) returned, walking, to the main road. The Coco-Nutters proceeded to dance again and momentum gathered as the number of followers increased the nearer the dancers got to the centre of town. They danced outside the fire station, situated on the road entering Mount Pleasant, and were served a cup of tea by uniformed firemen. They danced at two more venues, outside a block of pensioners' flats and a public house, before reaching the centre of town where a crowd of spectators waited expectantly for their arrival. A cheer was raised as the Coco-Nutters came into view and they danced, amidst applause and whistles, into the town centre. After a Garland Dance, on the newly paved area outside the Conservative Club, and a few poses for photographs, they divided into two groups. One group danced in the Conservative Club and the other in a nearby public house, after which they downed a

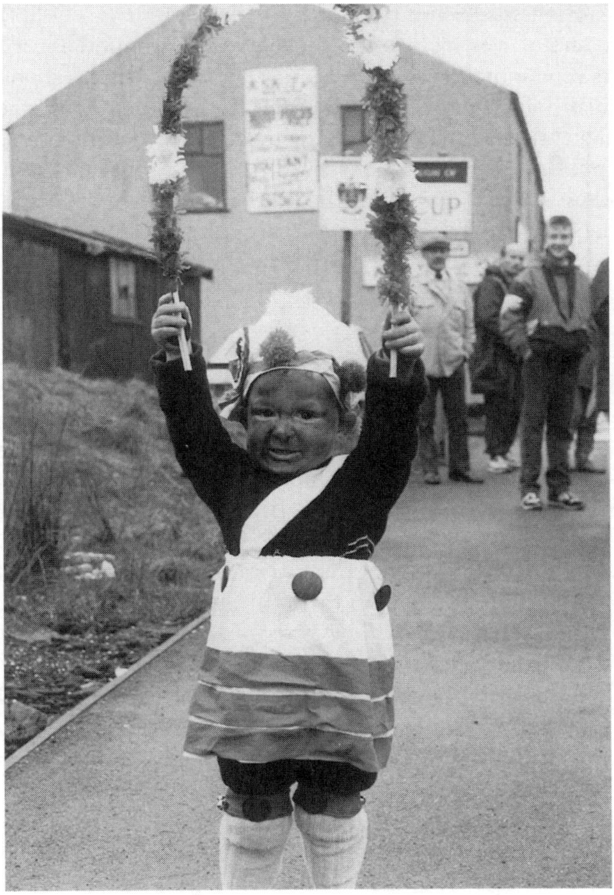

PLATE 14. Waiting for the Coco-Nutters

swift half and regrouped. They then proceeded on the road north from the town centre. Two Garland Dances were performed: one outside a public house straddling the river Irwell and the other in front of pensioners' flats, housing, amongst others, retired and elderly mill- and quarry-workers. From there, they backtracked at a walk, and the final leg of the journey proceeded westwards along the valley floor through to Stacksteads. Followers were shed from, and attracted to, the procession as the troupe danced intermittently along the route. And although the last stretch was long and the dancers tired, spectators were numerous and encouraging. Garland Dances were performed, and beer drunk, at a number of venues along the way, and the final dance of the day, with dancers mustering surprising reserves of energy (after ten hours), took place on the forecourt of a petrol station on the western boundary of Bacup. The few followers remaining raised a cheer and the Coco-Nutters shook hands with them, each other, and members of the band. Dancers and band members congratulated each other and cars belonging to friends or family transported them back to the public house from which they had begun that morning. The landlady had laid on refreshments and I heard that the celebration and retelling of the performance and the day continued through the evening and well into the night.

Origins—Local Lads?

In 1988, there were nine Coco-Nutters and two apprentices. Records show there were at least four groups of Coco-Nut Dancers in Rossendale at the turn of the nineteenth century and the present day troupe is said to be descended from the Tunstead Mill Nutters, who celebrated their half century in 1907.[8] In the recent past they were named the Bacup Coco-Nutters, but this caused ill feeling amongst certain residents of Britannia who argued that they ought to make explicit the fact that this group were from Britannia. Marilyn Greaves recalled being quite upset when, in the local press, they were called the Bacup Coco-Nutters. She was pleased they had now been given their 'proper title'. Aware of such criticisms and of the nuances of a name, the troupe is now officially called the Britannia Coco-Nut Dancers of Bacup. When I asked Mrs Jones what they did, she said she did not know, but told me 'they used to start at Stacksteads, but now they start at Britannia seeing as they're the Britannia Coco-Nutters'.

Any suggestion that Bacup be dropped from their title is also met with disapproval. Britannia might be included under the rubric of 'Bacup', but Bacup is not encompassed by 'Britannia'. The Coco-Nutters stand for Bacup and as such symbolize its well-being. The town's survival and continuation is imaged in the Coco-Nutters and in their dances which are unique to Bacup. In so far as the Nutters are claimed by Bacup people as 'belonging' to the town and thus to them, it is expedient for dancers to show evidence of appropriate Bacup qualifications. Consequently, when I asked individual dancers where they came from I was often answered 'Rossendale', rather than a specific place-name. The fact that, in 1988/9, three members of the group lived in Bacup (one in Britannia), four in Waterfoot, one in Rawtenstall, and the most recent member in Rochdale, is not something that the dancers themselves dwell upon. For them to draw attention to places of birth or residence outside Bacup would be to compromise the connection between Bacup and the Coco-Nutters.

[8] Tunstead is a neighbourhood that grew up around two mills of the same name, west of the town centre on the road to Stacksteads.

They do, however, emphasize the fact they are 'folk-dancers' *not* Morris dancers. They deny any similarity between themselves and Morris dancers. Such a distinction reinforces the link between the Coco-Nutters and Bacup. Mr Dearden explained that Morris dances originate from many parts of the country, and each group of Morris dancers performs a variety of dances which originate from different places. Folk-dancers, on the other hand, perform only 'their own' dances. The seven Coco-Nut dances—five Garland and two Nut Dances—are performed only by the Bacup Coco-Nutters. Dance and dancer belong to Bacup. Consequently the arrangement and steps of each dance, I was told, are guarded as secret. Place, person, and dance are implicated in each other. The Coco-Nutters know themselves to be unique and they emphasize this quality as a positive attribute. They acknowledge that their uniqueness makes them worthy of study and provides an imperative for them to continue dancing and recruiting new members.

Recruitment depends on several attributes: commitment, skill, and tenacity are said to be necessary qualities of neophytes. New members tend to be friends, relatives, or work partners of existing members. Mr Dearden, for example, joined from an advertisement in the press, although his brother was already a member and since then two of his brothers-in-law have also been members. A new member has to be proposed, the proposal supported, and the whole troupe has to agree. To be considered as an apprentice at all, men must be married. Mr Dearden explained that this is because the repertoire of dances takes at least two years to learn completely, so there has to be a strong commitment to learning and to practising, and men who are courting are easily distracted. There are also those who join and who find learning the dances too difficult.

> Quite a lot come to join and within two or three months find they're not going to be able to do it. Co-ordination between hands and feet is difficult. It's easier to learn the Garland Dances because you're in pairs. Every movement has a name and you have to learn all the movements. It takes about three years before you can dance without prompts.

The dancers with whom I spoke emphasized the enjoyment they got out of being a Coco-Nutter. Their performances at national and European dance festivals provide affirmation of their uniqueness and a forum where their skills are recognized and applauded. Locally they accrue prestige from their public role and visibility and have been the subject of numerous poems, articles, and features in the local newspapers. Here are the first four verses of a poem entitled 'Eawr Nutters'. It was written *c.*1952 by Bill o' Bows.[9]

> Eawr Nutter's are comin', they're dancin' in t'street,
> Ther's crowds standin' watchin' all havin' a treat,

[9] A fuller version of the poem can be found in *A Bacup Miscellany* (1972).

In red and white costumes, wi' faces all black
An' t' coco-shells beatin' a-crack-a-jack-crack.

Th'owd Lancashire clogs are tappin' eawt t'tune,
An' youngest to th'owdest familiarly croon

For year after year it's bin handed deawn,
This melody played when they're dancin' through t'teawn.

It coom first of all, well, so Ah've bin towd,
When th'owd Cornish miners invaded eawr fowd,
Areawnd Wit'orth valley an' o'er Tunstead way,
'Til 1907 showed a Jubilee day.

Fifty long year o' Folk Dancin' in t'street,
Fro' mornin' 'til midday, 'til lat' on at neet,
Fifty long years sin' Tunstead began,
A team wer then formed up at good owd Britann'.

The present group have also taken part in a number of television programmes and perform at a variety of national folk-dancing events and competitions. Dis-

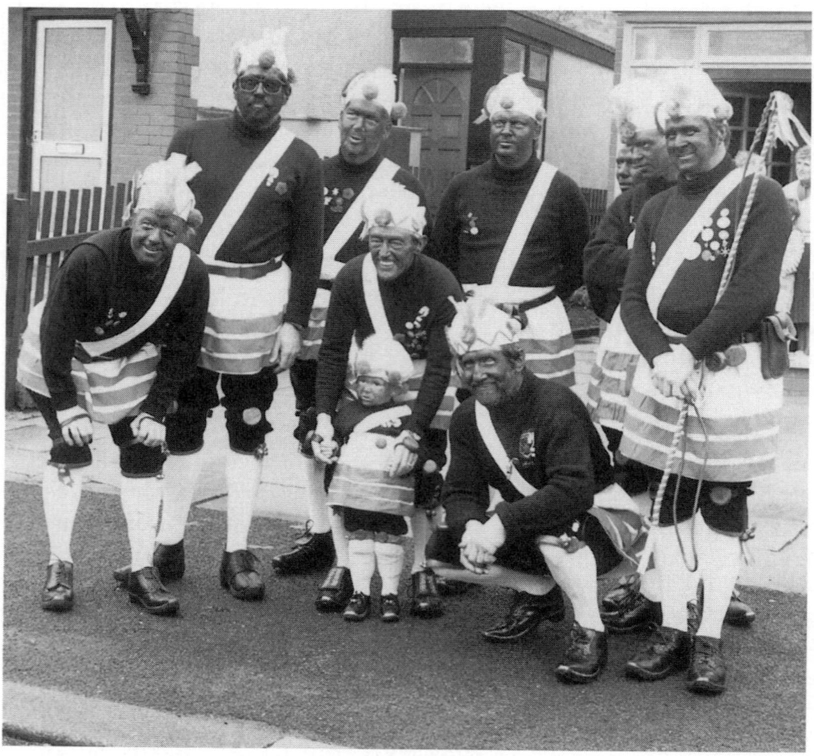

PLATE 15. The Britannia Coco-Nut Dancers of Bacup, 1988

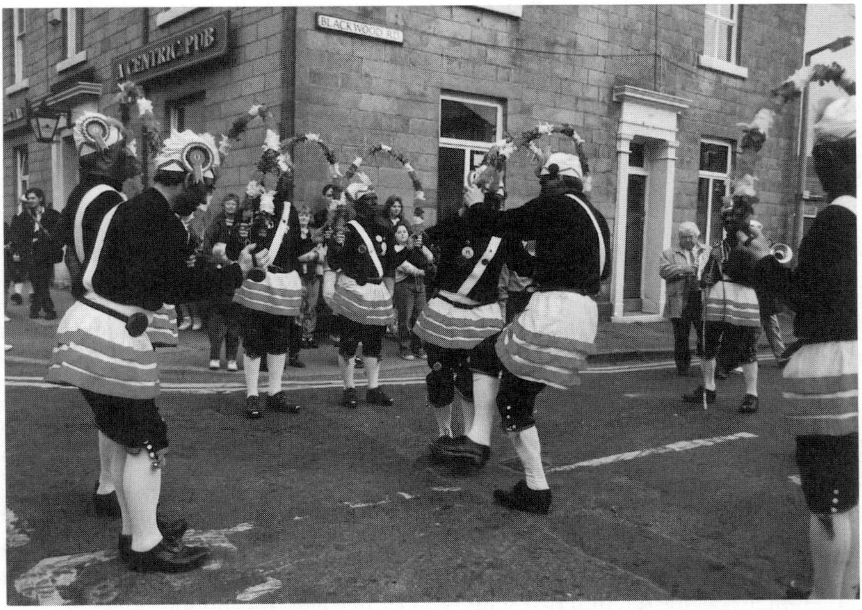

PLATE 16. A Garland Dance

cussing their role with me, several members of the team talked of preserving a 'tradition' which, without their efforts, would be lost. They were highly critical of the approach of one television presenter of a programme on which they were invited. They had been ridiculed, and one of them explained that, even though they knew the programme was billed as 'light entertainment', they had not anticipated nor predicted the mocking tone of the presenter. Given their role in preserving a 'tradition', he felt they deserved more respect. He could understand why a social anthropologist might be interested in them as not only were they keeping the past alive, but they were unique. The Coco-Nutters and their dances have been studied extensively by folklorists and *aficionados* of dance and they perceive themselves to be a legitimate focus of academic study. They expect experts to be interested in the complexity of their dances, in their role as preservers of tradition, in the ritual of Easter Saturday and, importantly, in their uniqueness.

In the face of what they perceive to be a decline in the 'thriving community' of Bacup, we have seen how some residents strive to make explicit the special and unique nature of Bacup and its people. The harsh physical environment, a distinctive dialect, idiosyncratic characters and unique traditions are among some of the hooks on which distinctiveness can be hung. Such explicitness counteracts what many people perceive as a trend towards uniformity. A uniformity said to be manifest in, amongst other things, dress ('everyone looks the same now'), the anonymity of supermarket shopping, and BBC English. Ennew (1980: 121), in her research in the Western Isles, also refers to features such as these as constitutive of 'bland English culture'. She shares with Bacup people a similar idea about what is distinctive and what is therefore worthy of anthropological study. Bacup might be considered an example of 'English culture', but it is far from bland.

A Private Club Sort-of-Thing

The lengthy apprenticeship needed to become a Coco-Nutter is given as reason for accepting only married men into the group. Young unmarried men, it is thought, are unlikely to show the commitment and tenacity required to become a Nutter. It also takes a great deal of commitment to teach the large number of steps and complicated sequences entailed. Hence the Coco-Nutters have to be sure that apprentices are keen and will continue. Practice sessions are held one evening a week in Stacksteads Conservative Club, where dancers are accompanied by two concertina players. The short practice session is preceded by a business meeting and afterwards some members leave and others have a drink together. I attended only one regular practice session but was invited to the annual pre-Easter practice which takes place at the public house in Britannia from which, on Easter Saturday, the procession begins and in which, in the evening, the celebration ends. Mr Dearden told me this would be more interesting for my purposes as the weekly practice sessions were a 'private club sort-of-thing'. 'It's the get together (that's important) . . . they're a fine bunch of people. There's never a cross word between us, might be disagreements but we talk about it and sort it out.'

There is evidence in the way in which members talk about their activities that they, like other Bacup people, place a positive value on self-help. Like Nat members, they say they are creating their own entertainment while contributing something to Bacup. They are helping both themselves and Bacup. 'Fun' is also a dominant theme running through Coco-Nut narratives: dancing is fun, as are the social relationships entailed, and there is also pleasure in giving pleasure. Mr Dearden is often asked 'what the heck do you do it for?' He supposes its 'a selfish attitude' that keeps him going. He explains: 'You're able to see the pleasure you can give other folk and you get pleasure out of seeing that.' He quotes from a song that used to be sung about the Coco-Nutters: 'If smiles and bright eyes are wages that they earn then they all must be millionaires.'

Contested Values

On Easter Saturday, the Nat opens its doors. An exhibition of photographs of 'owd Bacup' is mounted and members sell refreshments and provide guided tours around the museum. Nat member Bernard Thomas complained about the Nutters: 'They ought to play more. They dance today and at other gigs but they're not seen enough. People are proud of them.' This echoes Patty Cooper's remark that 'without the Coco-Nutters, Bacup would lose its pride'. Despite claiming quite different connections to Bacup, both Mr Thomas and Mrs Cooper agree on the effect and significance of the Coco-Nutters. They are a source of Bacup pride and their appearance affirms the place and its people. However, as in other symbolic resources, the value attached to them is not always positive. As 'traditionally' Bacup they can be used as evidence of both all that is good and all that is bad.

Before Easter of 1988, and before I had given the Coco-Nutters much thought, I went to visit Shirley Gray, Alan Gray's niece (brother's daughter). She is 21 years old, Bacup born and bred, and lives with her partner and child on the outskirts of town. Laura Gray had suggested I meet Shirley as, having 'opted out', she was bound to have different 'take' on Bacup.[10] Laura introduced me, in what were by now familiar (but still discomforting) terms, as somebody who was 'trying to find out about Bacup'. Shirley smiled knowingly, perhaps conspiratorially. Wordlessly she made it clear there was a great deal 'to find out about'. She asked if I had seen the Coco-Nutters yet, conveying in a few words, with a tone of voice and a look, what she perceived to be the bizarre nature of such a custom and such a group of people. In so doing, she appeared to distance herself from Bacup and its peculiarities and create for herself a category of distant observer. The next time I met Shirley was on Nutters' Day. She was walking with her child, like me, behind the dancers, and had been waiting for them, like many mothers with their children, in the town centre. She told me it was important to bring the children to see the Nutters, and suggested they would 'miss out' if they did not see them. Like many people that day, she also told me they were 'not as good' as last year.

On the same day, Jake Watson (Pam's son) stood on the doorstep of his house and watched the Coco-Nutters dance past. I stood awhile with him, changing the batteries in my tape recorder. After a while, he remarked loudly and with feeling: 'I hate them and their music.' There was little more he would say on the subject, but conveyed disdain in the way a teenager can with seemingly little effort. Although I was left in no doubt that Jake did not like the Coco-Nutters and their music, his hostility had as much to do with the way in which the Nutters are put to work as a potent symbol of Bacup continuity as with a matter of taste. Obviously Jake told me he hated the Coco-Nutters because he did, but the point is the Coco-Nutters are good to hate. Jake explicitly breaks the connection between himself and the Coco-Nutters and denies the unchanging and enduring tradition with which the Coco-Nutters are associated. The past of Bacup and its present-day boundaries, rendered visible in the activities of the Coco-Nutters, are too restricting for him and he needs to

[10] Opted out—elsewhere 'hippie'.

breach them. The Coco-Nutters, standing as they do for a quintessential Bacup, provide a readily available and identifiable image of all that is typically Bacup from which to exclude oneself.

Being an Audience

Speaking of the audience on Nutters' Day, Barbara Jones echoed an opinion often put forward by recent immigrants, but in a different context. Bacup people, she said, are not interested in 'preserving their heritage': 'People in Bacup—locals—don't support local things. They don't bother. They're not interested.' Pam Watson made a similar point, but this time to show up the idiocy of visitors who follow the Nutters around all day. She summed up the attitude of what she considered to be the majority of Bacup people in this way: 'Bacup folk don't give them a second thought. No one follows them the whole route. They see them in the town centre and don't think of them again.'

Both Barbara Jones and Pam Watson draw on the same evidence—Bacup people 'are not bothered'. 'Not to bother' is evidence of either apathy or pragmatism and which is evoked depends on the way in which speakers place themselves. The evidence that Bacup people do not pay the same kind of attention to the Coco-Nutters as visitors or incomers is put to work in different ways. Barbara excludes herself from a category of 'locals [who] don't support local things', while Pat includes herself amongst the pragmatic Bacup folk who do not *need* to follow the Coco-Nutters all day and the whole way. Like neighbouring, it is not that a fine line is drawn between bothering too much and bothering too little, but each is used inclusively or exclusively. Barbara went on to express a resentment towards what she called 'the professor-types' who were 'taking over' the dances. She explained how it was becoming increasingly more difficult to watch the Coco-Nutters on Easter Saturday as the view was often blocked by a growing number of visitors with cameras, tape recorders, and videos. She includes under the rubric of 'professor types' all visitors who, from this perspective, are attempting to appropriate that which does not belong to them. Outsiders, armed with trappings of technological status, are collecting a record of the event which will then be unhitched from its mooring and disconnected from where it belongs. Bacup people perceive themselves to have a prior claim on the Coco-Nutters, and consequently the Coco-Nutters (who stand for Bacup) have an obligation to them rather than to professor types.

Pam Watson also contrasts visitors with locals and she does so in terms of who *needs* to follow the Coco-Nutters from start to finish. She includes herself within a category of pragmatic Bacup folk who do not make the same kind of fuss over the Coco-Nutters (and other things axiomatically Bacupian) as the visitor or the incomer, both of whom are revealed in this formulation as unconnected to Bacup. A distinction is revealed between those who are interested in the Coco-Nutters academically (in the abstract) but have no claim on them (the visitor), and those who are neither interested in interpreting the dances nor in following their every move but who have an axiomatic claim on them and are thus inextricably connected (Bacup people).

Both Barbara Jones and Pam Watson use the Coco-Nutters to image a distinction between belonging and not belonging. The issue at stake is not about the women belonging to Bacup but about the Coco-Nutters belonging to Bacup and therefore about who can legitimately lay claim to them. They agree that the Coco-Nutters, as 'truly Bacupian', ought to be supported, but what that entails takes a variety of forms. As a Bacup person, one may express only mild or fleeting interest but still be attached to them. In fact to be too zealous (like the visitor) belies an axiomatic connection. Visitors, in showing a keen and undiscriminating interest, reveal their outside status.

One evening I attended a meeting of the Ladies' Fellowship at the Baptist church to which one of the Coco-Nutters had been invited as a guest speaker. He gave a short talk about the Coco-Nutters and described his costume, paying particular attention to the clogs. His talk provoked many narratives about the

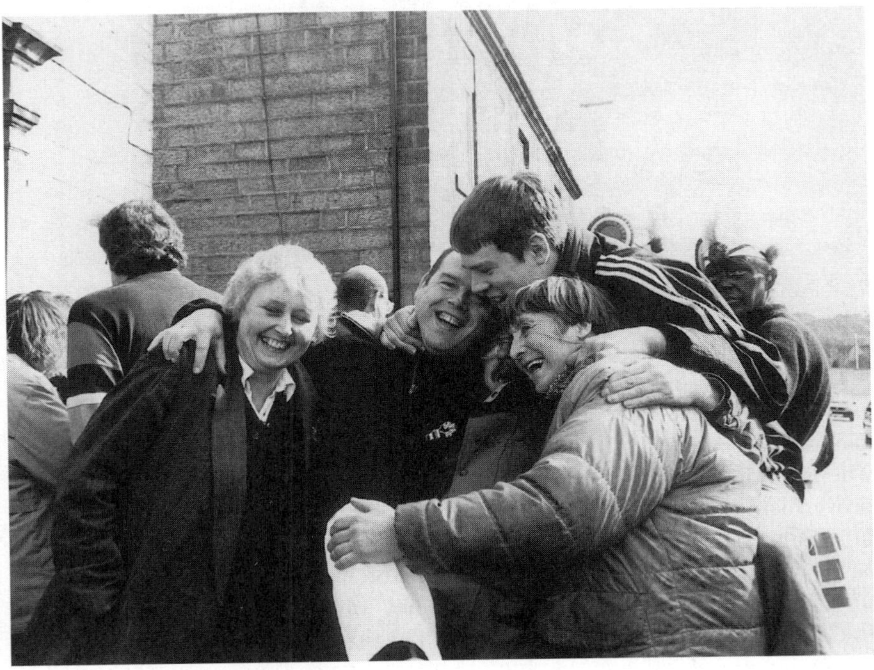

PLATE 17. Being an audience: 1

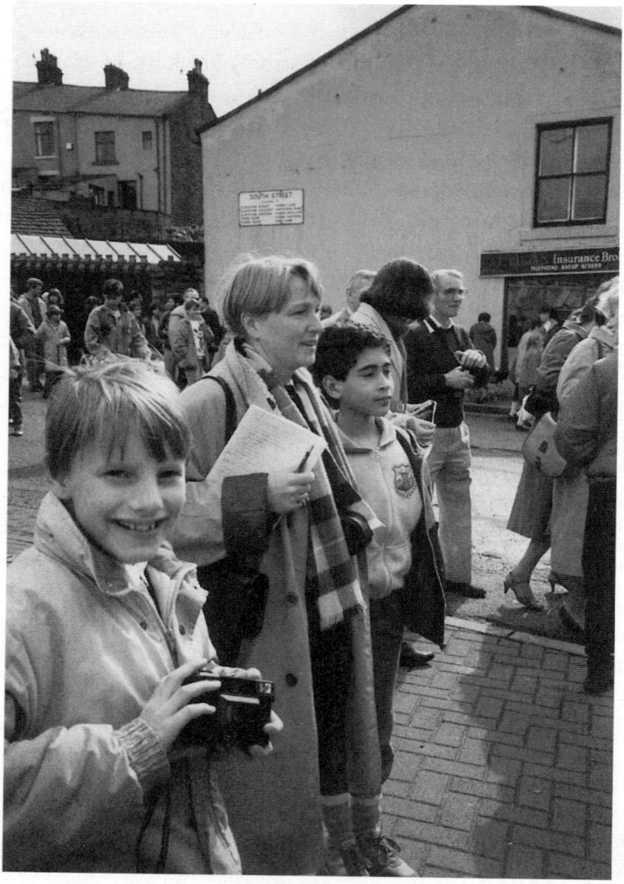

PLATE 18. Being an audience: 2

past and the women contributed with memories of past Easter Saturdays and their own experiences of and relationships with past Coco-Nutters. Their narratives were filled with pride and relatedness and many women traced connections to former dancers, through family, friends, and neighbours. I asked whether women had ever been Coco-Nutters. The question went down like the proverbial ton of bricks. It was ignored by some of the women and answered, in no uncertain terms, by others: women had *never* been Coco-Nutters and *never* would be, I was told. The women who engaged passionately with my question assumed it was not innocent. They interpreted it as a suggestion for the future and consequently as a criticism of the present. They were indignant at the thought of 'allowing' women to become Coco-Nutters, and their indignation was fuelled by the fact that such a suggestion had been mooted by an outsider; a person with neither present-day attachments to Bacup, nor connections with its past. An appeal to the continuity of tradition was made; one woman telling me the tradition should be kept as it was, and another explaining if women joined, 'the tradition would be spoiled'.

The Coco-Nutters provide an image of that which belongs exclusively to Bacup (no other dance troupe performs the Coco-Nut dances). In turn, they are claimed exclusively by Bacup (nobody else, anywhere else, has Coco-Nut dancers). The majority of today's dancers do not live in Bacup, and as outsiders looking in, they may draw on the same symbolic resources in placing themselves as other incomers. Hence they may locate Bacup on a periphery and call it 'the back of beyond' and impute to it those qualities associated with remote places such as parochialism, interrelatedness, and fixity. After the Coco-Nutters had passed through the town centre and were on their way to Stacksteads, one of the dancers remarked: 'They'll be fighting now in Bacup.' Earlier one of their supporters, who carried a collection box and cajoled spectators to contribute money, explaind they no longer included Mount Pleasant in their itinerary because of the risk of collection boxes being stolen. These stereotypical comments act to dissociate the Coco-Nutters and their supporters from Bacup. At the same time, however, it is crucial they maintain and make explicit their connection to the town: it is along those connections their credentials travel. In making explicit their connection to Bacup, they screen out other connections, for example, to places of origin (or residence). They bring into focus what they do—they do Coco-Nutting and the Coco-Nutters belong to Bacup.

I met Sylvia Conrad in the town centre. Sylvia was in her early twenties and she had brought her two young children to see the Nutters. She asked me, with evident pride, what I thought of them and, after listening to my enthusiastic response, told me they were not as good as last year and not as many people had turned out to see them. She invited me to join her and her friends later on in the day, explaining: 'It'll get better later when we can go on the pop.'[11] Nutters' Day is considered by many young women as a holiday and a good night to go out and 'let loose'. Many take their children to see the dancers in the town centre and then leave them later in the care of babysitters (often their mother or younger sister, occasionally a neighbour). Unlike many young men who spend weekend afternoons drinking together, usually after playing or watching football, young women are rarely found in public houses during the day. But Easter Saturday is unusual; it is marked as a day outside the normal run of things and women, as much as men, ensure they begin celebrating as early in the day as possible.

Later that evening, I met Kate Murray. She asked me whether I had enjoyed the Nutters. I said I had, and she expressed a similar opinion to that put forward earlier by Sylvia Conrad and Shirley Gray: This year, Nutters' Day

[11] To go on the pop means to drink alcohol.

had not been as good as usual. Kate explained that not as many people had turned out and the Nutters had not danced for long enough. Of course people may have been intent on telling me the event was better last year because it was; indeed my recent visit to Nutters' Day bore out their observation that increasingly fewer people were turning out to watch them. At the same time, by impressing on me this point, they also emphasized the fact that they were there and I was not. They made explicit their links to the Coco-Nutters and hence to Bacup and made manifest their expertise.

The women at the church meeting defended tradition in the face of what they saw as a threat to it in the form of my question about whether women had ever been Coco-Nutters. The young women with whom I spoke on Nutters' Day, neither fetishize the Coco-Nutters as preservers of tradition, nor consider themselves in need of preservation as truly Bacupian. Nevertheless, they made an effort to ensure their young children saw the Nutters, they assessed their performance, and spoke with pride of past performances. These young women did not offer an exegesis of the ritual nor speak explicitly about the need to 'preserve tradition'. They did, however, acknowledge their connection to the Nutters. They compared events and performances and presented an opinion on how well the dancers had performed, exhibiting their own connections to Bacup (through their knowledge) and throwing into relief the unconnectedness of incomers like myself. And while they may have smiled ironically at the folly of the Nutters (as indeed the Nutters do themselves) they are allowed to because the Nutters belong to them. Just as the Coco-Nutters lay claim to Bacup (they are *the* folk-dancers of Bacup), so Bacup people claim the Coco-Nutters, and such claims always entail the possibility of rejection. Stories about, and knowledge of, the Nutters, like th'owd characters, the Nat, yuppies, or troublemakers, serve to differentiate between categories of resident by making certain links and obscuring others. Links between people, between people and pasts, and between pasts and places, mark those who do, and do not, belong. Like th'owd characters, the Coco-Nutters also disconnect; they are drawn upon to dissociate oneself from what is considered to be uniquely or typically Bacup. Similar to th'owd characters, to tell of the Coco-Nutters is to provide evidence of familiarity which throws into relief the unfamiliarity of those who do not know. But the way in which evidence is mobilized differs according to the questions people ask of themselves and the context created in the question. Status can lie in either including or excluding oneself from the same moral category as the Coco-Nutters. The point to make is that either is possible.

The Gardens

In the early spring of 1986, the local authority initiated what they called a programme of environmental landscaping. This exercise and the resultant changes remained an issue of conflict throughout my stay in Bacup. The layout of an area in the town centre had been altered: 'landscaped' according to council officials and 'demolished' according to some residents. When I arrived in 1987, the controversy was still raging. One town planner told me the scheme was part of a much wider plan to upgrade the town centre. He informed me the materials used were to be in keeping with the stone of the buildings in the town centre, some of which were now listed. Speculative builders, he went on, who had successfully bid for and were now renovating a row of two- and three-storey eighteenth-century buildings, had to maintain the original style and use the same building materials from which the buildings were originally constructed. In this spirit, the new town square is paved with Yorkshire flag and the lamp standards, seating, and bus shelters have been designed to include 'Victorian detail'. The intended effect, he said, was to 'preserve the olde worlde charm' of the town. These architectural changes remained, during my stay in Bacup, the focus of acrimonious debate. There was by no means whole-hearted support for the re-creation of 'an olde worlde charm' and the feasibility and desirability of such a project was hotly contested.

The paved area in front of the Conservative Club used to be what local people called the Gardens. They described flower-beds which were surrounded by benches and the whole enclosed by privet hedges. The landscaping entailed removing the hedges and the benches and paving over the flower-beds. A barrier of evenly spaced railings, ornately decorated, now separated the paved area from the road, and benches also sporting decorative ironwork were arranged in a line, facing the road, just behind the railings. The detail on the railings and benches, as well as on the bus shelter and lamp standards is in what local politicians and town planners call 'Victorian style'. This style, they said, was 'in keeping with the traditional architecture of the town'. One irony of the controversy is that while council officials intended the improvements to replicate what they perceived to be the traditional style of the town (which had never existed before then[12]), many Bacup people expressed their distress at the changes in terms of the 'destruction of tradition'. One man told me he missed

[12] I cannot resist this quotation from J. Marshall Mather who, writing in 1888 of his 'Rambles around Rossendale' (cited in Water Marks n.d.), described the river Irwell as it ran through the centre of Bacup as 'A fouled and pestiferous stream, churned into a filthy foam and discoloured with the refuse of a hundred mills . . . smooth stones once the glory of the river's boulder bed, all stained with the flow of blackened waters: and bobbins, corks, fragments of broken skips and the decaying carcasses of domestic animals, chasing one another as in a dance of death, amongst the swirls and eddies. Thus, before me runs the once beautiful river, now an open sink of feculant deposit, a miasma of death, a blackened and despoiling stream.' A Government Inspector's report written in 1849 for the General Board of Health noted how pollution from the mills as well as household sewage had by then exterminated all aquatic life in the river Irwell. The report likened the town's water supply to 'liquid manure'. Beatrice Webb (1929: 154) also noticed the river. Of her first view of Bacup in Nov. 1883, she wrote: 'The place seemed deserted. There was a curious stillness in the air which overtakes a purely manufacturing town when the mills with their noise and their lights are closed . . . the small river Irwell splashed as merrily as it could, considering its free mountain descent, over bits of crockery, old boots and pieces of worn-out machinery.'

'the traditional layout' of the Gardens. While two opposing views are apparent in these brief comments, it is worth noting that both are couched in idioms of tradition and preservation.

One of the most vociferous voices of dissent in the conflict belonged to Jane Griffiths who had moved to Bacup five years before with her husband Malcolm. Jane worked as a care assistant in a residential home for the elderly. Malcolm was a civil servant in Rochdale, a profession that Jane labelled as middle class. She described herself as working class. Both she and her husband were active members of the Labour Party and the Peace Movement. She was a tireless campaigner and practised in utilizing media, petitions, and civil action in the courts to bring attention to issues that concerned her and to question decisions with which she disagreed.

One of Jane's major criticisms of what she referred to as 'the demolition of the Gardens' focused on the lack of consultation between decision-makers and residents. Jane placed the local conflict in a wider and national political arena where it was commonplace for politicians and policy-makers to act without consultation or a mandate from 'ordinary people'. To illustrate her point, she located the demolition of the Gardens in a sequence of events which included major 'catastrophes': 'First they dug up the Gardens. Then they bombed Libya. Then there was Chernobyl.'

While Jane perceived all politicians to abuse the power they held, she also accused ordinary people of accepting too readily their decisions. She told me a public meeting was called by the council in order to discuss the proposals, but it had not been well publicized and was not, therefore, well attended. She herself only heard of the meeting after it had taken place. Objections were raised at that meeting and Jane and others assumed because 'there was so much fuss' about the proposal, they would abandon it. One of the convenors, however, was reported to have said 'well we're going to do it anyway', thus vindicating Jane's opinion that those in public office 'see their position as a licence to do as they want'.

Jane described the Gardens as having been 'really peaceful'. The hedges which surrounded the area afforded protection against the wind, and people, she said, would take a bus ride to town and sit there all afternoon. It attracted many people, particularly the elderly, but also those who were unable to get out much, such as 'mothers with young children, the unemployed and young people'. In fact, mused Jane, there was a 'right good social mix'.

> Old age pensioners spoke to children. It was a place people used to go of all generations; used to sit there and talk to dozens of people. It was a right good place—such a peaceful little spot. If you sat there you were bound to see people you know. It was a community thing. I thought it was really important.

Jane went on to remark that now, since the Gardens have gone, there is no place for people to meet, sit, and have a chat. She associates what she (and many residents) call 'the breakdown of the community' with the demise of the

Gardens. 'It really did fulfil a need—not a need that's officially recognized. When people say "there's no community", it's because there's no meeting place. Nobody would come down on a bus to sit on that bloody thing. Some of the old people were heartbroken.'

Jane talked of how she herself took pleasure in the Gardens, she couched her objections and considered her efforts to be on behalf of the community. An aspect of community has been 'destroyed' in the destruction of a forum for communication. Community, in this rendering requires communication (the words also of members of the Bacup youth theatre). For Jane, the physical disappearance of the Gardens made 'the breakdown of the community' tangible. Losing a forum in which to conduct face-to-face social interaction prefigures a loss of those types of relationship. But exactly what kind of community was destroyed in these changes? For Jane, it was a community within which there was intergenerational communication, where people knew each other and created their own entertainment. Indeed, the same kind of community that Bacup people mourn the loss of, incomers come in search of, and hippies accuse yuppies of hastening the decline of.

Jane described how the bulldozers came during a period of particularly bad weather in the early spring of 1986. The shopkeepers were not warned and 'although they did it on the Tuesday, because of the weather it wasn't until the Thursday that most people got to see it'. When people finally realized what had happened, they were shocked. Furthermore, the flower beds, which had been replanted only several weeks before, were dug up and all the bulbs placed on the rubbish heap. That weekend, Jane and Malcolm initiated a petition 'to get the Gardens back'. They collected 300 signatures in three hours and Jane tells of how angry people were about the 'waste and destruction'. While they were on the street collecting signatures, Malcolm was accused by a local councillor of being 'naïve and ill-informed'. Malcolm levelled the same accusation at the councillors who, he said, did not 'communicate with the electorate' and, not using the town's facilities, 'haven't a clue' about what is actually needed. In his words, 'Their view is that it looks tidier. The fact that people don't meet there any more isn't important. The same councillors who called me naïve and ill-informed [*pause*] they have money to socialize elsewhere.' Recall the observation 'the posh don't drink in Bacup', and Mrs O'Brien's scorn of local authority workers who 'make their own tea'. Incomers, local authority employees, and town councillors are each accused of not reciprocating in an appropriate manner; of not forging those ties of sociability which require effort and time to sustain.

Many Bacup residents talked of their discontent with changes to the town centre and with decisions made by councillors and local government officials. Some dwelt on the destruction of what one woman called, 'the most beautiful flower gardens for miles around'. Ideas shift, however, and not only over time but also according to contexts in which they are expressed. Several residents told me although they had not initially agreed with the change, they now felt it was probably for the better as the area was, at least, 'tidier' now. Others situated the 'landscaping' of the town centre as one element in an ongoing project of general 'improvement'. One woman put it this way: 'Bacup's gotten much better. The estate [Mount Pleasant] used to be terrible but they're doing it up, and they've done up the bus stops and moved the forms. It's a bit better than what it was.' From another perspective, the paving of the Gardens is but one element in the inexorable decline of Bacup. In the words of another woman: 'Everything's run down [it's] not like it were. I don't like the centre. Changing it has spoilt it. It looks cold.'

Talk about the demise of the Gardens is couched in idioms which resonate with other contested spaces. As well as representing the loss of community, which is itself an image of rapidly occurring social change, the loss of the Gardens symbolizes an erosion of autonomy and self-rule which many residents know to have taken place since the abolition of Bacup Borough Council. According to a number of my co-conversationalists, the flower gardens were beautiful but they were never adequately taken care of. 'If they had been in Rawtenstall', pointed out one woman, 'then they would have been looked after.' She also thought the decision to pave over the Gardens would never have been made if 'members of the community' had been consulted. The Gardens, it is said, would have been looked after if Bacup had remained autonomous and responsible for its own affairs (including its own entities). The loss of the Gardens also provided an image of the pragmatic and common-sense qualities of Bacup folk by throwing into relief the fickleness and short-sightedness of councillors.

A local councillor described the Gardens as having been 'just an untidy scrap of grass'. He spoke of how difficult it had been to maintain the area adequately, especially with continual damage wrought through vandalism. While he realized many people were unhappy with the changes at the time, he believed they had now 'come around' and realized that 'it's much tidier' than it was. An adviser in Bacup's Citizen's Advice Bureau is more emphatic and declares the Gardens to have been 'a disgusting mess'. Now, he said, the area was much easier to keep clean. He described the way in which litter used to collect in the hedges and how this made the whole area look scruffy. But according to Jane Griffiths, the hedges not only sheltered visitors from the wind but collected the rubbish—without the hedges, she said, 'rubbish just blows everywhere'. Meanings attached to the same phenomenon are flipped: 'a patch of dirty grass' is 'a splash of colour', and hedges that collect rubbish are either an eyesore or diminish the eyesore. Recent immigrants, particularly those who arrived after the alterations, invariably pointed to how attractive the town centre was.[13]

[13] A colleague visiting from Manchester remarked that the town centre was 'pleasing to a middle-class eye'.

While many Bacup people hold the Local Authority responsible for not looking after the Gardens, councillors placed the same responsibility squarely on the shoulders of 'the people'. They argued that vandalism (by local inhabitants) prompted the local authority to do something. They accused Bacup of not looking after its own. Similarly, recent immigrants commented on the regrettable amount of rubbish in Bacup town centre (post-landscaping) and, suspending for a moment their knowledge of not-so-distant city streets, expressed mystification as to why, in the words of one woman, 'local people just don't seem to care'. Aware of vandalism, several Bacup people proposed a causal relationship between it and a decision to demolish the Gardens. Bacup was being punished, they suggested, for the actions of a 'selfish minority'. If the local authority was acting punitively, they told me, then it explained the stealth with which the deed was carried out.

Council officials were also criticized for their wastefulness and an analogy was made between the Gardens and the car park. I was told the council had granted planning permission for a new supermarket on exactly the same site on which they had recently built a car park. The story of the car park was told as further evidence of the improvidence of local politicians. This, together with the wastefulness of digging up 'hundreds of pounds worth of bulbs' (which had only just been planted) are examples drawn upon to portray the fickleness and wastefulness of local government: those traits which are not Bacup's. 'The Bacup character', you will recall, is consistent, thrifty, and straight-talking.

Narratives about the Gardens connect up a number of preoccupations. The paved area is a concrete example, to many residents, of what happens when autonomy is lost: when decisions are imposed from outside the town, first, without reference to the wishes of those who lay claim to Bacup and its belongings and, second, in a manner that presumes to know better, which is either patronizing, or punitive, or both.

Common Sense

A 'common-sense' approach to conservation is advocated by Bacup people. Such an approach is related to the pragmatics and practicalities of living in Bacup and of requiring and using its facilities and services. A common-sense approach stems from experience, and councillors who have no experience of living, communicating, working, bringing up children, and 'going out' in Bacup are said not to know what is needed. Some residents conceded the paved area is tidier than the Gardens but added that, now, it was dangerous. Barbara Jones said she disagreed vehemently, at the time, with the conversion and the way in which it was implemented. Consequently she boycotted the opening ceremony. She told me her objections still stood and, what is more, it was clear the changes had made the town centre a more dangerous place. The paving stones, she explained, were slippery when wet and readily froze in the winter, thereby presenting a hazard for pedestrians, especially the elderly. The area was much colder now, she observed, after all, the river Irwell ran right underneath it. She implied that if one *knew* Bacup, one would have predicted these consequences. 'Bacup folk are not environmental conscious', Barbara explained, 'we want it looking nice, but we want it sensible and practical.'

The way in which opposition to the landscaping transformation of the town centre was framed is familiar from other Bacup forums. The neighbourhood in which Mrs Jones lived, and where I was her neighbour for a year, is still made up of five parallel streets which rise steeply from the river at right angles to the main road. The streets were originally cobblestoned, and a decision was made in the early 1980s to renovate the houses and upgrade the area. In order to create more space one row of houses was demolished, thus widening the street. The area was landscaped, which consisted of removing the cobblestones, paving the sidewalks, planting trees and shrubs, and creating car-parking spaces. One of the end streets is commonly used by cars as a throughway between the main road at the bottom and a top road. The street is still steep and negotiating the junction at its summit provides a telling test of the effectiveness of a vehicle's handbrake and a driver's clutch control, especially in snow or ice. The major primary school in the town is located on the top road which means the street is widely used by parents and guardians dropping off and picking up children at the school gate. Its dangers were the focus of much conversation and concern and it was often pointed out that the improvements to the area had made it more dangerous.

On the top road there was a corner shop, which was filled (before and at the end of the school day) with children putting together a selection of sweets from those displayed either in large jars or compartmentalized trays. The proprietor of the shop used to talk often about the difficulty of driving up the steep street and negotiating the junction at the top (which he could see from his shop window). He berated the council: 'I think they should have left the cobblestones. It was safer when it was cobblestoned. You couldn't go so fast up that hill then.' Similar rationales, couched in idioms of safety and common sense, were given when questions arose about the preservation of the mills. Bacup people locate middle-class incomers, who express an interest in conserving 'Bacup's heritage' (in the form, say, of its factories), outside the moral community in which they situate themselves. Incomers, like the councillors in examples above, are said to lack relevant experience of Bacup. They are not, therefore, qualified *to know* what is best for the town or its people.

A conservation society based in Rawtenstall was campaigning to preserve a disused mill in that town. One elderly Bacup man, commenting on their activities, remarked that it was highly unlikely that members of this group had any experience whatsoever of working in 'satanic mills'. The fact that he had never worked in a mill either was beside the point, or maybe it was the point: his connection to mills could be traced via Bacup, he need not have actually worked in one to be related. In claiming Bacup's history as his own he also claimed attachment to, amongst other things, its factories. Questions around the conservation of mills is another domain in which the pragmatic and 'down-to-earth' character of Bacup folk can be made explicit. One Bacup woman made the observation, 'They say the mills are our heritage, but there is no point preserving them if they don't look after them. Then they may as well pull them down.' What was the point, she asked, of conserving merely for the sake of conserving.

Conservationists, like Nat members, wish to preserve a past they perceive to be embodied in the town's edifices and relics. They consider themselves to be acting on behalf of local people whom they deem to be unconcerned, perhaps even apathetic. But local people are far from unconcerned. They question the reasons for conserving particular things and not others, suggesting that if it is, in fact, *their* heritage being preserved then mills are not axiomatically, or always, appropriate items to keep. Nor do they consider incomers to be appropriate guardians of Bacup's heritage and culture. From this perspective, incomers have little or no experience of the town and therefore do not *know* it adequately. Furthermore Bacup's past is not theirs to keep, just as the mills, back-to-backs, th'owd characters, and the Nutters are not theirs to preserve.

Derelict mills, a single remaining factory chimney, drystone walls, and scars left by quarrying are just some testaments to an industrial and industrious history. A past that, on the one hand, is an integral part of Bacup today and, on the other, has been left behind. People move on even if they stay in the same place. Many Bacup people would wish neither to work in the harsh conditions of textile mills, nor live in back-to-backs; they have bettered themselves and wish for better things for their children.

Of Knowledge and Experience

Architectural changes to the town centre are said, from one perspective, to be part of a Victorian conservation programme and, from another, to be an element in the destruction of tradition. When Henry Frazer related the story of the newcomer and his search for a bit of history, he revealed the newcomer's lack of connection to the town, its past, and its people. The newcomer could only acquire a fragment of history: a disembodied and disembedded 'bit'. Similarly, to preserve a mill of which you have little or no experience (are unrelated to) is to guard a disembodied and disembedded piece of heritage. Tradition is located not only in artefacts but also in social relationships. And for some people the demise of the Gardens, when flower gardens were replaced with paving (which is either tidier or messier), was also the destruction of everyday social relationships. The paving, as well as the new 'Victorian' bus-shelters, railings, and benches, were seen to place a wedge in quotidian communication.

Criticisms levelled at those who oppose and those who support the transformation of the town centre were couched in the very same idioms of common sense and practicality. Council officials expressed puzzlement as to why Bacup people should want to preserve the Gardens, and Bacup people as to why newcomers should want to preserve the mills. Each accused the other of lacking common sense. Common sense stems from the experience of daily life and is contrasted with knowledge gained in chunks through education or study. Common sense is common knowledge gained communally. It is practical and pragmatic and, for particular purposes, is privileged over education; so that, for example, the fussy, abstract, and unrealistic goals of 'professor types' are the antithesis of the practical, down-to-earth aspirations of 'ordinary people'. When either (experience or education) is brought into relief it screens out (denies) the other. Each, however, depends on the other for its purchase; for its hold on the imagination. Local politicians are said to lack the common sense gained through experience and the expertise of Nat members stems, partly, from their experience of Bacup. But the Nat, no less than the council, are also considered to be 'out of touch'. From certain vantage points within Bacup, Nat members may be seen to lack the necessary everyday experience which would qualify them to know what is best. To be out of touch is to be disconnected, and as we have seen, to be connected to some things is to be disconnected from others.

The contrast between knowledge gained through experience and knowledge gained through education mirrors a central theme of this book, namely, the relationship between being born and being bred. In a cultural imagination which mobilizes a dichotomy between birth and breeding (nature and nurture), it is as if one's birth is a given (although it is not as fixed and immutable as we might imagine at first glance) and one's upbringing a variable. Central to such ideas about the reproduction of persons is the separation of two different domains—what one is born with (nature) and how one is brought up (nurture). Each relies on the other and each cuts off (screens out) the other. The final chapters of this book explore these ideas further as they are revealed in conversations about NRT. I have argued thus far that idioms of relatedness emerge in domains other than those readily identifiable as kinship. So when residents of Bacup talk about social change as they perceive it they mobilize and put to work ideas about the way in which persons are connected not only to other persons, but also to places and pasts. In Part 3 I explore what happens when they talk specifically about kinship; when they think explicitly about, for example, how they are connected or not in families, what is transmitted through generations and how, what is required for 'the growing of babies' and what makes and breaks intimate social relationships. NRT provoke people to make explicit what would otherwise remain implicit. They also provoke people to talk about the ways in which they are related to each other as well as to places and pasts.

PART 3

In Kinship

8

An Expertise in Kinship

I WENT to visit Laura Gray in the autumn of 1990. It was the kind of light, bright October day in Bacup when a watery sun shines weakly through a thin, translucent layer of cloud. We sat on her front doorstep with a cup of tea and talked of things that had happened since we last met. She told me she had recently been working in a shoe factory, but had to give it up because by the time she paid for child-minding 'it wasn't worth it'. She also told me about her son's debut at school, her mother's house move away from Bacup, and a quarrel with her neighbour; and she asked me about my son, my ex-partner, and my work. We talked about these continuing and broken relationships in our lives and I told her I was now working on a project about NRT: 'things like sperm and egg donation, IVF, surrogate motherhood, things like that'.[1] Laura's response was swift and laden. She had already told me who should and who should not be 'allowed' to donate eggs or sperm, to whom, and why, before I thought to make a note of what she was saying.

She immediately raised the question of whether 'sisters should be allowed to donate eggs to sisters', and went on to explore, from different angles, the implications for those involved in such a practice. She considered it in terms of its potential advantages and disadvantages, looking at it, in turn, from the vantage points of the father, the baby, and the sisters. She explained, first, that the father of a child conceived from the ovum of his wife's sister 'won't be bothered—because it's his sperm—its *his* child'. Second, 'it won't bother the baby' because 'it'll *know* where it came from'. Finally, as far as the sisters were concerned, it would all depend on the way in which the 'donating mother treats the baby'. Laura explained: problems would arise if the donating mother (elsewhere 'the baby's auntie') tried to tell the baby's mother (her sister) 'how to look after it (the baby)'. She implied that the mother (the woman ultimately responsible for the child) would not appreciate this kind of intervention from her sister and that such interference in bringing up children was bound to be a source of conflict. The danger, left unsaid, is that such conflict has the potential of fracturing the link between sisters; a link through which care and

[1] Idioms of donation (and by extension donor) in the field of NRT are not self-explanatory. For Ken Daniels (1998: 76), the term 'semen donor' is unsatisfactory, especially since in many cases money is exchanged for semen. He prefers 'semen provider' and draws attention to other terms used in the literature such as 'vendor' and 'consignor'. I retain the idioms of donation and donor mainly because they are terms Bacup residents use, but also because they are culturally loaded and are not self-explanatory. The same should be said for 'infertility' and 'surrogacy'.

intimacy proceeds and which itself may have motivated the transference of ova from one to the other in the first place.

That Laura should have focused on whether sisters should be allowed to donate eggs to sisters when initially thinking about NRT is itself germane. She was reminded in NRT of kinship and of the intricacies in maintaining and sustaining intimate relationships in an appropriate manner. She explored not only the implications of NRT for kinship, but also of kinship for NRT, and with an alacrity which was unexpected. Looking back at the first page of fieldnotes made on Laura's doorstep in October 1990, I am struck not only by the amount of detail packed into the page but also by the obvious celerity with which Laura moved from one perspective to another. The page is replete with what look like mini-genealogical diagrams. They are marked not only by abbreviations for kin terms, but also sweeping arcs, double-headed arrows, dots, and circles indicating both the direction of gametes and passages and culs-de-sac of relations.[2] Laura related some of what she knew to be difficulties of sustaining familiar social relationships in an appropriate manner. She posed her own questions and in answering one was led to another; each answer creating the context from which the next question emerged. Like other Bacup residents with whom I spoke about NRT, Laura drew upon and put to work an expertise in kinship. I return to this conversation below, but first I introduce some of the ways in which Bacup residents deploy what they know from their own experiences of kinship to shed light on unfamiliar territory such as NRT.

Tied and Tied Down

I met Judy Wilder again at a conference on 'The Environment' organized by Rossendale Groundwork Trust and held in Rawtenstall, in a converted and renovated mill. It was a Sunday, not long after my conversation with Laura Gray. The conference comprised workshops on landscaping, land conservation, and environmental sculpture. In one of the workshops, participants learnt how to make elegant weavings from willow, while in another they created haunting stone sculptures and placed them strategically in nooks in the hillsides surrounding the mill. Another workshop was devoted to making lanterns from paper and bamboo. I joined this workshop and talked with a fellow participant about dexterity which seems to atrophy through lack of practice, and artistic visions which are innately limited, nevertheless we all managed with kind encouragement to produce something that was named and displayed. The lanterns were hung along the edges of the path leading away from the mill. They were lit at dusk and, swaying in the breeze, cast an enchanting light over the moorland. There were also exhibitions, seminars, and speeches and the

[2] I am grateful to Mary Bouquet (pers. comm.) for being curious about whether anthropologists draw genealogical diagrams in the margins of their fieldnotes these days, and, if they do, what goes into them.

conference ended with music from, and dancing to, the Radio Bacup Band, a local rock-group featuring Sam Watson on lead guitar.

Judy told me she was in charge of the catering and, as I stood in a noisy but orderly queue for food, she explained she was only 'helping out' and, as she was not getting paid, she was not to be blamed for the quality of either the service or the food. We caught up briefly on some news of each other and I told her in a few words about the 'new' project. Her first response was to tell me forcefully that, as far as she was concerned, they ('things like egg and sperm donation and test-tube babies and surrogate mothers') were no different to things that had always been going on: 'Look at Mark [her partner]—he's the guy who *looks after* Rachael [her daughter]—*he's* dad to her.' 'In the same way' she said, when a child is conceived with donated sperm 'its dad is the man who looks after and cares for it, not the sperm donor'. The analogy Judy made between Mark and Rachael and children conceived with the help of a sperm donor is interesting in the direction it took; a sperm donor, who only provides sperm, is clearly not a dad. The point Judy underlined is that Mark was dad to the children with whom he lived and for whom he cared. She then quoted her own father as saying: 'I have five grandchildren, and no two have the same father.'[3] Her father overstated his case, in so far as Mark was the father of two of his five grandchildren, nevertheless Judy repeated his comment to convey the authority with which she spoke about these things. For Judy, NRT raise recognizable issues and dilemmas (albeit in novel ways) which have familiar resolutions. 'The most important thing', Judy concluded, was the way in which individuals involved 'deal with it'. She believed this to be the crux of the matter. 'What happens afterwards' was all-important. She drew on another example from her own experience to further illustrate this point. Years ago she had to terminate a pregnancy but, she told me, nowadays she hardly ever thought about it. There were other women, however, who could not forget: maybe they counted the years, saying things like, 'I would have had a son who would have been 12 now.' Judy was not like that—'what is done, is done'; 'these things', she said, 'don't bother me'. Judy drew on both these examples to impress upon me (and herself) that, for her, as opposed to others, NRT were not 'a big deal'. They raised the same dilemmas as had always been raised in creating, sustaining, and curtailing social relationships.

In her commentary, Judy provided evidence of a nonconformist attitude to life: an eschewal of 'mainstream' values and a worldliness born from a diversity of intimate relationships. Yet her nonconformism was belied by the kind of things she missed from her own childhood. For example, she told me she missed 'sitting down, as a family, to eat': when she was a child, she said, they all *had* to sit 'at the table together', and if her father was late from work then he might have his meal later when the children were in bed, but normally they

[3] Judy's sister has one child and Judy four (three of whom live with her and Mark).

sat down together 'at the table'. She mused out loud, more to herself than to me, 'I should try and get mine together more often—as a family unit' (with the stress on unit, rather than family).

Judy continued with her conference catering tasks and the queue for food grew more disorderly as well as longer. I asked if I could visit her at home and talk about these things more. She said, 'of course you can'. She had no doubt that her varied and unique experience of kinship thus far provided her with an expertise with which to address questions raised by NRT.

It was in fact, two months before I saw Judy again. I arrived on her doorstep with, amongst other things, a bag of doughnuts and a tape-recorder. She welcomed me with characteristic warmth and a cup of tea. We were pleased to see each other. Judy's way into talking about NRT, which in fact she barely spoke about directly (which is my point), was to describe her own life. She told me of her childhood, which she thought was a 'good one'. She spoke of her relationship with her father, who was very protective and of her relationship with her mother, who was one of those who 'can't quite understand why people just don't get on with their lives, properly', and of her relationship with her sister, who 'makes rules for other people, but breaks them all herself'. She talked about her life with her first husband: 'he was nice', American, wealthy, 'I suppose I had it dead cushy . . . but he had to put up with hell with me.' She told me of the times she was *truly* in love and the times she only thought she was; the times she was happy, like when she bought forty tickets for Pink Floyd for her friends just because she had the money; and the bad times when 'you cry until there's not another tear left in your head'.

Here, from the transcript of our conversation, are some of her reflections starting with her childhood:

JUDY: I think it was a good childhood. I think I was me dad's favourite. I think I was me mum's in a way as well. Catherine always had just funny ways about [her] all the while, you know what I mean? Like, me mum admitted it to me once, she said, 'I always liked you better than Catherine', you know? 'I didn't love [her] any less', but Catherine always was a bit—she's like me dad. She takes after me dad more than—I take after me mum. Let alone, I was more—my dad used to take me on the building sites every Saturday—I laid bricks for him, you know what I mean? . . . always had that sort of life. From a young age. Bought me a pony when I was 7. You know what I mean? I had it, when I look back, I had a smashing childhood. I wouldn't want to change any . . . He was in demolition and I used to go into big houses that're being pulled down and there'd be all stuff left in the attic and pots and vases and all sorts and I really, you know, the things that must have happened to me were once in a lifetime's and they happened more than once. When I look back, I often look back at me childhood and think, 'god it was a good one'. My dad was very protective.

JEANETTE: Was he?

JUDY: Mmmm. Little things. Like, it's come through with me, like, he would never let anyone babysit for us. There was only one girl was allowed to babysit and he even didn't like her having her boyfriend there, he'd come home early and mum said, you know, he'd leave somewhere early, he'd say he'd be back at one and he'd come back at half eleven, you know? And little things like that and he'd come in quietly. Not to catch them at it but just to make sure.

JEANETTE: Just to check you were all right?

JUDY: The girl's were all right, *his* girls, you know?

JEANETTE: Right.

JUDY: So that come through, protecting the children on that level.

Judy identified the protectiveness of her father as a positive strand in her life. She drew on it here as evidence of his care and commitment to her and her sister. It had been 'passed on' to her and she too is protective of her own children. She dwelt on time spent with her father, accompanying him to work and learning his trade. She took after her mother but took up with her father. His protectiveness was clearly a sign of his care for her, and evidence of his attachment to 'his girls'; not any girls—'his girls'. Later in our conversation, she put her father's behaviour and his relationship with his daughters to work again, but now dwelt on the downside of the same behaviour. Now she interpreted it as his attempts at control.[4] She told me about when she left home for the first time:

JEANETTE: Did you still have a good relationship then with your mum and dad?

JUDY: Well me dad was a very domineering person in the sense that we weren't even allowed to slam a door and go up to our bedroom. He'd make you come back down. You know what I mean, he controlled me very, very severely. In the sense, 'where was I going', 'where was I'—I mean, I had to work like a trooper to get out. You know what I mean? And that was why marriage was [*pause*] I think why—I honestly believe, looking back, why I can't handle marriage. Because I will not—I got told what to do by my dad and then I got married and then I'm told what's got to be done by my husband. And I couldn't—I can't handle it.

JEANETTE: What age was you when you got married?

JUDY: Seventeen. Pregnant.

JEANETTE: Was, um [*pause*] did your parents mind?

JUDY: No. This was the crack. This was one of the most amazing things. All the people I were knocking around with were like into drugs—hippies. And, I'd gone to, I'd gone out horse-riding and I turned up at this American's house who I knew. And there was a wedding on. And at this wedding was this guy called Frank Wood, and he took a shine to me, even though I didn't really notice it.

JEANETTE: Was he the same age as you?

JUDY: No. He was eight years older than me. But he was very well off. I mean related to the—there's an inherited title through him.

JUDY: I fell pregnant when I was 17. Got married when I was 18. That's right—'cause I married in May and I was 18 in February before it.

[4] Control and protectiveness, like the friendliness and nosiness of the tight-knit community, are flip sides of the same coin. The same behaviour is assessed either positively or negatively according to the purpose of invoking it, and without contradiction because the contexts formulated in which different assessments of the same thing are made do not overlap.

JEANETTE: So what did you make of having a baby?

JUDY: Well, you see, remember, I had a daughter who was perfect. She slept for hours. She never woke up of a night. After the first two nights, she slept all night, she did every[thing] by the book. She was the most adorably good child. And I thought all children were like her. They're not, you know what I mean? I mean I'd take her off to Spain, hitchhiking when she was 3 years old. Ran away with her. We ran away to Spain. Hitchhiked right through, down into Ibiza. Know what I mean? [*pause*] never looked at it as dangerous. Mind you, I think maybe things were different then.

JEANETTE: How did Frank relate to the baby?

JUDY: Oh he was good. Yeah he was good. Yeah, you couldn't have wished—really I couldn't have wished for a better marriage. It's just, 'cause it was too young to be told what to do again, and be tied. I think that was the trouble.

The connection Judy identified between her and her father was both protective *and* constraining. From the retrospective of marriage, being connected to her father also meant being tied down: it meant being 'told what to do' whether one did it or not. She married but was too young—it was too soon—to be tied in the same way again. Judy continued: after she ran away and travelled in Spain, she returned to make a living in London. She worked in night-clubs in Soho, managed to make a good living, and revelled in being untied (at least partially and temporarily).

Judy told me more about her life and work in London, and then she was reminded of a time she was in a village just outside London, where her mother had lived as a child:

I went to a little pub. And this bloke, these old boys were sitting there and I happened to be sitting near. They got talking to me and they said 'where you come from—these bleeding outsiders'. I say 'I belong here'. They said 'what do you mean?' and I said, 'I bet you know my grandmother—Phoebe Frost'. He went, 'then you've got to be one of Phoebe's, you're not Sophie's, and you're not the eldest son's' [*pause*] and like, from that minute, it was, 'bloody hell, one of Phoebe Frost's—I remember her playing the old piano down the Old Grey Mare'. They all knew her. It was great. 'Cause I was one of the, you know what I mean, I wasn't an outsider in this funny little pub, I was Phoebe Frost's granddaughter [and] she was a character, [a] strong character of the town, in her day, you know.

What is it about NRT that reminded Judy of her grandmother and of her visit to her mother's place of birth? Like belonging to families, belonging to places is not only positively valued but also achieved through making explicit one's connections through persons. Phoebe Frost mediated Judy's connection to her mother's place of origin. In participating in the identity of Phoebe Frost, Judy belonged to the village which she had never known. It was connected to her and she to it and furthermore the connection was recognized (known) by the locals who, in this context, *truly* belonged. Significantly, Phoebe Frost was a character and, like th'owd characters of Bacup, she embodied the idiosyncratic and the unique. She had strength of character, unmistakable and unforgettable. Judy was not connected to this place by 'any old person' but by Phoebe Frost, her grandmother, a character in her own right, remembered with fondness and respect.[5] It was Phoebe Frost who mediated Judy's connection to the village in which she had never lived, but to where she could now trace her origins. The historical figure of Phoebe Frost rendered Judy's connection to the village tangible.

Mary Shaw was also reminded, by NRT, of the past, and more specifically of her childhood in Bacup. She recounted the house moves she and her family had to make when she was a child and the way in which local people still called her 'George's lass'. Mary had always been called 'George's lass', but when she was a child she hated being identified in this way and wanted to shout 'no I'm not!' 'It's funny', she said, but now she liked it when people call her this. She now felt proud to be known as 'George's lass'.[6] It was no longer necessary for her to reject the public explicitness of this relationship. It was couched in an idiom of ownership: belonging to George, she was placed both in a past and in a place as well as in a family. 'When you're a kid', Mary said, 'you want to assert your individuality—cut off your ties.' She used this example to give voice to concerns she had about whether the way in which children were conceived affected the ways in which they were related. Her question hung in the air between us: Would children born through surrogacy arrangements, or conceived with donated gametes, be connected to people and to places?

In an earlier chapter, I borrowed selected items from Mary Shaw's narrative to illustrate a point about housing histories and the diminishing status of council houses (Ch. 5). But Mrs Shaw had a different motive for selecting, and telling me, these particular scenes from her past. She was telling me about her father and about how the loss of their home, when she was child, was due to her father's addiction to alcohol. Her mother suffered terribly. Thinking about NRT, she thought about relationships of her childhood: she thought about her parents, as well as neighbours and peers. And while I borrowed from what she said to make a point about housing trajectories, Mary was in fact talking about NRT. She was reminded of what it meant to belong to people and places and wondered how firmly children born from new reproductive arrangements would be connected to these things.

[5] Ethnographers of Britain have focused on the use of nicknames both as marker of familiarity and as forms of abuse, jocular or otherwise. Ch. 6 introduced *th'owd characters* with names such as Ailse O'Fusser, Mad Ab, and Robert the Devil which are familiar: nicknames not only act to individuate persons, but also to collectivize. *Th'owd characters* represent a quirky, idiosyncratic Bacup and in telling of their exploits narrators provide evidence both of knowing the place and its past, and of they themselves being part of it.

[6] George and Phoebe Frost were prominent characters, known and knowable. They were neither bland nor nondescript and, similar to *th'owd characters,* they exhibited certain noticeable and idiosyncratic characteristics. Furthermore, they linked Mary Shaw and Judy Wilder to places and pasts in ways that were both liberating and limiting.

What we Leave Behind

I sat in the kitchen of Agnes Swift' s house. I had been introduced to her at the NSPCC Christmas Fair which took place one Saturday morning in late November at the A, B & D (Aged, Blind, and Disabled) Centre. Mrs Swift was a committee member of the local branch of the charity, an ardent golf player, and an active member of the Soroptomists; she professed to knowing nothing about 'test-tube babies' but agreed to let me visit her at home. She lived in a detached house built in the 1970s, in an area of town that several people over the course of fieldwork identified as where the 'local posh people' lived. I told her a bit more about the project. She told me something about her background; she talked about the housing and occupational histories of her parents, and in so doing classed herself. She provided me with what she considered relevant autobiographical detail within which to place herself in Bacup. She hardly talked about NRT at all, or perhaps that is just how it seemed. What she did talk about were her parents and her children and what is inherited and how.

Agnes Swift was born in Rawtenstall, in 1939. Both her mother and father were from Rawtenstall and, until she was 11 years old, they lived in a terraced house rented from a private landlord. When her parents first got married they had had to live with her father's parents, but by the time Agnes was born, they had managed to set up a home of their own. They did actually own a house at the time (it had been inherited) but they were never able to live in it as it was occupied by protected tenants. According to Agnes, her mother was 'determined to be independent and property owning' and 'determined to better her standard of living'. She saved, diligently, from the money sent by her husband who was 'in the forces'. When he was demobilized, he became a fitter and turner in an engineering firm and her mother took a course and got a job in a factory nursery. Eventually Agnes's mother left the nursery and 'went into slippers' because it paid more. With Agnes's encouragement, and further education classes and training, both her parents eventually became civil servants. This was the first job either of them had ever had which entitled them to sick pay; it meant they could build up a pension and, by the time they retired, her mother and father had, respectively, nine and eleven years pensionable salary. When they retired, they went to live in St Anne's,[7] not long after her father's brother moved there, in 1966.

Agnes trained as a calculator operator and after leaving school had a series of jobs. Eventually, much to her mother's dismay, she went to work in Manchester. Her mother

[7] St Anne's is on the Lancashire coast (sometimes referred to as the Fylde Coast—see Jade's comments in Ch. 5). It has had strong connections with Rossendale since the mid-19th cent. According to local historian Chris Aspin, St-Anne's-on-the-Sea was, before 1870, a square mile of 'wilderness' on the sand-hills between Blackpool and Lytham. It was transformed through Rossendale enterprise into 'The Opal of the West': 'Rossendale stone as well as Rossendale money helped to build the new resort; it gave—and still gives—a feeling of solid affluence found in no other stretch of the Lancashire coast. The infant town was fortunate in capturing the interest of William John Porritt, a Helmshore woollen manufacturer, who not only built splendid houses, but also took charge of the venture at a critical moment; more than any other person he was responsible for the success of St Anne's' (Aspin 1983: 37).

argued that working in the city was 'giving her big ideas', evidence of which was the fact that Agnes went to work each day in her 'best clothes'. She changed jobs and went to work for a company in Haslingdon. She got married when she was 19. Her husband was three years older than she was and he was born just outside the Rossendale Valley. They met at the local grammar school and by the time they got married he had returned to the same school as a teacher. At first they rented a flat near Rawtenstall and Agnes went back to work in Manchester. Two and half years later they moved to Nigeria, where her husband taught and where they lived for almost four years. Agnes returned briefly to England for the birth of their daughter in 1962, and then permanently just prior to the birth of their son in 1964. Living in Nigeria, she tells me, was a 'wonderful experience', and it enriched her life enormously.

When Agnes and her husband returned to England they temporarily moved back into the flat in which they had lived before going to Nigeria, but after six months her husband found a teaching job in Manchester and they bought a house on the north side of the city. By May 1975, when their son was 10 and their daughter 12, they had decided it was 'too dangerous' to bring up teenagers so close to the centre of a city. There was, recalls Agnes, a big drugs problem in Manchester, and it was time to move back to a 'slow lifestyle'. They bought the detached house in which they now lived partly because they could afford it. It was amazing, Agnes told me, how, for the price, houses in Bacup were much better quality than anywhere else. Had they been able to afford it, they would probably have moved to Bolton, but the same kind of house would have been prohibitively expensive there. Agnes's husband took early retirement from teaching at 53, and had since gone back to work on a temporary contract for Rossendale council. Her daughter was now 29, married, and a civil servant. She lived near Preston, owned her own house, and, said Agnes, would probably start a family soon. Her son was 26 and worked in a bank in Bacup. The weekend after our conversation he was due to move away from home. Agnes had been 'encouraging . . . nagging . . . him to buy a house for the past three years'. Although he did not, in her view, need to live away from home he ought, by now, to be investing in property, particularly as he could benefit from low mortgage rates because he worked in a bank. He had bought a large mid-terraced house within two miles and Agnes expected that he would still spend quite a bit of time at home with them.

Agnes Swift told me about her house moves; the autobiographical detail she presented was filled with movement; not only her own but also that of her parents and her children. Like many recent incomers, she talked about the attractiveness (compared to the city) of Bacup as a place to live in terms of its safety for children, particularly adolescents, and of how affordable decent housing is compared to nearby places, one did not have to come from afar to acknowledge that a move to Bacup is as driven by the low cost of property as any other reason. She described how her parents 'bettered themselves' in terms which resonate with the way in which other Bacup residents talked of their own social trajectories. She elaborated upon the help and support she provided her parents in their upward mobility. Agnes participated in the identity of her parents in the present as much as she participated in their success in the past. Later in our conversation she described the encouragement she and her husband extended to her husband's mother. Thinking about NRT, then, she thought about parents and being a parent, and what it was that parents transmitted to their children and children to their parents. She told me she would not expect anything from her parents: 'children, once they're set up, should stand on their own two feet'. She was aware, however, that her parents would like her and her sister to inherit their house. They would like them to share the proceeds from its sale and thought this was rightfully their due. But Agnes thought her parents may well need to sell their house in order to be looked after later in life: savings and investments were easily eaten away if some kind of residential care were required. She cited the example of her great-auntie who had always hoped to leave something to her nephew, but she now lived in a residential home for the elderly which cost £1,200 per month. This was obviously diminishing the nephew's inheritance and Agnes thought there would probably be nothing left for him in the end which was very upsetting for her great-auntie. Without a formal system of inheritance, there is nevertheless a desire on the part of elders to contribute material substance, in this case money, to a surviving generation. Connections are not fractured on death, and nor is money only part of the world of commodities. The assets of elders, in Agnes Swift's formulation, belong to their inheritors, and her great-auntie was spending on her care what is already her nephew's.[8] But this is not, of course, the full story: as in many of the cultural understandings explored in previous chapters, there is an ambiguity in inheriting things (in this case assets). Because children should 'stand on their own two feet', Agnes herself expected nothing (materially) from her parents, despite their desire to give.

Agnes explained that for her parents property meant security, but they were now disillusioned. They thought the benefit system[9] unfair and this was reason enough for them to switch from Labour to Conservative; they had been Labour all their lives prior to retiring. Agnes pointed to friends of her parents who, from marriage, have never been 'as careful' with their money, but who were now eligible for state support: 'at the end of the day, they live in a council house which is paid for' (she referred to their eligibility for housing benefit and rate rebate), whereas for her parents, 'their hard-earned money will end up keeping them'. She thought about her husband's parents: they owned a shop and when her father-in-law died her mother-in-law sold it and moved into a council house. Agnes and her husband encouraged her to spend the capital from the sale of the shop which meant 'at least now' she would not fall into the same trap as Agnes's own parents, who had had to spend all their

[8] I am reminded of a documentary film made by the BBC's *Under the Sun* series called 'Spending the Kids' Inheritance'. It reported on an increasing number of elderly people in the United States who were selling their static homes to buy mobile ones (Winnebagos). They settled for periods of time in different areas of the country forming new communities and spending what they would otherwise have passed on to their children.

[9] She was referring predominantly to income support and housing benefit.

savings and investments on day-to-day-welfare. Having money (tied up in property or otherwise) in old age was, from the distance of this relative, ambivalent. Even if, as most people agree it is extremely difficult to have to rely solely on state benefits for subsistence after the age of retirement, from the perspective of not having to, it has its upside. Carried with assets is the expectation of being able to *pass them on*. Money and property, from this perspective, do not fully belong to a person but are part of what they hand down to following generations.

Thinking about NRT, Agnes talked about her own and her husband's family. She drew on notions of thrift and resourcefulness and in noting that these qualities did not always pay, she rendered them all the more valuable. Her comments resonate with ideas about self-help which, as we have seen, emerge in quite different contexts: ideas that have as much to do with making tangible social class than they have with prudence. Portraying a feckless class places in relief a respectable and industrious class (both middle and working), showing it for what it is. Agnes found it difficult, she said, to predict what the future may hold for her and her husband. They may have to sell their home in the future in order to pay for their own residential care. But in the end, she said forcefully, property and material things were not very important. The things she valued were 'mementoes' of a personal nature which had little economic value. 'What we leave behind', she concluded, 'is how we've brought up our children—their ideals and moral standards—that's what we leave behind.'

In NRT, Mrs Swift is reminded of the responsibilities of being parent and offspring. As the child of a parent one should grow up and be independent, and as the parent of a child one's responsibility is to instil appropriate values to enable children to grow up and be independent. The fact that children grow up into independent, successful adults is evidence of the effectiveness of parenting. How children are brought up is all-important, then, not least because values endure: they are the traces of oneself left in offspring whether they look like their parent or not. Recall Judy Wilder who had been left a legacy of protecting her children: her father *passed on* to her this imperative. What is left behind, and how, are central elements in kinship thinking. In the kinship thinking I am calling Born and Bred, one leaves behind actions and intentions (as well as genes). Parental demeanour is made manifest (emerges) in offspring. The potential is always there, however, to adumbrate values instilled by other elements that are passed on and particularly those passed on in 'the blood'.

Made and Made-up

Mrs Lawson wondered how donated semen was 'screened'. Being healthy was not, she thought, a reliable indicator of the suitability of a sperm donor: 'There could be healthy criminals—in fact, there are plenty of them. In America criminals can sell their blood. Why not sperm? That's the next step. I mean, they could ask somebody on death row then.' It is not just medically compromising conditions that can be passed on in sperm then; so too can socially compromising conditions. A disposition to criminality was as likely, according to Mrs Lawson, to be passed on as a propensity to illness. She provided examples from her own experience of kinship to further illuminate for me the complexity of inheritance. The autobiographical details with which she provided me illustrate and concretize the abstractions with which NRT deal.

Wendy Lawson was born in Bacup but moved away from the area when she married. Her first husband was violent and unsupportive, and eventually she left him and returned to Bacup alone with three young children. After a few years, she met and married a man—'a local lad'—who also had three children, and they had a child together. This man, her second husband, died, tragically, twelve years later. Mrs Lawson told me with pride that she was 'mother' to all seven children.

'I have got myself two families, haven't I? One set of stepchildren and one set of children. We've got two different mothers who are totally different, personality-wise. And the children out of one family, they've definitely got characteristics of their father. I mean, the eldest son's a spit for what his dad was at that age. But they've taken the characteristics of the mother as well as the father and not necessarily good characteristics—you know the good part of the character . . . Now my family—they're a funny mixture. Because I've got one boy, the eldest lad actually, is slightly retarded because he had glandular fever when he was a baby, nearly died. And then James, I think he's like me. And Ellen is like me, looks like her father but the only thing she remembers about her father is him beating me. So she takes after me insomuch as [she] follows my example. Having said that James takes after me, but he's been in trouble with the police—I mean he hasn't done it for years now, but I mean, as a teenager, you know?—if it were loose, he lifted it. I think it was a case of him being easy with life—having said that, his father did a stretch for arson.'

Mrs Lawson was mother to seven children, divided into two families. Her two families were separated by the mothers (her husband's first wife and herself) and united by their mother (herself). She dwelt on characteristics her stepchildren shared with their father (her husband) and while acknowledging they had some characteristics of 'the mother' they were not, necessarily, she said, the good ones. What Mrs Lawson sees in her children is selective and itself makes and breaks connections. Certain characteristics are chosen as significant. Plucked out from myriad possibilities, these characteristics provided visual (concrete) evidence of abstract connections. She told me that her children from her first husband are mostly like her, and in so doing screened out similarities between them and their father. However, there is one thing she thought he had passed on, fortunately to only one son, and that was a tendency towards crime.

Mother to seven children, Mrs Lawson is stepmother to three of them.

There is no contradiction in being both: both are true. She has, she said, 'two families'. The different characteristics, as she saw them, exhibited in the two families and between individual children in the same family, provide evidence of the variety of possibilities embedded in and emerging from inheritance; both good and bad traits can be *passed on*, as can disease and criminality, and they come from the mother or the father, or both, and are transmitted in shared substance (be it blood or genes) or by example. Mrs Lawson drew on the example of her own family to highlight the complexity of inheritance and in order, eventually, to make the point that anonymous semen donation is not a good idea: 'unless they could guarantee it was only from people without criminal records and no hereditary defects'. Donated sperm, from this perspective, should be screened for all kinds of possibilities; and to scrutinize only sperm, and not the person to whom it belongs, is to get only a fraction of the picture.

Judy Wilder also dwelt on the complexity of inheritance. She reminded me again she had 'four children' with 'three different fathers', and that *to her* this made no difference whatsoever. She thought, however, for some women (perhaps in 'different circumstances') there would be more of a problem.

> Three fathers, isn't there? I don't think of it as any different. You see I don't hate any of their fathers. And I really do think it has a lot to do with it. You know? Really. A lot of women don't—I'm not saying all of them—but some girls are, some people have got such weird—narrow—weird minds, the way they look at things. I could imagine, quite easy, that a girl would go against a kid because she didn't like the father. Especially when you can see the traits come through. Yeah, I think you could, you know.

Judy identified a danger in women recognizing in a child those things she disliked in the child's father. In turn this may influence the way in which they behave to a child who turns out like the man she no longer likes, if she ever did. Several Bacup men told me, as fathers, they did not want to be like their own fathers: they were determined to bring their children up in a manner different to the way in which they were raised. Their inheritance included the very experiences they rejected.[10] There are also the unpredictable and

[10] I am reminded of a conversation with two young Bacup people who fashioned themselves, in the late 1980s, as Goths. (Goths are striking for their extraordinary appearance. Both male and female Goths usually wear black clothing, with flowing shirts and much jewellery; they also dye their long hair a very deep black. They line their eyes and paint their lips with black which contrasts dramatically with white, or very pale, face make-up.) Our conversation had meandered towards racism in Bacup, and the young man, identifying what he called 'a Bacup clan', said: 'If their parents are racist they grow up to be racist for the rest of their life. Me mum and dad are very racist, but I'm not. I'm totally against it.' This example seals a point I hope to have made by now, which is that seemingly contradictory views emerge as responses to different questions. Prior to the specifics of racism is a cultural understanding of inheritance which relies on an interplay between the given and the mutable; between genes and background; between nature and nurture, which allows both to be evoked at the same time, by the same person, but to address different questions: for example why the 'Bacup clan' are racist and why I am not.

immeasurable ways in which offspring are interpreted and acted upon by parents who are reminded, for example, of their own parents, or of a former lover, or of a past ever-present. In the words of Marilyn Greaves: 'It's hard to tell, isn't it, what's been made and what's in their make-up'. It is difficult to discern what is fashioned by the constant chipping and moulding (not only from primary carers but also from geographies and histories) and what is given or there from the start and will inevitably show through. The question requires no answer, but of interest here is that it is asked at all and furthermore that it is asked frequently, in many different ways.

People in Bacup with whom I spoke about NRT put to work different elements of inheritance. Exploring inheritance in the context of NRT, they revealed the kind of characteristics passed on and the routes they took. Bacup exerts its influence as do parents, and the past is ever present. We have seen how being brought up in the town, or near the moors, or in the north of England, is constitutive of particular characters and certain characteristics. Not only are there inherited items passed on in 'the blood' or in 'the genes' and said to be given and immutable, but also characteristics imbued through example. There is not, however, a measurement of each in each person, but different elements of inheritance are congealed (purified) for different purposes. Different aspects of a person's make-up are made up (put together as in a prescription) according to the question being asked and the reasons for asking it.

Blood Lines

Blood is ubiquitous in Bacup formulations of kinship; there are *blood relatives* as opposed to in-laws and step relatives; blood *is* said to be thicker than water (although there are as many exceptions to this edict as there are examples); and the *blood line* is a common idiom of inheritance and connection.[11] Thinking about whether sperm donors would be related to ensuing children, Sam Watson described the way in which he was connected to his own children. He explained that he was connected through a 'microscopic blip' which was 'a definite blood line'. But the microscopic blip alone, he went on, was not enough to connect him to his own children. For Sam, the blood line required other kinds of connection (physical and mental) to be active. Thus sperm donors, without these connections to children conceived from their sperm, would not be fathers. In his words: 'Without the mental and physical connection, the microscopic blip will become lost on the floor of the laboratory. . . . There is no mental and physical connection between the donor and the baby . . . there is a huge gap. However microscopic there's got to be a connection.'

[11] Blood is, of course, a key cultural symbol of relatedness in what scholars have identified as Euro-American or Western kinship (e.g. Schneider 1968 [1980]; 1984; Wolfram 1987; Delaney 1991; Strathern 1992*a*; and see Bouquet 1993 for alternative Portuguese key symbols of kinship).

I asked Pamela Watson and Marilyn Greaves, one afternoon, who was to be included in the family. Pamela told me 'it's the blood line'. Later in our conversation I asked what that meant.

JEANETTE: So what's the blood line, then?

PAMELA: I would see it as a line through which genetic characteristics are passed down—so a purely biological thing.

MARILYN: You can *feel* for one another though. You can feel, because—like my two lads they're not twins, but it has happened—our Tony never ailed a thing in his life and then Edward had to go in to have his tonsils out. Oh god, Tony were ill, he could hardly talk. He went to the doctor and he said 'I can't understand this', he says 'you've all symptoms of tonsillitis, but it looks all right.' The minute Edward's tonsils were ripped out, Tony were as right as a bobbin. Edward goes in to have his gland removed . . .

JEANETTE: How old was he then?

MARILYN: Twenty-two, Tony were. Edward were 19. Two years since, Edward went in to have his gland out, Tony were *exactly* the same. Couldn't talk. Oh he *were* ill. Goes to doctor and doctor says 'it sounds like throat trouble but it look all right does your throat'. Minute Edward's gland were out and back home, no problems again, you know? I said, 'it's psychosomatic'. 'Is it hell' [said Tony]. But, they're alike, they seem bound together. And it happened twice and he were right as a bobbin as soon as the operation were over, no lingering illness or owt like that.

PAMELA: He must have been really worried about him, mustn't he?

MARILYN: Oh yeah. Their uncles talk about them, up there, about that—being so close. Auntie Jean was saying, 'Alec's always remarking—Marilyn—on how you've brought your lads up close.' I just said, like you, 'have I brought them up close, or are they close?', you know? And she said, 'well it must be something to do with upbringing', and I said, 'well, I don't know, they might have been close anyway', you know? They have, they've always stuck together [*pause*] It's hard to tell, isn't it? what's been made and what's in their make-up.

The blood line might be genetic connection, but it goes further even as it embraces it. While Pamela initially wanted the blood line to be confined to a 'purely biological thing', Marilyn was reminded of intangible and immeasurable links between kin. She was unsure whether the closeness of her sons had been forged through the way in which they were brought up or axiomatic connections binding them as siblings. Either or both are possible: the question of which, or in what combination, is again not a question which requires a definitive answer. It is another version of a culturally significant and perennial opposition, sometimes couched in terms of nature and nurture, that has no resolution: each is implicated in the other. Being connected to families, like places, requires sociability as much as shared elements, be they biological substances of blood or genes, or community substances of back-to-backs or the slipper works.

Blood is also, however, a potentially dangerous substance; all kinds of things, good and bad, can be passed on via blood. Thinking about bio-medical technology generally, Sam Watson wondered whether we were not expecting too much from it. Perhaps, he pointed out, there was an expectation of 'immortality—a dream of staying alive'. This led him more specifically to organ transplantation. 'Not sure about organ transplant. I've got a kidney donor card. I'd like it to be specified—to go to a young adult . . . preferably a 16- or 17-year old. If they were healthy—they're not much use to me—then they should be used. I wouldn't like somebody to volunteer me for it though.' For Sam, the autonomy of the decision both to donate an organ and to specify to whom it should go is of paramount importance, and there are categories of people who are more appropriate recipients than others. I asked him about the donation of blood: 'Blood's a bit dodgy. Blood carries things. I wouldn't like my blood to go to anybody. Shouldn't be swapping blood, there's a risk of AIDS, especially to kids. Wouldn't like to pass on something naff.' Sam had an inherited respiratory condition which, although minor, could, he thought, be passed on in his blood. He hated the idea of inadvertently transmitting this disease and likened the possibility to the transmission of AIDS through the transference of blood. In turn, he 'wouldn't expect blood or organs off anybody'. It was unclear whether this was because of the danger of disease being passed on through substituted blood or organs, or because if one did not donate these things then one could not expect to receive them. I suspect the latter. Embodied in the donation of body substance is an expectation of reciprocity, and a reciprocity linked with altruism—so that if one takes an organ one should be prepared to give one, but not necessarily vice versa. This led him on to the donation of gametes and he told me he found 'the whole idea of sperm donation abhorrent'. For Sam, there were good reasons why gametes should not be alienated from bodies, not least the potential for their manipulation by 'scientists'. There were also, for him, imponderables about how children born through techniques of assisted conception were connected and disconnected to the providers of gametes, or in the case of surrogate arrangements, the providers of wombs.

Analogies between gametes, blood, and organs in narratives about donation were frequently made. One theme that constantly emerged was the potential for their exploitation once they were disembodied. Jane and Malcolm Griffiths wondered about what would be done with surplus gametes and embryos. Jane assumed 'to do something' with them one had to own them.

JANE: When you get to this, you suddenly realize that the whole thing is not very nice. When you start to talk about who owns living things.

MALCOLM: . . . if you didn't have enough room to put them away to be frozen, what do you do? You throw them in the bin. Well you know, I mean that is the—to me, that epitomizes what I feel about the whole thing. When I heard the National Health Service was selling blood, I stopped donating for a time, until I got this reassurance that they weren't. And that's because it's my blood and been given for humanitarian purposes and not to fill the pockets of private medicine.

JEANETTE: What about organs?

MALCOLM: I wouldn't do it. I'm sorry, I don't think I would feel like either donating or receiving an organ.

JEANETTE: You see a difference between organs and blood, in that sense?

MALCOLM: Yes I do. Because blood reproduces itself, doesn't it? And I give a pint and, within a couple of hours isn't it—well, its made up again. But organs are an irreplaceable part of me. And whether I be dead or not, I don't feel like giving them. And I certainly wouldn't want to receive them.

I asked Malcolm if there was a difference between blood and sperm: 'sperm is a starting point of life', he told me, therefore he '*would* distinguish between the two'. Like Sam Watson, he said he would neither donate nor receive sperm.[12]

Both blood and gametes are packed with the potential of kinship: if gametes are the precursor of new human beings, blood is the substance of relatedness. Blood transports and transfers microbes at the same time as it links kinsfolk both collaterally and from one generation to another. It is thought to be potentially dangerous, carrying, amongst other things, viruses from one person to another and transmitting traits which might include criminality and violence. It becomes doubly dangerous with the addition of a hint of commercialization. In late twentieth-century Britain, blood and organs are inappropriate objects of commercial enterprise and financial profit ought not be accrued from them.[13] Originating as parts of persons, organs, blood, and now gametes are thought not to be completely alienable. The two, the inalienability of blood as a commodity and blood as a medium of inheritance, when conflated, provide a potent analogy for the donation of gametes.

The idiom of 'the gift' in narratives of assisted conception has been noted in the literature: the way in which gamete donors, surrogate mothers, and clinicians, amongst others, are described as providing 'the gift of life' has been analysed (see e.g. Ragone 1994; Strathern 1992*b*; Price 1998; Daniels 1998). But the gift of life embodied in, for example, organs, blood, and gametes may carry with it part of the giver (literally), but it cannot compel a return.[14] In NRT, the transference of gametes, or the legitimation of claims to children, also means breaking connections, or at least particular kinds of connection to gamete donors and surrogates.

[12] To borrow a favourite English homily: 'never a lender nor a borrower be'.

[13] Just as babies ought not to be exchanged for money and financial criteria ought not to be used in assessment of who is an appropriate parent, so too love, like hearts, should neither be bought nor sold.

[14] In its Maussian sense, gifts carry the giver with them and hau ('the spirit of things') demands a return (Mauss 1966: 8; but see Strathern 1992*b*; Parry and Bloch 1989; Cheal 1988). In Daniel Miller's (1998: 131) formulation hau is 'the cosmological principle that the Maori use to define the inalienable element in the gift that creates reciprocity'. However, there is no obligation to return the gift of life: social relationships are not necessarily created and maintained through this particular act of gift giving.

Close and Too Close

'Closeness' is an idiom which emerges again and again in Bacup ideas about assisted conception. Here I look at two aspects of closeness central to the way in which relatedness between persons is conceptualized. The first, imagined in idioms of biology (or to borrow one woman's expression 'scientific things') designates categories of relatedness in terms of the strength or dilution of shared substance. In this formulation, siblings are more closely related to each other than cousins, and parents more closely related to their children than grandparents to their grandchildren. The second refers to the quality and quantity of social interaction, particularly in ideas of mutual support. One woman, for example, described her family as close knit mostly because they all 'get on smashing', but importantly, 'if anybody needs anything then we are all there'. The frequency of contact, as well as the kind of interaction, between siblings and between parents and their offspring, begets closeness. But then it is because families are close that they are mutually supportive.

Bill Cooper told me that although he is not close to his brothers, 'the family itself is close'. He and his four brothers and sisters are all close to his mum and dad, but he thinks he is 'a bit out on a limb' in relation to his siblings. He thinks they are more closely related to each other than he is to them and says this is probably due to his being the eldest. 'As you know', he remarks, 'when you're growing up' there are different expectations of the eldest: 'we had to set the norms and standards, didn't we?' The role of the eldest works against (cuts across) the intimacy shared by brothers and sisters. But the fact that he perceives himself not to be as close to his brothers and sisters as they are to each other does not compromise the closeness of his family.

Closeness is not a privilege of kin. I was invited to the creative writing class held at the UWC on my return to Bacup. I was asked to talk about my thesis and class members (all women between the ages of 40 and 75) engaged with relish in the topic of my 'new research'. I asked a member of the class what she meant when she described her friend as 'close'. She told me: 'they know everything about you—all the skeletons in the cupboard—[she's] somebody who has known me all my life and I know her life and all her children's'. This reminded Mrs Moore, another class member, of her friend whom she was visiting every day. She and her friend were very close, she told us, they had known each other 'from being born'. The other face of being close, however, is being too close. The close-knit community, for example, is both a source of support and gossip, and cousins are too close to fight and nearly too close to marry, although they do both.

Jane Griffiths, thinking about children born through techniques of assisted conception, was reminded of her own family. She talked about the way in which the lads in her family—her son, her brothers, and her nephews—were alike: 'Bring all the lads together and sit them down in a room and you *know* they're all from the same family and they've all got the same bits of traits and looks.' According to Jane, this sense of similarity created a sense of inclusivity, which went beyond day-to-day interaction: 'when they all get together, they all think—they feel they're all part of the same family'. Her strategy of inclusion required marking shared characteristics which connect up in 'one family' individuals who also had families of their own. Including 'the lads' as members of the same family meant not making the connections which would delineate the other families to which they belonged and which they created.

Mrs Griffiths evoked her own family to talk of children born through egg or sperm donation or surrogacy arrangements. She wondered if they ever felt totally connected to the families in which they grew up if they did not share the 'same traits'. It would be easier, she thought, for them to exclude themselves, or to be marginalized. For the same reasons of connectedness persons who share origins, for example, those born of the same surrogate mother or from the semen of the same donor, were linked. Of children born from the same 'batch of sperm', Jane predicted: 'one of these days, they'll go to a football match and they'll sit next to each other on the terrace, and they'll look at each other and they'll say "You're my brother!" and they'll say "Yes I am!" I bet you a million quid. I bet you they will.' A positive recognition, a sense of familiarity, but not unambiguously good. What happens, Jane asked, if these people were different sexes. If, rather than two brothers meeting up for the first time, it was a brother and a sister: 'that's where you are going to have a problem. I mean if they do get together like that, and they start marrying each other and . . .' She left the sentence unfinished: enough had been said, and elaboration was unnecessary. Jane assumed we all 'knew' the implication of such a union was incest. In her example, boys from the same batch of sperm would recognize (be familiar with) one another—they would 'know' each other. For Jane, the same familiarity between a man and a woman would inevitably result in a sexual attraction—they would 'know' each other with much more dire consequences. We have seen the way in which statements about the tight knit community (where cousins marry cousins) or big, close-knit families (who interbreed) are mobilized in strategies of social differentiation. When people with whom I spoke about NRT thought about the possibilities of substituting the gametes of kin, they brought to the fore notions of 'closeness' and 'distance'. Some relationships were too close to allow for the transference of gametes because, with or without marriage, and with or without sexual intercourse, the connection would be incestuous. Hence, for a brother to provide his sister, or a father to provide his daughter, with sperm, would axiomatically constitute incest; as it would for a daughter to provide her father, or a sister to provide her brother, with ova. It is the prior relationship between father and daughter, or sister and brother, through substance they already share, which makes the transference of gametes between them incestuous. The strangers who meet on the terraces and turn out to be brothers, or who meet through Dateline and turn out to be brother and sister, are already related.

Further elaboration on the union of kin who are too close was made through frequent and detailed analogies with non-human animals. Mrs Lawson, thinking about whether a woman could receive sperm from her brother, drew on her expertise of breeding goats.

That would be bad breeding. I mean you don't even do that with animals It's *too close*. I mean, you don't do that with animals do you—fathers to daughter, or brothers to sister—because it's just bad breeding. Did I tell you I used to breed goats? You don't do it with *any* animal. You don't do it with dogs even, if you can help it . . . whether it's human or four-legged. I mean, that's what they did with white Alsatians. They put—they had a white father and then they had a white daughter, they put them two together, hoping for pure white offspring, and they ended up with a load of mad Alsatians—really unbalanced and things like that.

A similar point emerged when Jane and Malcolm Griffiths and I explored the possibilities of relatives donating gametes to relatives:

MALCOLM: And really when you think about it, I don't care what your geneticists say, it's sound genetic sense really. I mean, let's face it, if you want to breed a runt in the line, you breed with the same stock don't you? If you want to inbreed certain weaknesses . . .

JANE: Well, what they've done in breeding dogs.

MALCOLM: Yeah, yeah.

JEANETTE: But don't they also do that with strengths as well?

MALCOLM: What?

JEANETTE: Don't they also do that with strengths? If they want to breed a particular strength in something, a particular positive trait, don't they interbreed then?

JANE: Yeah.

MALCOLM: But they also, at the same time, breed in the worse aspects. I mean, let's face it, look at bulldogs. They've bred for the short nozzles so they could grip tight on the bull's throat, and they've finished up with a breed of asthmatic dogs.

Contradictory examples coexist (and side by side) but one neither dislodges nor raises doubt about the validity of the other. Serving different purposes, they are not contradictory in their use, but only appear contradictory as I juxtapose them in analysis. Malcolm rejected the expertise of geneticists if they contradicted what everybody knew: if, in other words, their practice contradicted the common-sense knowledge of those who knew anything about breeding animals. He had, in his example of bulldogs, as had Mrs Lawson in her example of white Alsatians, evidence ready to hand of the folly of interbreeding.

But of course not all kin are restricted as far as the substitution of gametes is concerned. Distinctions are made between those who might be allowed to donate sperm and eggs and those who categorically cannot. In certain contexts, keeping gametes 'in the family' is seen as advantageous, not least because 'children know where they've come from'. People perceive there to be advantages in substituting the ova of sisters or the sperm of brothers, after all, from one perspective, children are related to their grandparents via one son in much the same way as another and the reproductive substance of siblings, originating as it does in the same parents, is similar enough to be substitutable. Furthermore, there is safety in *knowing* the origins of children. Now, the 'closeness' of the relationship between two sisters and between two brothers is foregrounded as good reason for allowing such procedures. If the provider of gametes is already related then there is less of a disjuncture between origins and birth. 'Keeping it in the family' mitigates the separation of component parts of relatedness. Furthermore, these relationships have the potential of becoming even closer through the assistance given. The support shown, for example, by a woman who provides the ovum from which her sister conceives a child is, it is said, an ultimate act of love and the interest they share in the ensuing child will strengthen their relationship: will bring them closer. However, their closeness is also a disadvantage and a potential source of difficulty. Their shared interest in a child (in its upbringing, for example) is just as likely to jeopardize their relationship as strengthen it.

Knowing has its downside. One can know too much. If a woman *knows* that the father of her child is reprehensible, there is a danger she 'sees' similar characteristics in the child. Or if an egg donor *knows* the woman who adopts the baby that was conceived from her ovum, or a surrogate mother *knows* the couple who adopt the baby she has gestated, they may be reminded of connections along which claims cannot travel. And why, people ask, is it always beneficial for children to know their origins. For children who are too young to understand 'seeds', one woman told me, they only had to hear it once—'I am not your father' and it would destroy them. They need not know.

Family Claims

To return to my conversation with Laura Gray: 'What about the husband's family?' she asked, referring to the husband of a woman providing the egg (the donating sister's husband). She thought about her question: '*They* will be bothered. They'll think the baby is theirs. And even though it's not connected to them, they'll want it.' This led her to surmise that it would be better all round if the donating sister were unmarried ('and younger'): 'Then', she said, 'there'd be no husband to connect the baby to his family.' For the same reason of connectedness, Laura thought the substitution of ova between sisters would not be a problem for 'their family', referring now to the family of the sisters. If a woman donated an egg to her sister, she explained, '*their* family isn't bothered [because] they're still connected—its still their grandchild'. Here Laura had the women's parents represent 'their family' and they were related to both their daughter's children in the same way. For Laura, it was obvious that grandparents would want to claim their grandchildren as their own. The problem lay in the claims of those not designated grandparents but in a similar structural position. Parents of the husband of the donating sister would be both connected and not connected to the ensuing child.

Next Laura told me to imagine two sisters, one of whom could not have a baby because her husband was infertile: 'What if her sister's husband donates sperm?', she asks. He would 'do it for his wife', she thought, and the other husband would also do it (that is, receive sperm) for *his* wife. The point she made was that a man would agree to provide sperm for his wife's sister, or receive sperm from his wife's brother, for his wife's sake—to please or to help her and because she desired it for herself or her sister.[15] Sperm is transferred via prior relationships between spouses and siblings. Laura thought this configuration would present a problem for 'the family' of the donating husband: 'The baby will *look* like the husband's dad, but it won't be connected to him and his family.' Links are made manifest in family resemblance and although the father of the man providing sperm, who was now a son (a consanguine) rather than a sister's husband (an affine), had no claim on the child, the child would look like him. In this example a man mediates a connection between his family (his parents) and his wife and by extension between his family and his wife's family. As a son he connects his parents to a child conceived from his sperm. And to be connected and not to be able to claim connection is problematic.

Laura then invited me to imagine two brothers, one of whom was infertile. She asked, what if the fertile brother donated sperm to the infertile brother? This would be less problematic, she said, especially for their family: 'it [the baby] will look like them', and it would be 'still theirs'. Here family resemblance and claims fortuitously coincided. Laura also pointed out that 'the woman's family won't be bothered—because it is her egg, and she gave birth'.[16] She did not mention a wife of the sperm provider but, again, thought it better if the donating brother was *not* married, then 'there is no *other* family to get annoyed'. Family resemblance renders visible (makes explicit) links already present. Thus, Laura surmised, a child conceived from the gametes of a woman and her husband's brother would look like her husband's family, and a child conceived from the gametes of a woman and her sister's husband would look like her sister's husband's father. The former is a generic rather than a specific 'look', while the latter—'like his dad'—provides a more potent image of the potential for conflicting claims. The provider of sperm, in this last

[15] Whether it is eggs or sperm, Laura spoke here of the donation of gametes as if it were to women not men.

[16] Here, the making explicit of a double attachment (ovum and birth) images a firmness of attachment.

example, was already linked as an affine to his brother's wife and now he mediates a link between his parents and the child which, in turn, is made evident in the child's looks.[17] But the problem as Laura saw it, in this example, was that his family could not legitimately claim the child as their own, despite the fact that they were, from another angle, inextricably linked.

If a child conceived from the gametes of a woman and her husband's brother looks like the husband's 'family', a correspondence between looks and claims is intact. But connection does not require both; one or the other will do. If the donating brother is not married there is 'no other family' to which connections (without looks) can be made. If married, he mediates a connection between the child and his wife's family, who will inevitably want, although be unable, to act on the connection. In both these examples, Laura portrayed vividly a sense that children are valued and that connections, however mediated, will be made because families will *want* to appropriate *their own*. Who is to be included in 'their own' depends on the mediators through which connections are traced.

Let me pull out four strands from Laura's narrative about the substitution of gametes between kin. They are themes which emerged in other Bacup conversations and are strands which I pick up in the final chapter. First, Laura emphasized the fact that families will *want* to claim children to whom they can trace connection. Her conviction that both individuals and families covet children is striking, and she constantly returned to the problem posed of not being able to claim (include in one's family) a connected child. Second, connections are traced through affines as well as consanguines, hence a potential chain of connections (mediated by the gamete provider) is cut off if the donor is unmarried—there will be no other family (affines) who will inevitably wish (but be unable) to claim connection to the child. Third, the concept of family is mobilized more or less inclusively. Boundaries of family shift to designate the family you were born into (represented by your parents), the family you create (in the reproduction of children), and the family you trace through affinal as well as consanguineous connections. Fourth, gametes are transferred to women rather than men, which may be literal in so far as it is women who gestate a pregnancy, but is symbolic in so far as the desire for children is in this model located primarily in women—men co-operate and act on behalf of their wives.

Laura raised what she saw as dilemmas common to brothers donating sperm to brothers, and sisters donating eggs to sisters. She talked of the implications of such reproductive innovation for families, embedding the specifics of NRT in wider social relations and mobilizing idioms of kinship in thinking about specific forms of conception. Laura foresaw no conflict of

[17] At the same time the child's looks are evidence of the link between the child and the sperm donor's family. The child has the potential of making a consanguine out of an affine.

interest for parents of brothers who substitute sperm, or for parents of sisters who substitute ova. From this perspective, one is related to the children of all one's sons, or all one's daughters, in the same way. Consequently affective ties, if you are a grandparent, are not necessarily compromised if gametes are provided by another of your offspring. A puzzle is posed, however, by the spouse of the gamete provider who is already connected as an affine. By extension his or her family is also already connected. This family is now both a problem (will want to claim the child) and is presented with a problem (is connected to a child it cannot claim). It is self-evident in Laura's discussion that families will *want* to claim children they consider their own and children are desired not only in themselves but also in their capacity to mediate connections.

The connection Laura narrated between the donating sister's husband (or the donating brother's wife) and the ensuing child evocatively portrays the hybridity of the kind of kinship on which I have focused in previous chapters. A man's family (in this case, his parents) would normally claim all *his* offspring as also belonging to them. They may also claim his wife's children by tracing their connection to them via their son. A son mediates a connection between his parents and his wife and by extension his wife's children. The concept of family is mobilized exclusively to include only relations in which some kind of substance (be it imaged in terms of blood or genes) is shared, or inclusively to cover connections forged through care and intimacy. (And indeed family may jettison members however they are related.) The substitution of sperm between brothers, or ova between sisters, presents similar kinds of advantage (close) and drawback (too close). The success or otherwise of both these innovations depends ultimately on the way in which pertinent social relationships are conducted. It all depends, Laura concluded, on *the relationship* between 'the donator and the receiver'. Now affective ties between, for example, same-sex siblings determine whether substituting their gametes (in order for one of them to conceive) is advantageous or disadvantageous. The kind of intimate social relationship same-sex siblings are supposed to enjoy cuts across links inhering in shared substance either augmenting (adding to the notion of shared substance) or displacing it (providing an alternative).

Our conversation continued and I asked Laura about the anonymous donation of gametes. She considered it in the light of her previous examples: 'if it is kept in the family, they [the children] will know where they're from', whereas there could be problems, she suggested, 'if sperm and eggs are unrelated'. She explained: '*All* children want to know where they come from—it's a natural instinct to look for your real parents.' Here, gametes are already related (before, that is, a relationship is forged).[18] Other Bacup residents I spoke with about NRT made comparisons between known and unknown sources of eggs and

[18] They are both discrete and alienable entities, and carriers of relations and identities.

sperm and while I return to this, the point to make here is that the gametes of sisters (or brothers) are already related and in their substitution their relatedness is revealed.

While the closeness of certain family members might make the substitution of their gametes not merely possible but preferred, the closeness of others curtails the possibility making it not merely impossible but abhorrent. Like the close-knit community assessed both positively and negatively as either friendly or parochial, or close-knit families who are either the backbone of Bacup or its scourge, so prior relationships, implicit in the use of NRT, can be suitably close or far too close for comfort.

9

Gametes Need Names

PATTY COOPER and her friend Sarah Daley were neighbours and partners in their own business. After leaving school, both women worked in shoe factories and became skilled sewing machinists. In their early thirties, they were each married with two children, and since becoming mothers had mostly continued working either from home as outworkers or in local shoe factories in shifts that fit in with the school day. When I returned to Bacup in 1990, they were self-employed and working from Patty's house making and fitting elegant and ornate domestic 'window wear'. They designed, sewed, and assembled sumptuous curtains and window blinds from bold, Laura Ashley-type, printed fabric. The prints were often larger than life-size flora and fauna in designs and colours reminiscent of the late nineteenth century. Patty and Sarah skilfully and creatively dressed windows by hanging and draping large quantities of ruched fabric from pelmets covered in matching or contrasting material. The curtains were held in required places with tasselled tie-backs and/or rosettes, while blinds were opened by threaded ribbon which pleats the material neatly and elegantly. Patty and Sarah designed and made all the accessories and trimmings (such as pelmets, tie-backs, and rosettes) by hand, and did the fitting themselves. I used to visit them when the children were at school and chat with them while they were working or taking a break.

Rooting for You

PATTY: It is a good thing to know where an egg came from. The same rules as adoption should apply—the child has a right to know. It will want to know 'who do I look like—who is this other person?'—it will be curious to know where its *roots* are from.

SARAH: The donor should be quite pleased to see the result of donation. Say there are twenty-five children—that is lovely, great—all the more people you have helped. You have no ties to these people, no obligations. No real moral ties.

PATTY: You have done the family as a whole a favour.

This interchange highlights a central ambiguity with which this book is concerned: roots are both axiomatic (given) and require sustenance (develop). Patty looked at the substitution of gametes from the perspective of a child conceived from an egg provided by a donor, and suggested its roots (origins) were revealed in the egg and that the child (like everybody) would want 'to know' its origins. From the perspective of the donor, however, there are no ties to ensuing children because there is no relationship with them. The ties to which Sarah referred are not only about a special kind of attachment (moral), but are forged in interaction: ongoing and characterized by reciprocation. Sarah applauded the action of donors who had no ties and no obligations to children resulting from their donation. Both women assumed successful techniques of assisted conception would benefit not only individuals or couples but 'the family as a whole'.

The notion of moral obligation also emerges when people talk about the vulnerability of detached entities such as gametes and embryos. A danger that clinicians or scientists will have no moral obligation towards such things is identified. Responsibility goes with connection and clinicians, for example, are unconnected to the embryos and gametes with which they work and are not therefore axiomatically responsible for them. These reproductive substances are not, in other words, 'their own'. A commonly expressed concern is that without curbs on the scientific endeavour children could eventually be conceived, gestated, and born exclusively in a laboratory. As conception and the growth of an embryo can now take place outside the body, it is predicted that the next step is for a foetus to be nurtured outside the womb and ultimately for an infant to be reared outside homes and apart from intimate social relationships. We miss the point if we dwell on whether or not this will or can actually occur. The idea of laboratory-reared people reveals certain cultural understandings of how persons are created and related. If NRT addresses and draws on such understandings then it is not surprising they both intrigue and alarm. Bacup residents, whether they are knowledgeable or not about technologies of assisted conception bring to them certain knowledge, which includes the idea that to be disconnected from people and places, both past and present, is to be without roots, and to be without roots is to be unprotected. 'They need a moral bond—it's down to *roots* again—*roots* of a person', one man told me, when thinking about people born with the help of NRT.

Roots connect places, persons, and pasts. In popular usage, one's roots, refer to both family of origin and attachment to place. Many Bacup residents at some point, in one or other of our conversations about NRT, wondered whether children conceived from donated gametes or born of a surrogate mother would have roots. 'Everybody needs *roots*', I was told by one man, 'these children do as well.' Not knowing one's roots means, as one woman put it, 'having no real beginnings, no family and no ancestors'. These comments beg the question of why children conceived from donated gametes or gestated in the womb of a surrogate mother might lack roots.

One answer lies in the inability of the gamete donor or surrogate mother to mediate connections to other persons. A potential avenue of relatedness is curtailed. Again the emphasis is on knowing. In the anonymous donation of gametes, donors are unknown: they cannot therefore act as a link (a node) in a chain of connections. But, of course, from another perspective this is irrelevant, as adoptive or commissioning mothers and fathers equally mediate chains of connection. We might be tempted to read a commentary on roots as claims about genetic connections and disconnections, perhaps as statements about the inability of individuals conceived with gametes from anonymous sources to trace their genetic origins. But roots both axiomatically connect persons (it is merely a case of revealing them) *and* are only made manifest in moral obligations engendered through interaction. An alternative set of connections can be traced through, for example, adoptive or commissioning parents who also effectively root children in places and pasts, as well as in families.

The substitution of gametes in assisted conception renders visible, then, core ideas of what I am calling Born and Bred kinship. Gametes are both discrete entities *and* contain and transfer past social relationships which make up a person in the present; they are, on the one hand, alienable and, on the other, irrevocably attached. And that is why, as we shall see, 'gametes need names'. Roots are not only about linking a person to the past but also about locating them in the present.[1] The concerns people express about clinicians or scientists having no responsibility for children born through the conceptive technologies they control addresses an interest in kinship. The danger is that children born with the aid of NRT are disconnected from those relationships which root them in places and pasts. Children could be born, one woman said, without anybody taking full responsibility for them. To be disconnected from your roots, then, is to have fewer people rooting for you.

Previous chapters have highlighted ways in which the past is rendered visible today and how current preoccupations are aired in selective and selected elements of the past. Thus selected items of history are mobilized to portray a resilient and resourceful Bacup character which is contrasted with the fickleness and fecklessness of city folk. In this way present-day distinctions between categories of resident are rendered visible. At a personal level, the bits people tell of their lives, and the way in which they order and reorder the pieces, do not root them in soil but in relation to other persons. Persons are not only connected to the past, but are constituted of the past. The present then is formulated not merely with reference to the past but with the past on board. Just as

[1] Liisa Malkki (1992) explores English botanical metaphors such as those referring to roots, the soil, and the land which powerfully represent identity and territoriality. She notes the earthy etymology of idioms, such as native, culture, autochtonous, and indigenous and shows how they serve to fix people to particular lands or to the soil. It is a sedentary thinking, she writes, which fuses natives to their forests, or 'incarcerates them in primordial bioregions'. Her concern is to show how, in the light of these metaphors, displacement and homelessness is viewed as pathological, particularly by Western scholars writing about refugees. Malkki identifies ways in which these metaphors are used tragically and powerfully to the terrible disadvantage of particular populations and she shows clearly how there is a need to unravel the hegemony of particular meanings imposed on heterogeneous peoples. How do we understand those same metaphors when they are part of the cultural repertoire of self-definition? Some of those very same metaphors that are as damaging when imposed upon certain populations are put to work in Bacup. But here roots are not only about fixing people to places or tracing connections to the past (although the idiom of roots embraces both of these things) but are also about making tangible the prior relationships that constitute persons in the present. A scrutiny of the meanings packed into such idioms sheds light on the way in which only certain, and not all, meanings are unbraided and given prominence for political and partisan purposes.

the history of Bacup is said to have moulded a particular character, so roots are a connection to a past we carry with us. The past is put to work to provide a voice and a form for significant relationships of, for example, kin, friends, enemies, and neighbours. To want to know one's roots is not a romantic ideal which purports that in the past, that is, before technologies of procreation, roots were more prolific or deeper. Rather it draws on a cultural understanding of kinship where prior relationships make up a person and where persons are constituted by, and constitutive of, those relationships.

Naming and Placing Gametes

I return to a conversation with Patty Cooper and Sarah Daley. They told me there were advantages and drawbacks in knowing sperm and egg donors. They talked of the advantages of 'keeping it in the family'. Sarah said she would have been willing to donate an egg to Patty had the need arisen. They were, she said, *close* friends and both agreed they would do 'anything for each other'. Neither Patty nor Sarah seemed keen on the idea of donors being anonymous. Thinking of anonymous sperm donation led them to wonder who owned the sperm. Clinicians or laboratory workers were not connected—they had no ties to it. Turning her attention to eggs, Patty thought that if it was necessary to freeze and store them then 'they would be safe in her [the donor's] name . . . she would have the right to say they were to go to someone else. They are still hers. They have still got her name on.' She concluded that everything, in fact, should not only be named but also addressed: 'they should have a name and address on every egg and sperm'.

The danger inherent in unattached and disembodied gametes is made explicit in her commentary. Unconnected gametes are vulnerable: they have nobody rooting for them. They are perceived as matter out of place, belonging neither to the donor nor the recipient; liminal and disembodied, exposed and in need of protection. Perhaps if 'on loan' they are safer than if relinquished. The stored embryo generates a similar kind of concern. You will recall for Mr Griffiths, the disposal of 'spare embryos' symbolizes many of the anxieties about technological intervention in human reproduction more broadly. Patty Cooper disliked the idea of storing frozen embryos, according to her it was tantamount to storing frozen lives. Her friend defended the practice, 'it is for ease', she pointed out, 'imagine your life without a baby, then you'd agree'. She concurred with Patty, however, that embryos should not be 'owned' by clinics: 'it is dangerous if they belong to an institution', and again the solution is to name them until they are 'allocated to another couple'. By putting a name and address on gametes and embryos they are located in relation to people and places; they remain, in other words, connected to their origins until they belong elsewhere.

I wish to dwell for a moment on the notion that gametes need names in the light of ways in which other entities are named and what such naming strategies do. The way in which people make sense of NRT is of a piece with the ways in which they make other kinds of connections. If culture is constituted of connections made between different domains of social life, then my concern is with a cultural analysis of NRT. The views of Bacup people about, for example, the naming of eggs and sperm, or whether sperm donors should be named or remain anonymous, or the naming of children born of surrogate mothers, need to be understood in relation to the significance of naming in other spheres of social life.

Kin terms gave Bacup respondents pause for thought. Mrs Moore exclaimed vehemently in our discussion in the creative writing class: 'I don't believe in this step. I have never been a lover of step-anything. Not a step-gran. I won't be a step-grandma. I'm a grandma not a step-grandma.' She explained: 'some of my grandchildren are not my blood', but they are 'accepted exactly the same'. For Mrs Moore, there was a drawback in being called 'step-grandma': it implies a different kind of relationship from 'grandma'—a once-removed (distant) grandma, which she refused to be. One young woman told me she would 'fight anyone' who said her brother was her stepbrother. While he might have a different father from her, he was, in her eyes, her brother without qualification. 'Step' implies a qualified connection, not a real one. It is in the denial of a difference, however, that difference lies and these examples suggest a resistance to the privileging of biological connection while reaffirming biological connection. The point to make is that in order to emphasize shared substance, often couched in idioms of 'biology', an alternative, such as shared sentiment, is needed. Sentiments are evoked and connections embraced in the use of kin terms, whether substance is shared or not. One woman felt strongly that had her daughter-in-law's two children from an earlier marriage called her and her husband 'grandma' and 'grandpa' instead of calling them by their first names, they would have been differently and more closely related. Kin terms are not sluggish; they do more than fix and locate people in relation to each other, they also connote special types of relationship and are thought to create particular kinds of ambience, with or without (or with more or less) shared substance.

Another question arising frequently in Bacup discussions of NRT, was how to name a child born through surrogacy arrangements. In the words of one man: 'What name will it have when it is born; what name will go on the birth certificate. It is not so simple.' Naming gametes or embryos or infants born of surrogate mothers acts to connect them to persons and thus renders them safe. It is not acceptable for them 'to belong' to clinicians or scientists, who being unconnected are perceived to have no moral responsibility for their well-being.[2]

[2] Sam Watson made an analogy between the treatment of embryos and the treatment of indigenous peoples: 'The same scientists buggering around with embryos, it's the same as those going to the Amazon giving tribes the flu.'

The naming of gametes makes explicit to whom they belong. There is also, however, a matter of intentionality. One woman talked about the difference between donating sperm for somebody else's use, and loaning ova in the hope that fertilization (on your behalf) occurs in the clinic. She talked about the ownership of gametes in this way:

It's a bit of a problem really, isn't it? Because it's—it depends—I mean if it, like you say, it was sperm taken from a student—I mean, he's given his for no purpose. [Whereas] she's given hers for a reason—she hasn't given them actually—she loaned them to them to see if they can fertilize them. They really still belong to her don't they? I can see they're [clinicians are] saying 'well really they don't belong to either donor they belong to whoever is *doing* it'. Which could be very dicey, couldn't it?

On the one hand, the man who donates semen anonymously does not intend for ongoing connections to be forged via his sperm: to attach his name to his gametes would create a link he does not seek. On the other, the intention of a woman undergoing fertility treatment is to conceive, consequently her ova whether in the clinic, or not, are still connected to her and naming them will render that connection and her intention explicit. The idea of naming gametes is to attach them to their origins rather than to 'the clinic' or 'the clinician'. But there are other, perhaps more pragmatic, reasons given for recording the names and addresses of gamete donors. Children born through such procedures, it is said, *should* be able to trace their origins if they so choose in the future. The suggestion is that unconnected children, like gametes, are vulnerable—they require protection. One woman asked: 'what if kids get brought into the world by scientists and get passed about between scientists and families'. She made an analogy with fostered children who, she said, were often passed around between social services and families, but belonged to neither. She argued that many, unsurprisingly, became drop-outs because:

They don't have a permanent home. They have nobody to take full responsibility . . . They just think 'who cares?' If they had a mum and dad, their mum and dad would *care* if they robbed a bank or killed somebody. . . . They can't say 'can't do that because what would me mum say? she'd kill me'. Or 'what would me dad say? he'd kill me'. [They] need somebody there to say 'that's not nice', or 'I'm proud of you', or 'that's not on'.

This woman was not talking about the ability or otherwise of foster-parents, nor was she suggesting that foster-parents and children in their care never forge intimate attachments. (In another conversation she told me how an adoptive or foster-parent is, in many cases, 'more of a parent' than a 'real one'.) But she had to hand an example which confirmed the danger of persons being unattached and unconnected. Free-floating gametes, like free-floating children, are in a precarious place: detached they are unconnected to persons and the danger is they have nobody fully responsible for them.

Incest in a Petri Dish

There is an additional reason given for recording the names of sperm and egg donors. If records are kept, it is said, then the possibility of incest occurring in the future is reduced. Incest loomed large in many Bacup conversations about NRT. There were many variations on a particular theme which, broadly speaking, focuses on children conceived from gametes of the same donor who meet up in the future and, not knowing they are related, marry and reproduce. Mrs Griffiths, you may recall, asks what would happen if children born from the 'same batch of sperm' met up on the football terraces. Again we miss the point if we dwell on the chances of this actually happening. Such a preoccupation derives from a cultural understanding of the prior relatedness of those who share substance, be it 'genes' or 'blood'. It also draws on a common notion that 'like attracts like'; the intangible affinity set up through relatedness will be made manifest when those who do not know they are related meet. Roots trace genetic connections to the past but they also make explicit who a person is related to in the present. Incest, like the spectre of children reared in laboratories, or of cloning human beings, acts as a conceptual brake on challenges NRT present to kinship: to the unhitching of being born and being bred, which elsewhere are inextricably linked. The concept of incest delimits who can donate gametes to whom and images a limit to technological intervention in reproduction.

The combining of gametes from different-sex siblings, or from a father and his daughter, or a mother and her son, is incestuous. It matters not that fertilization takes place in a Petri dish. Sexual intercourse is not a requirement for the brakes of incest to be applied. Incest is not only about prohibited sexual intercourse, it is also about the mixing of shared substance. Siblings already share blood and genes, it is therefore deemed unproblematic for their parents if their gametes are substituted (in examples of sister-to-sister egg donation, or brother-to-brother sperm donation): ensuing children will be grandchildren in much the same way. But different-sex siblings cannot *combine* their gametes. The possibility of men donating sperm to their sisters or to their daughters might seem obviously problematic, and it is problematic in a different way from their donating sperm to sons or brothers. In the latter gametes of kin are substituted, in the former they are combined. The union of substance that is already shared (between a father and daughter, or a brother and sister) is incestuous. Ideas about incest which emerge in conversation about NRT are of a piece with ideas about cloning. They both raise a question about whether a unique and new individual can be created from such procedures. Both incest and cloning, like laboratory-reared children, compromise the uniqueness of individuals.

Putting Names to Work

I have wanted to show that unnamed and disembodied gametes are betwixt and between, liminal entities—vulnerable and dangerous. But to do so I have needed a context. Earlier chapters of this book have provided that context. Naming strategies feature large in my analysis of Bacup. I remark on the disdain with which Bacup readers of my thesis treated my use of pseudonyms. Those who criticized me about my use of them thought that not naming people was a wasted exercise. First, if you *know* Bacup you can identify residents, and second, to understand Bacup and to make meaningful comments about present-day life there, then the identity of those about whom you speak is crucial. Bacup residents know there to be a variety of perspectives within the town, and they know your background influences not only what it is you know, but how you know it. My co-conversationalists contextualized their ideas about a topic such as NRT in relevant details about their own background. They know that the way in which you are connected to people, places, and pasts is integral to your understanding of NRT, as it is to your understanding of Bacup. And names are one way in which connections are revealed.

I touched on the etymology of 'Bacup' and noted that by far the favourite origin story featured frolicking deer running 'back up' the hill. This particular story, I argued, is popular for its charm—not any old history will do. The past, relevant today, is one peopled by idiosyncratic characters who exhibited fortitude in the face of adversity, as well as a resilience and distinctiveness. They moulded the present-day sensible and pragmatic Bacup character. While many residents lay claim to the status 'Bacup born and bred' the notion of real Bacup people carries further weight, and particular patronyms are evoked as real Bacup names.[3] Whether such names are assessed negatively or positively the import of them rests on the image they portray of bounded and discrete groups of kin. Names may individuate—a particular combination of a first name and a family name does mark a unique person—but, at the same time, they carry with them the significant relationships that constitute a person. Hence actual names can be ignored as irrelevant to the task at hand: Mrs Miller

[3] Accounts of Bacup's industrial history, both written and oral, underline the fact that labouring families who settled in the town during the 19th cent. came predominantly from Leicestershire, Cambridgeshire, and Norfolk, despite the fact that many older Bacup people trace their ascendants to Lancashire, Yorkshire, and Ireland. In the abstract, original Bacup people come from rural central and southern English counties. I note parallel ideas concerning contemporary immigration: a common stereotype is that all recent incomers are yuppies, come from Manchester, and commute back there to work. But not all and not only incomers are yuppies, and as we saw, many new households in the recently built speculative housing in Bacup are established by people from the nearby towns of Rawtenstall, Todmorden, Rochdale, and Burnley.

is really a Murphy, and Mr Smith a Leary. Just as changing the name of a housing estate (Mount Pleasant) will not transform the relationships it houses, so changing your name will not change the social relationships of which you are constituted.

I have explored the work of names in Bacup. It could be argued I have jerked from one arena of naming, the etymology of place-names, to another, the connotations of surnames, to yet another, the ambience of kin terms. It might be argued they are different orders of naming and, as such, incomparable. And they are, of course, both similar and different. The idea that gametes need names is of a piece with the way in which names are put to work in all kinds of different spheres of English social life. In narratives of origin, connections are made between family names and places, and between kin terms and types of relationship. Names also connect vulnerable entities (e.g. gametes) to persons. They have a life which outlives their demise (such as Mount Pleasant). While names might be given to places, people, and gametes as if they were entities, their power lies in the connections they make explicit. Names in industrial, secular society are active.[4] They are far from inert, and perhaps the idea they are has been but a strategic device with which comparisons between Western and non-Western societies have been made.

Consumer Procreation

I have remarked elsewhere that the views of Bacup residents with whom I spoke about NRT were marked by ambivalence (Edwards 1993; 1995*b*; 1998*a*). On the one hand there is an empathy with what is often referred to as the heartache of infertility and on the other a call for limits on possibilities presented through medical and scientific intervention. Some techniques are more problematic than others, and there is a general agreement that 'science' can go *too* far and its excesses need to be curbed; there are some ways of conceiving and growing a child deemed not only inappropriate but beyond the pale. But limits are not fixed points. It is not possible to discern, from what people say, a line between appropriate and inappropriate intervention. The same criteria are not applied to every instance and what is relevant in a particular context depends on the question formulated in interaction and itself provides the context for subsequent ideas.

One common theme running through many of my conversations in Bacup about NRT is the distress of wanting a child and not being able to conceive. Many Bacup residents describe the stigma attached to infertility and speak of ways in which it is understood by family, friends, colleagues, or neighbours as a failing and a failure. The stigma of infertility is gendered: in the case of men, connections are made with virility, and in women with femininity. There are

[4] Contrary to Lienhardt's (1988) assertion that names in the West are adventitious and arbitrary.

common expressions and euphemisms for infertility, often spoken in jest, but with barbed messages. It might be said of men they 'have no lead in their pencil', and of women they are not 'proper women'. One woman told me she was convinced that if her husband had been infertile he would have been impotent: as if he had been 'castrated', she said. The men with whom I spoke, imagined what it would be like not to be able to have a child. They acknowledged they would, more than likely, be the butt of a great deal of teasing; they also linked infertility with sexual drive, but not necessarily in a predictable way. Bill Cooper, for example, thought about the similarities between being infertile and being sterilized. Having recently had a vasectomy (in his words 'the snip') he pointed out he was, actually, 'clinically infertile': 'but it doesn't make me feel like I am not a man, in fact quite the opposite, its great—you can throw away the rubbers'.[5] Alan Gray talked about what would happen 'if a bloke couldn't have kids'. He imagined if it were him, he would 'think something were missing'. Although he thought that yearning or longing for children came from women rather than men, he imagined it would be very difficult for him: everybody 'around here' has kids, and 'a couple, thirty years old, without kids, has never been known'. He thought if he and his wife had been unable to conceive, they would have argued a great deal. There would have been 'rows': 'shall we do this?—shall we do that?' For Alan, a vasectomy was not the same as being sterile: with a vasectomy you still '*know* you can—you have already fathered children'.

Knowledge has its own effects: the damage lies as much in the knowledge of infertility as in the fact. This view was echoed by Sam Watson from a different angle: 'It's man-made traditions that make people feel bad', he told me. If people were infertile they saw themselves as 'lacking', but really it was 'just the luck of the draw': 'In Western civilization people have to be morbid. Ignorance is bliss. The more you have got to worry about, the more you will. If people are ill and can't get a transplant, it will make them more anxious.' Mrs Shaw put it this way: 'It's more the fact that they can't [have children] and *know* they can't. When you are married, if you can't have one then you probably *definitely* want one. When you are told you can't do something then you want it more.' For Sam, demand was generated by the scientific endeavour itself and with demand came an attendant expectation of fulfilment. New anxieties followed. The whole thing, he argued, was tantamount to 'consumer procreation', and in pursuing the theme of consumption he remarked, 'technologies will destroy themselves'. They would, he suggested, consume themselves.

Bacup residents talk about infertility as a source of great personal suffering. One man, raising the question of whether he would, were the need to arise, donate semen to either of his sons, predicted that if his son and his

[5] Rubbers: slang for condoms.

daughter-in-law were infertile, they would be in 'a desperate situation—horrendous', and consequently he would have no qualms about 'helping them out'. One woman thought, before the birth of her fourth child, that she was unable to conceive again. It was, she said, her experience of wanting to be pregnant but not being able to get pregnant that allowed her to understand the feelings of 'infertile couples'.

> You see I've been through the stage where I didn't think I'd have any more and I wanted them. I do know what it's like to go up to the toilet and see blood in your knickers and that feeling of 'aaw', you know?—You see, I thought I'd have the coil taken out. I'd worked [it] out like on a watch, you know? 'I'll have a baby in nine months.' Because I always fell pregnant so quick, and I'd had to have abortions, so I believed it. And as time went on, one year went by, I think it went on to nearly two years. I understood. I started to think babies all the time and I did start looking at prams—I can understand. I'm lucky to have experienced that, so when people go, 'oh she keeps on going on about it', I know what it's like. I know the feeling.

For this woman wanting a baby and not being able to conceive was obsessive: 'it eats you away—it eats them away wanting a baby'.[6]

The majority of Bacup residents with whom I spoke about NRT expressed an empathy for those unable to conceive. They thought that not being able to have a child would, for most people, be extremely distressing and would attract a great deal of unwanted attention. They identified pressures on young couples to reproduce. I was told family and friends *expect* pregnancy to occur within two years of marriage, and if this does not happen, it is automatically assumed there must be 'something wrong'. In the words of one woman, 'People who have chosen to be childless—[other] people assume they must be infertile. They say, "I can't have any" to shut people up. It's not seen as normal for women not to *want* a child.'

Acquaintances assume there are fertility problems when couples do not start a family within two years of marriage, and people can invoke infertility to put a stop to prying questions about their reproductive future. While many Bacup residents note that voluntary childlessness is not a positively valued option for married, heterosexual couples in Bacup, recent literature suggests infertility is increasingly no longer considered a sufficient reason for involuntary childlessness. In other words, there is an increasing expectation that one can and ought to overcome infertility through medical intervention and thereby have a child of 'one's own' (see e.g. Franklin 1997). In early-1990s Bacup, there appears to

[6] I am intrigued by idioms of eating and consumption emerging in discussion of NRT. I was often told that the experience of infertility 'eats' people away; one man, talking about the rapidity of technological developments, argued it was getting out of hand and it would, eventually, 'eat itself'; and scientists are said to be 'feeding their own egos'. Images of cannibalism, like cloning and incest, symbolize, from this cultural perspective, things beyond and out of control. They are images that make explicit what are perceived to be limits to the scientific endeavour or to technological and medical intervention in social life.

be more ambivalence surrounding 'the need' to have a child of one's own. Bacup residents in 1990 were aware that 'needs' can be manufactured, encouraged, and marketed and that 'needs' do not necessarily come ready-made. They may identify a pressure on young women to reproduce, but they also talk of how difficult parenthood, particularly motherhood, is and of how promises of 'fulfilment' are broken.

Biological Imperatives

As well as social pressures to have children, Bacup residents identify a 'biological need' to have children. But such an imperative is not absolute. It is moderated and mediated by such things as careers or well-paid jobs. As one woman put it, 'it comes in different strengths'. Hence, despite the fact that biological needs are said to be innate—one is born with them—they are not necessarily switched fully on. Mrs Moore thought about her niece who, she said, is ambitious, has a good job and a nice home, and does not want children. This view was echoed by other Bacup women. It is more likely, they suggest, for women with careers not to want or need children. 'Want' and 'need' are juxtaposed in this formulation. As one woman put it, 'with a fantastic career you don't *need* children'. A career can intervene: it cuts across what is elsewhere perceived to be an unyielding, inbuilt drive to reproduce that cannot be assuaged. Most men I asked about a 'need to reproduce' suggest they never really thought about whether they wanted children or not. In the words of one Bacup man, 'I always assumed one day I'd get married and have children.' Another told me, 'only the most stupid of men *want* children'. I asked him what he meant: 'If I had known, I would not have wanted them. I am short-tempered with them. I feel guilty all the time. A lot of women deal better with kids, but all women with children are in prison.' Alongside an empathy for 'infertile couples', then, is an acknowledgement that having children, particularly for a woman, is not necessarily the end-all and be-all it is made out to be. In the words of one woman, now a grandmother several times over:

> It's a terrible thing, isn't it, motherhood. You want it so desperately, and if you can't have it, they don't feel complete without it and . . . they'll do *anything* to get it, you know, won't they? Yeah, you stand back and look at it when you've got your own and you think, 'oh my god, I must need my head tested'.

This woman identifies a common, and to her mind erroneous, idea that motherhood completes a woman: that somehow a woman is unfinished—not a proper woman—without a child. If a woman think this then it is clear to her why infertility should cause such suffering and why women are 'desperate' to have children. From the retrospective gaze of experience, motherhood is known to be difficult: fraught with doubt, anxiety, and hardship. From this perspective, motherhood is not all it promises. Mary Shaw professed to feeling unusually 'hard' about NRT. She explained:

> If I were 20 now I wouldn't have any kids. Women who haven't got children don't know that motherhood's not all it's cracked up to be. There are limited resources, and nobody's died through not having a child. Hip replacements are more effective—they help more people. We really need to look at the positive aspects of being childless.

For Mrs Shaw, as for other Bacup women who spoke about NRT, a major problem is the way in which women continue to think fulfilment lies in having children. They acknowledge the difficulty in remaining childless, but suggest the difficulty stems from a false sense of what motherhood actually means in practice. From this perspective, retrospective knowledge, born of experience, questions assumptions of fulfilment: it cuts across other kinds of imperatives, especially imperatives to reproduce.

Anna Brody told me her friend had been attending counselling sessions prior to embarking on a course of IVF: 'She's been told that she has only got three chances. She's paranoid and she's going against everything she believes in. Even though she is a friend of mine, I don't condone it. I think its kidology—they're fooling the public. There are loads of kids who need adoption.'

At the same time, many people with whom I spoke conceded they would feel differently if there were someone *close* to them who required fertility services. Mrs Shaw told me she would 'talk differently if there were somebody infertile in the room'. It is the knowledge of how upsetting and traumatic infertility is for those experiencing it that makes people cautious of bringing it up in certain conversations and, in particular, of criticizing the desire for children at any cost. Involuntary childlessness is experienced vicariously from different perspectives, of which there are many as it is seen to be a problem not only for individuals or infertile couples but for families as a whole.

In Chapter 2, I remarked on the kind of non-conversations I had in Bacup about NRT and argued that they stemmed as much from a knowledge of the reproductive histories of those present (either physically or virtually) as they did from taboos surrounding explicit talk of sex and reproduction. However much people question medical intervention in conception, and wherever they place limits, there is an assumption they would feel differently if they knew somebody who required fertility services. Talking of those 'who oppose it', Mrs Greaves said, 'if it was their families they'd understand'. You can never really *know* unless you, or those close to you, have experienced infertility, another woman old me. Participating in one another's fertility, kin also inevitably participate in each other's infertility. The idea that 'knowing' is achieved through experience is central to the way in which people make sense of NRT. Such an idea is put to work in myriad ways and used to explain seemingly contradictory sets of ideas. For example, it is only through the experience of infertility that one can truly know the distress it causes and, likewise, it is only through the experience of bringing-up children that one can *know* 'it's not all its cracked up to be'. An understanding of the implications of involuntary childlessness is not gained through discrete items of information, although they have their part to play, but is achieved through experience transferred along axiomatic links between those who are already *close*.

During fieldwork the so-called 'virgin-birth controversy' hit the news headlines.[7] Its focus was single women requiring access to clinical services such as donor insemination. As well as being reported extensively in British newspapers, a number of television and radio discussions addressed the topic and many of these were brought to my attention by Bacup friends and acquaintances. Although, in the context of the research, the subject of 'virgin births' was raised, I am left with the impression that it did not generate the same kind of interest as, say, the substitution of gametes between kin or surrogate motherhood. Single women having access to donor insemination was perceived to *affect* fewer people. First, because it was assumed not very many women would want children *without* sexual intercourse, and second because there is no immediate third party, such as a surrogate mother or a *known* gamete provider, to take into consideration. Those with whom I spoke seemed to trace fewer links between single women requiring fertility services and their own experiences of intimate social relationships. Remarking on the kind of publicity 'virgin births' had attracted, and on the way in which single women requiring fertility services and the clinics providing such services had been criticized, one Bacup woman echoed a view put forward by many others: 'If it happened in *their* family they would change their point of view, because they would be able to talk it out and understand. If it was somebody they loved, they would see what they needed and they'd stick up for them, against others—until they believe it themselves.' Bacup residents are convinced people feel differently about assisted conception depending on who mediates it for them. If a member of their family, or a person close to them (that is, already connected) requires fertility services, then they are linked differently to the technologies, and they are more likely to understand feelings generated by involuntary childlessness, because feelings travel between people already connected. Connections, then, between those already close allow for the passage of experience, and empathy travels well-worn routes, which in turn brings people closer.

[7] It is telling that the idiom 'virgin birth' was applied to unmarried women (heterosexual and lesbian) who required fertility services. One theme the media picked up was whether women who had never had heterosexual intercourse were suitable candidates for assisted conception. The virgin-birth debate in social anthropology also focused on narratives of conception that did not privilege heterosexual sex as a cause of pregnancy (Malinowski 1929; Leach 1966; Spiro 1968; Delaney 1986; 1991; and see Barnard and Good 1984 for a concise overview of the debate), and parallels have been drawn between this debate and so-called virgin births in the context of assisted conception (Franklin 1997).

Knowing and Knowing Too Much

One danger people are reminded of in their explorations of NRT is that children born through technologies of assisted conception will be socially marked as different, and the way in which persons are conceived will become a means of marginalization. One young woman asked me to imagine 'a family of donated children': 'You will get situations where people will say "they're donated—don't play with them". It will be like twenty or thirty years ago when people said "don't play with them—they're bastards".' For this woman, the facts of assisted conception might replace illegitimacy as a means of stigmatizing certain families. Of concern here is not the question of whether or not this will be the case (a question which I am not qualified to address) but the kind of analogies she is able to make.[8] Connections made between illegitimacy and assisted conception, like connections made between adoption and surrogacy, cloning and IVF, or incest and donor insemination (to name but a few), juxtapose phenomena which from one angle belong to different domains of social life and are, in one sense, incommensurable.[9] But connections across these domains can be made because each draws on similar cultural ideas about how persons are made and relatedness between them constituted. Bacup explorations of NRT draw on understandings of, amongst other things, what comprises a parent, 'the needs' of foetuses and infants, ways in which significant social relationships are reproduced, maintained, and curtailed, and what gets passed on and how. Such understandings are rendered visible in the personal histories people tell, the connections they narrate, and the analogies they make; all of which portray both the resilience and the fragility of social relationships. The need, identified in Bacup, for children to know their origins is counterbalanced by their need to be fully attached to the families in which they find themselves. Knowledge is not unambiguously good, it is also dangerous. It can rupture intimate relations. The presence of shared substance, in the form of, say, blood or genes, is not essential to enduring attachments of love and care. Talking of genetic fatherhood, Mrs Moore was provoked to complain to fellow members of the creative writing class 'well, we're talking about scientific things now'. In her subsequent comments she implicitly contrasted 'scientific things' with the day-to-day imperatives of social relationships:

my uncle was adopted, for instance, and I don't know how much he wondered about his real mother but his adopted mother was always his real mother, from his point of

[8] From social policy perspectives, the stigmatization of children born through assisted reproductive technologies is raised and often explored through analogies with adoption (see e.g. McWhinnie 1993; Haimes 1988; 1993). While my aim is not to downplay the very real and thorny issues of marginalization and family support in either adoption or assisted reproduction, my interest here is in ways in which ideas about stigmatization emerge in explorations of NRT.

[9] Connections are made across different domains which are also separate (independent) because of another sphere of connections in which they are placed. Strathern calls this kind of link merographic: 'difference . . . is a connection from another angle' (1992*a*: 72–3).

view. . . . It's more to do with relationships than it is to do with birth, I think; and the relationships what you build up. And I had a discussion with me mother some time ago and something to the effect that it wasn't blood necessarily that counted, it was the relationship that you'd built up between you, which I think does count for more. But that can always be disturbed by, as you say, adopted people growing up and wondering and trying to find out where they actually come from. Which I can imagine will also take place with those who want to find out what laboratory [they came from].

For Mrs Moore, the pragmatics of daily relationships, the quotidian connections, were privileged over substantive entities which she glossed on one occasion as blood and on another as genes.[10] She said her uncle's *real* mother was the woman who looked after him. She also noted that adoptees may attempt to make explicit, to find out, where 'they *actually* come from'. Both the origins of adoptees and the parent who looks after them are 'real' together, and there is no difficulty holding two 'reals' together. If unhitched, however, one can pose a threat to the other, threatening to cut it off. Thus Mrs Moore knew that relationships between adoptive parents and their children, forged through effort and care, could be disturbed by adoptees making explicit (looking for) connections through birth. Tracking one possible set of connections through, say, shared substance has the potential of cutting across another, tracked through, for example, interaction. Acting on one set of links (looking for your birth mother) has the potential of screening out another (looking after your real mother).

Thinking about bureaucratic state and health systems, some Bacup residents were reminded of the danger of not being able to provide what they called 'full medical histories'. They pointed out that if the source of gametes is unknown then the incidence of diseases that run in the family would also be unknown. *Knowing* is central to what constitutes a person in late twentieth-century English thinking. It is said that people need to know, for example, their roots, their family history, their place in networks of kin: where they come from. How a person comes to know these things is a constant source of speculation. Knowledge is conceptualized, on the one hand, as items of information, bounded and discrete, which might be imparted, acquired, or appropriated but in whatever way, is learnt. On the other hand, knowledge is unbounded and nebulous, assimilated through a process akin to osmosis and gained through experience. Knowing in one way always entails unknowing in another.

In the previous chapter, I noted the way in which 'common sense' is invoked positively; it has class connotations and provides a reference point for differentiation between *ordinary people* and experts. A person might be said to be

[10] 'In terms of the real world in which we live and where we try to cherish our dear ones, Oedipus does escape his fate, he does not murder the man who saved him from death, nurtured him, gave him a bicycle, had his teeth straightened, paid for driving lessons, etc. Nor does he impregnate the woman who wiped his bum, taught him to sneeze, and catered to all the indignities of childhood that effectively de-eroticise the relationship between mothers and sprogs. Oedipus's genuine filial feelings are not outraged. His biological parents are perfect strangers' (Angela Carter, *Expletives Deleted*).

clever or formally qualified, yet have little or no common sense. Common sense comes from experience and is positively valued, while being clever is not always a useful thing.[11] But knowledge gained through experience requires an alternative, such as knowledge gained through study, for its hold. Like kinship, knowledge is a hybrid.

Cohen (1987: 70) makes a comparison between knowing someone in Whalsay to knowing someone in urban society. In an urban setting to know someone is to be acquainted with them—to have met a person is adequate criteria for stating that one knows them. In Whalsay, however, where everybody is acquainted, to know someone means much more: it means to know of their connections through, for example, families, boats, and houses.[12] Distinctions are made in Whalsay between 'wir folk' and 'the unken' (ibid. 71). Wir folk are related through kinship, and are neighbours, they are also associated with particular fishing boats and their crews. In islander narratives the concept of 'wir folk' is prominent or fades into the background; it is, as a social category, more or less significant depending on the reason it is invoked. For Cohen the category 'wir folk' is cognitive rather than structural and an idiom through which islanders distinguish close associates from a large number of acquaintances (ibid. 70). Such a process of differentiation need not be confined to the small-scale or the rural. Bacup residents towards the end of the twentieth century also connote more than acquaintanceship in their talk of knowing. They trace significant strands which link persons to Bacup and to other residents, and as we have seen, links run through, amongst other things, patronyms, houses, slipper works, and pubs.

To reveal the distinctiveness of Whalsay, Cohen retains a distinction between urban and rural and the kinds of relationship they embody. Bacup residents do the same, they characterize 'the city' as cold and anonymous, replete with single-stranded, utilitarian relationships. In so doing, they construe Bacup as warm and friendly, full of relatedness and connected to its past. But we have also seen the flip side to this, and the same qualities are assessed as parochial, backward, and far from friendly. It is a similar strategy of comparison, I suggest, which purports that in contemporary Western society kinship is diminishing in importance and rationality is replacing myth. The material from Bacup, at the heart (and, for some residents, the start) of industrial England, shows that 'to know' someone entails a whole lot more than merely having met them. 'Knowing everybody' is a significant criteria of belonging in Bacup. However, while it is a commonly used idiom which images the interconnect-

[11] A colleague dismissed my interest in common sense. He argued that common sense is merely a colloquialism and is of no significance to the anthropologist. Perhaps this is another example of the difficulty in identifying what is of anthropological interest in items of information which are to greater or lesser degrees familiar.

[12] Cohen maintains a distinction between rural and urban, suggesting in Whalsay it is the multiplexity of relationships which allows islanders to emphasize different avenues of acquaintanceship.

edness of the town as a whole—'everybody knows everybody else'—acquaintanceship has its limits. Hence the 'everybody' to whom Judy Wilder referred is a different, albeit overlapping, 'everybody' from that to whom Barbara Jones referred. But value attached to 'knowing everybody' is not axiomatically and always positive; it is also deployed to image a place that is parochial, interrelated, and backward.

A knowledge of Bacup is gained by a self-conscious activity of finding out, of unearthing the facts (to borrow a Nat idiom), and/or through the experience of living there. Likewise, a knowledge of kinship is found in the physiological facts and biological detail of procreation. But kinship is also known in the experience of intimate social relationship. Persons need to be grown as well as born. A Bacupian interest in the roots of children born through techniques of assisted conception refers not merely to the tracing of genetic origins but to the positioning of persons in the past and the present; it refers as much to their ability to trace a history as an ancestor. If persons cannot trace what are called their roots they may not be linked firmly. Furthermore it is through known links that reciprocal care travels. Mrs Watson commented she could never fully know her two grandchildren from her daughter-in-law's previous marriage because they had a separate family on their father's side—a family she did not know. To know her grandchildren fully Mrs Watson suggested, required a knowledge of those to whom they were connected. This is what it means to be *close*. A close relationship does not merely refer to services exchanged, or frequency of contact, or residential proximity, it means knowing how a person is connected: it means knowing 'the skeletons in their cupboard'. To know a person fully requires more than a knowledge of them as an individual, it requires knowledge of them as a person embedded in, and embodying, kinship. Closeness results as much from knowing as from relating.

Being Born

Perhaps it is fitting I conclude with 'being born'. I am intrigued by answers to the question, 'where were you born?' It is striking the number of times people said Bacup, then added a caveat—'well actually it was' and then gave me the name of a hospital—Burnley, Bury General, Birch Hill, or Rossendale. I had assumed I was asking a different question; about where people came from rather than the precise locality of their birth. My version of 'came from' had included parental identities and places of birth, and I had sidelined actual places of delivery. But again what, at first glance, appears incontrovertible—where a person is born—has an exploitable ambiguity. I asked Joanne Leary if she was born in Bacup. She said she wasn't, she was born in Rossendale Hospital, near Rawtenstall. In treating it as a question about the place of delivery, kinship appeared to take a back seat. Discussion about the impending closure of the maternity ward in Rossendale Hospital turned on the fact that it would no longer be possible for 'Rossendale babies' to be born in Rossendale. One man, an incoming spouse, told me his children were not born in Bacup, they were, he said, born in Rochdale and Burnley (which turned out to be the location of the maternity hospitals in which his wife gave birth). From another perspective his children would be considered Bacup born and bred, but in his commentary he distanced himself and his children from Bacup. Although he is connected to Bacup via his wife he had the option, through his own place of birth, to curtail that connection, interestingly he was able to do the same for his children. Another man told me he was born in Manchester. It turned out that because of a potential complication in his mother's pregnancy, she was encouraged by her doctor to attend the maternity unit of one of the larger teaching hospitals in Manchester. Judy Wilder told me she was from Hemel Hempstead, and at a different moment, when I remarked on it, she corrected my assumption: 'Well I was only *born* in Hemel. That was where the maternity hospital was, but I—it's always got Hemel Hempstead [on the birth certificate]—but I actually lived from a child—from a baby—in Keal.'

The duality of 'birth' (where one comes from and where one was born) like 'child' (both a young person and offspring), or 'community' (a place and a set of relationships), or 'family' (nuclear and extended) are central to English ideas about relatedness. They are consonant with the ways in which all kinds of connections are made and unmade across different domains. The idea of the individual as a separate entity from the relationships that constitute it, is analogous to the event of birth (in Rossendale General) as separate from the context of being born (to particular parents).[13] In delineating a place of birth as the place in which birth took place, people screen out relationships that beget and are begotten by the birth of a child. That is precisely the power of Born and Bred kinship. One or other—born or bred—can be brought into focus, momentarily screening out, but never fully replacing, the other. But only to be born (anywhere) does not on its own make a person: the experience of growing up and being grown is vital. One needs to be born *and* bred, no matter where or by whom, and not necessarily both in the same place.

My interest has been in the kind of things kinship begets, as much as its begetting. Take the example of 'community' which seems to have bedevilled

[13] Of merographic connections, Strathern (1992: 78) writes: 'persons connected through kinship are regarded as of a different order from the kinship that does the connecting'. She goes on: 'Kin relationships are about how individual persons are connected to one another, yet not as whole individuals, only as kin, so that kin ties appear as but a part of that unitary entity, the individual person. Kinship connects unique individuals with the constant proviso that kin roles are only one among a constellation of roles.' If, in English kinship thinking, a person is a unique individual and/or a kinsperson depending on which set of connections are mobilized, then the point I would wish to emphasize is that they (the ideas of a unique individual and a relative) require each other.

the anthropology of Britain.[14] For Cohen (1987: 13), the boundaries of community are symbolic and the power of symbols derives from their lack of inherent meaning: 'whilst the *form* of symbols may be common to those who bear the same culture, the *meanings* of the symbols, their contents, may differ. . . . they do not carry their meanings inherently: in using them we impute meaning to them'. It is in their use, then, that images are conjured.[15] But, I want to argue, within parameters: parameters set by the way in which relatedness is conceptualized. Symbols are not infinitely pliable. If residents in Bacup talk about 'preserving the community', they also mourn a loss of 'community spirit'. Some draw attention to 'the sense of community' that initially attracted them to the town, and 'the loss of community' which drove them away from the places they left. As in Whalsay, where 'community' refers either to the people who live there, or 'suggests that its putative members have something in common' (Cohen 1987: 14), it is used both inclusively and exclusively. When residents mourn the 'loss of community spirit', they reflect on what they perceive to be a loss of particular kinds of social relations. As Green (1997) notes, common idioms of community in contemporary Britain such as 'the gay community' do not fix categories of person to particular localities, but make explicit connections between persons, and thus distinguish them. She describes how the London lesbian community, in the late 1980s, was neither tied to locality nor internally homogeneous, and divisions within the community mirrored divisions in wider society. For her the symbolic boundaries of community enclose 'representations' and 'ideas' rather than 'people and their beliefs' (p. 132). But ideas are as leaky as beliefs and, as Green remarks, it is contestation as much as agreement which perpetuates and enables the notion of community. Inhabitants of Bacup, who from an outside perspective (which is also found inside) are sometimes described as if they were a homogeneous community, constantly differentiate between each other. This continuous process of differentiation belies the idea of a single Bacup community, despite it being conceptualized from some perspectives as if it were. It is my contention that a particular kind of kinship thinking informs the generative possibilities of

[14] There has been, it seems to me, an overemphasis on 'community studies' and a reluctance to say something that cuts across them. Rapport (1993), however, makes a virtue out of this and dwells on idiosyncratic meaning disguised in recognizable forms of communication. He argues that mutual misunderstanding between people is as likely as understanding. His ethnography warns against the imposition of neat analytical frames in the description and analysis of contemporary social life which in reality is 'chaotic, multiple, contradictory' (p. ix).

[15] '[A]ll knowledge, and in particular all knowledge of the social world, is an act of construction implementing schemes of thought and expression, and that between conditions of existence and practices or representations there intervenes the structuring activity of the agents, who, far from reacting mechanically to mechanical stimulations, respond to the invitations or threats of a world whose meaning they have helped to produce. However, the principle of this structuring activity is not, as an intellectualist and anti-genetic idealism would have it, a system of universal forms and categories but a system of internalised, embodied schemes which, having been constituted in the course of collective history, are acquired in the course of individual history and function in their *practical* state, *for practice* (and not for the sake of pure knowledge)' (Bourdieu 1992 [1984]: 467).

community. It is both an entity and a set of relations; it is both fixed and fluid. Community is mobilized to designate an inclusive set of people and to exclude others; who belongs to it shifts according to the reasons for formulating it. The concept of community is mobilized in similar ways in, for instance, Bacup, Whalsay, and amongst London lesbians. Rather than being 'very much less like each other than we may popularly suppose' (Cohen 1982: 9), it may be the case that the ways in which we conceptualize our social worlds and locate ourselves within them are much more alike than our constant strategies of differentiation would suggest (see also Macdonald 1997).

The creation of community is itself a creation of the context in which common cultural resources are deployed—in which, as it were, culture 'is done'. The perception of the unique locality is itself a function of the way in which idioms of relatedness, by no means exclusive to Bacup, are put to work. And the resonances between Bacup and other British localities are to be found in the ways in which idioms of kinship fashion places and pasts as well as persons and, of course, relationships.

The power of Born and Bred kinship is in its hybridity, and the kinds of connection made through the interplay between being born and being bred are robust and ubiquitous. Focusing on the way in which idioms of relatedness, such as birth and breeding, are put to work by residents in the north of England towards the end of the twentieth century reveals the cultural repertoire from which different kinds of expert select. As experts in kinship, the people whose words I have borrowed in this book mobilize different strands of connectedness: strands they trace through such things as blood, or genes, or care, or love and which together make up kinship. Perspectives (vantage points) are created when one set of connections is made instead of another. And perspectives can be congealed and often are for particular political purposes. Thus for another kind of expert (say in science) it may be instrumental to emphasize one set of connections over and above another. But to do this—to extract just one strand of kinship thinking and present it as the whole story—is partisan. The kind of kinship on which I have focused is generated from the interplay between born and bred perhaps couched in terms of nature and nurture, or the biological and the social. It not only makes fine differentiations between categories of person and relationship, but also lumps them together in broad encompassing categories. It formulates 'communities' as well as 'families', and it connects people to, and disconnects them from, places, pasts, and each other. And it is not confined to Bacup.

REFERENCES

Abelman, N. (1997), 'Narrating Selfhood and Personality in South Korea: Women and Social Mobility', *American Ethnologist*, 24 (4): 786–812.

Agar, M. (1973), *Ripping and Running* (New York: Seminar).

Ardener, E. (1987), 'Remote Areas': Some Theoretical Considerations', in A. Jackson (ed.), *Anthropology at Home* (London: Tavistock).

Arensberg, C., and Kimball, S. (1940 [1968]), *Family and Community in Ireland* (London: Peter Smith).

Aspin, C. (1983), *Mr Pilling's Short Cut to China* (Helmshore: Local History Society).

Bacup Publications

BNHS (1978), *Bacup Natural History Society: Centenary 1878–1978* (Bacup: Howard & Hargreaves).

BNHS (1987), *Bacup in Times Past* (Chorley: Countryside Publications).

Borough of Rossendale Official Street Atlas (1986) (Gloucester: British Publishing).

Bowden, K. F. (ed.) (1972), *A Bacup Miscellany* (Bacup: Bacup Borough Council).

——(1975), *A Second Bacup Miscellany* (Preston: Lancashire County Council).

——(1982), *Samuel Chadwick and Stacksteads* (privately printed and sold on behalf of Stacksteads Methodist Church).

Goldthorpe, I. (1985), *Rossendale Rambles* (Rossendale Groundwork Trust).

Grass Routes (n.d.), The Changing Faces of Rossendale (Rossendale Borough Council and Rossendale Groundwork Trust).

Water Marks (n.d.), The Changing Faces of Rossendale (Rossendale Borough Council and Rossendale Groundwork Trust).

Balsamo, A. (1996), *Technologies of the Gendered Body: Reading Cyborg Women* (Durham, NC: Duke University Press).

Barnard, A. (1994), 'Rules and Prohibitions: The Form and Content of Human Kinship', in T. Ingold (ed.), *Companion Encyclopaedia of Anthropology: Humanity, Culture and Social Life* (London: Routledge).

Barnard, A., and Good, A. (1984), *Research Practices in the Study of Kinship* (London: Academic).

Barnes, J. A. (1973), 'Genetrix : Genitor :: Nature : Culture?', in J. Goody (ed.), *The Character of Kinship* (Cambridge: Cambridge University Press).

Bateman Novaes, S. (1998), 'The Medical Management of Donor Insemination', in K. Daniels and E. Haimes (eds.), *Donor Insemination: International Social Science Perspectives* (Cambridge: Cambridge University Press).

Behar, R. (1996), *The Vulnerable Observer: Anthropology that Breaks your Heart* (Boston: Beacon).

Bestard-Camps, J. (1991), *What's in a Relative? Household and Family in Formentera* (Oxford: Berg).

Bloch, M. (1988), 'Interview with G. Houtman', *Anthropology Today*, 4 (1): 18–21.

Boissevain, J. (1974), *Friends of Friends: Networks, Manipulators and Coalitions* (Oxford: Blackwell).

Bott, E. (1957 [1971]), *Family and Social Network* (London: Tavistock).

Bouquet, M. (1993), *Reclaiming English Kinship* (Manchester: Manchester University Press).
Bourdieu, P. (1992 [1984]), *Distinction: A Social Critique of the Judgement of Taste* (London: Routledge, Kegan & Paul).
Bowen, E. S. (1954), *Return to Laughter* (New York: Harper & Row).
Briggs, J. (1970), *Never in Anger: Portrait of an Eskimo Family* (Harvard: Harvard University Press).
Bromham, D. R., Dalton, M. E., and Jackson, J. C. (1990), *Philosophical Ethics in Reproductive Medicine* (Manchester: Manchester University Press).
Bromham, D. R., Dalton, M. E., Jackson, J. C., and Millican, P. J. R. (eds.) (1992), *Ethics in Reproductive Medicine* (London: Springer-Verlag).
Buckland, T. (1986), 'The Tunstead Mill Nutters of Rossendale, Lancashire', *Folk Music Journal*, 5 (2): 132–49.
Carsten, J. (1995), 'The Substance of Kinship and the Heat of the Hearth: Feeding, Personhood and Relatedness among Malays in Pulau Langkawi', *American Ethnologist*, 22 (2): 223–41.
——(1997), *The Heat of the Hearth: The Process of Kinship in a Malay Fishing Community* (Oxford: Oxford University Press).
Cheal, D. (1988), *The Gift Economy* (London: Routledge).
Clifford, J., and Marcus, G. (1986), *Writing Culture* (Berkeley: University of California Press).
Cohen, A. (1987), *Whalsay: Symbol, Segment and Boundary in a Shetland Island Community* (Manchester: Manchester University Press).
——(ed.) (1982), *Belonging: Identity and Social Organisation in British Rural Cultures* (Manchester: Manchester University Press).
Daniels, K. (1998), 'The Semen Providers', in Daniels and Haimes (1998).
Daniels, K., and Haimes, E. (eds.) (1998), *Donor Insemination: International Social Science Perspectives* (Cambridge: Cambridge University Press).
Delaney, C. (1986), 'The Meaning of Paternity and the Virgin Birth Debate', *Man*, 21: 494–513.
——(1991), *The Seed and the Soil: Gender and Cosmology in Turkish Village Society* (Berkeley: University of California Press).
Dening, G. (1988), *History's Anthropology: The Death of William Gooch* (Washington, DC: University Press of America). Republished (1995) as *The Death of William Gooch: A History's Anthropology* (Melbourne: Melbourne University Press).
Dennis, N., Henriquez, F., and Slaughter, C. (1956), *Coal is Our Life* (London: Eyre & Spottiswoode).
Denzin, N. K. (1989), *Interpretive Biography*, Sage University Papers on Qualitative Research Methods, 17 (Beverly Hills, Calif.: Sage).
Douglas, M. (1992), 'Governability: A Question of Culture', *Millenium: Journal of International Studies*, 22 (3): 463–81. Also in Douglas, M. (1996), *Thought Styles* (London: Sage).
Edgar, I., and Russell, A. (eds.) (1998), *The Anthropology of Welfare* (London: Routledge).
Edwards, J. (n.d.), '*Ordinary People*: A Study of Factors Affecting Communication in the Provision of Services', Ph.D. thesis (Manchester, 1990).
——(1993), 'Explicit Connections: Ethnographic Enquiry in North-West England', in

Edwards, J., Hirsch, E., Franklin, S., Price, F., and Strathern, M., *Technologies of Procreation: Kinship in the Age of Assisted Conception* (Manchester: Manchester University Press). 2nd edn. with add. material (London: Routledge, 1999).
——(1994), 'Idioms of Bureaucracy and Informality in a Local Housing Aid Office', in S. Wright (ed.), *The Anthropology of Organisations* (London: Routledge).
——(1995*a*), 'Parenting Skills': Views of Community Health and Social Service Providers about the Needs of their 'Clients', *Journal of Social Policy*, 24 (2): 237–59.
——(1995*b*), 'Imperatives to Reproduce: Fertility in the Light of Infertility', in R, Dunbar (ed.), *Reproductive Decisions: Biological and Social Perspectives* (London: Macmillan).
——(1998*a*), 'Donor Insemination and 'Public Opinion': An Anthropological perspective', in Daniels and Haimes (1998).
——(1998*b*), 'The Need for a 'Bit of History': Place and Past in English Identity', in N. Lovell (ed.), *Locality and Belonging* (London: Routledge).
Edwards, J., and Strathern, M. (1999), 'Including Our Own', in J. Carsten (ed.), *Cultures of Relatedness: New Directions in Kinship* (Cambridge: Cambridge University Press).
Edwards, J., Hirsch, E., Franklin, S., Price, F., and Strathern, M. (1999 [1993]), *Technologies of Procreation: Kinship in the Age of Assisted Conception* (London: Routledge).
Eller, J. D. (1997), 'Anti-Anti-Multiculturalism', in *American Anthropologist*, 99 (2): 249–56.
Emmet, I. (1964), *A North Wales Village: A Social Anthropological Study*, Dartington Hall Studies in Rural Sociology (London: Routledge & Kegan Paul).
Ennew, J. (1980), *The Western Isles Today* (Cambridge: Cambridge University Press).
Favret-Saada, J. (1980), *Deadly Words: Witchcraft in the Bocage* (Cambridge: Cambridge University Press).
Finnegan, R. (1992), *Oral Traditions and the Verbal Arts: A Guide to Research Practices* (London: Routledge).
Firth, R. (ed.) (1956), *Two Studies of Kinship in London* (London: Athlone).
Firth, R., Hubert, J., and Forge, A. (1969), *Families and their Relatives: Kinship in a Middle-Class Sector of London* (London: Routledge & Kegan Paul).
Foucault, M. (1979 [1975]), *Discipline and Punish* (New York: Vintage).
Fox, R. (1967), *Kinship and Marriage: An Anthropological Perspective* (Harmondsworth: Penguin).
Frankenberg, R. (1990 [1957]), *Village on the Border: A Social Study of Religion, Politics and Football in a North Wales Community*, 2nd edn. with add. material (Prospect Heights, Ill.: Waveland).
——(1966), *Communities in Britain: Social Life in Town and Country* (Harmondsworth: Penguin).
Franklin, S. (1990), 'Deconstructing 'Desparateness': The Social Construction of Infertility in Popular Representations of New Reproductive Technologies', in M. McNeil, I. Varcoe, and S. Yearly (eds.), *New Reproductive Technologies* (London: Macmillan).
Franklin, S. (1997), *Embodied Progress: A Cultural Account of Assisted Conception* (London: Routledge).

Freeman, E. A. (1871), *Old English History* (London: Macmillan).

Froome, D. (1953), 'The Britannia Coconut Dancers', *English Dance and Song*, 17 (6): 209–10.

Geertz, C. (1993 [1979]), *The Interpretation of Cultures* (New York: Basic Books).

Gellner, E. (1973), *The Concept of Kinship and Other Essays* (Oxford: Blackwell).

——(1992), *Postmodernism, Reason and Religion* (London: Routledge).

Gluckman, M. (1955), *The Judicial Process Among the Barotse of Northern Rhodesia* (Manchester: Manchester University Press).

——(1965), *The Ideas in Barotse Jurisprudence* (New Haven: Yale University Press).

——(ed.) (1969), *Ideas and Procedures in African Customary Law* (Oxford: Oxford University Press).

Gonzalez Echevarria, A. (1994), *Teorias del parentesco: Nuevas aproximaciones* (Madrid: Eudema).

Gow, P. (1991), *Of Mixed Blood: Kinship and History in Peruvian Amazonia* (Oxford: Oxford University Press).

Green, S. (1997), *Urban Amazons: Lesbian Feminism and Beyond in Gender, Sexuality and Identity* (Basingstoke: Macmillan).

Gudeman, S., and Penn, M. (1982), 'Models, Meaning and Reflexivity', in D. Parkin (ed.), *Semantic Anthropology* (London: Academic Press).

Gullestad, M. (1992), *The Art of Social Relations: Essays on Culture, Social Action, and Everyday Life in Modern Norway* (Oslo: Scandinavian University Press).

Haimes, E. (1988), '"Secrecy": What Can Artificial Reproduction Learn from Adoption?', *International Journal of Law and the Family*, 2: 46–61.

——(1993), 'Do Clinicians Benefit from Gamete Donor Anonymity?', *Human Reproduction*, 8 (9): 1518–20.

Handler, R. (1988), *Nationalism and the Politics of Culture in Quebec* (Madison: Wisconsin University Press).

——(ed.) (1995), *Schneider on Schneider: The Conversion of the Jews and Other Anthroplogical Stories* (Durham, NC: Duke University Press).

Haraway, D. (1989), *Primate Visions: Gender, Race and Nature in the World of Modern Science* (New York: Routledge).

Harris, R. (1986 [1972]), *Prejudice and Tolerance in Ulster* (Manchester: Manchester University Press).

Hartouni, V. (1997), *Cultural Conceptions: On Reproductive Technologies and the Remaking of Life* (Minneapolis: University of Minnesota Press).

Hastrup, K. (1995), *A Passage to Anthropology: Between Experience and Theory* (London: Routledge).

Hauser-Schaublin, B. (1989), 'The Fallacy of "Real" and "Pseudo" Procreation', *Zeitschrift für Ethnologie*, 114: 179–94.

Herzfeld, M. (1987), *Anthropology Through the Looking Glass: Critical Ethnography in the Margins of Europe* (Cambridge: Cambridge University Press).

——(1992), 'History in the Making: National and International Politics in a Rural Cretan Community', in J. Pina-Cabral and J. Campbell (eds.), *Europe Observed* (London: Macmillan).

——(1991), *A Place in History: Social and Monumental Time in a Cretan Town* (Princeton: Princeton University Press).

Hewison, R. (1987), *The Heritage Industry: Britain in a Climate of Decline* (London: Methuen).

Holy, L. (1996), *Anthropological Perspectives on Kinship* (London: Pluto).

Holy, L., and Stuchlick, M. (1981) (eds.), *The Structure of Folk Models* (London: Academic Press).

Horowitz, I. L. (1969) (ed.), *Sociological Self-Images: A Collective Portrait* (Beverly Hills, Calif.: Sage).

Howarth, P. (n.d.), 'Aspects of Educational, Cultural and Leisure Provision in Bacup and the Surrounding Area 1860–1910', MA thesis (University of Manchester, 1979).

Hymes, D. (1974), *Foundations in Sociolinguistics: An Ethnographic Approach* (Philadelphia: Philadelphia University Press).

Ingold, T. (1986), *Evolution and Social Life* (Cambridge: Cambridge University Press).

——(1990), 'An Anthropologist Looks at Biology', *Man* (NS), 26: 208–29.

Inhorn, M. (1993), *Quest for Conception* (Philadelphia: University of Pennsylvania Press).

James, A., Hockey, J., and Dawson, A. (1997), *After Writing Culture: Epistemology and Praxis in Contemporary Anthropology*, ASA Monograph, 34 (London: Routledge).

James, W. (1988), *The Listening Ebony: Moral Knowledge, Religion and Power among the Uduk of Sudan* (Oxford: Clarendon).

Kuper, A. (1983 [1973]), *Anthropology and Anthropologists: The Modern British School* (London: Routledge).

Latour, B. (1987), *Science in Action: How to Follow Scientists and Engineers through Society* (Cambridge, Mass.: Harvard University Press).

Leach, E. (1966), 'Virgin Birth', *Proceedings of the Royal Anthropological Institute for 1966*, 39–49; repr. in *Genesis as Myth and other Essays* (London: Cape, 1969).

Lienhardt, G. (1988), 'Social and Cultural Implications of some African Personal Names', *Journal of the Anthropological Society of Oxford*, 19 (2): 105–16.

Loizos, P. (1992), 'User-Friendly Ethnography', in J. Pina-Cabral and J. Campbell (eds.), *Europe Observed* (London: Macmillan).

McDonald, M. (1987), 'The Politics of Fieldwork in Brittany', in A. Jackson (ed.), *Anthropology at Home* (London: Tavistock).

Macdonald, S. (1997), *Reimagining Culture: Histories and Identities in the Gallic Renaissance* (Oxford: Berg).

——(ed.) (1993), *Inside European Identities: Ethnography in Western Europe* (Oxford: Berg).

Macfarlane, A. (1978), *The Origins of English Individualism: The Family, Property and Social Transition* (Oxford: Basil Blackwell).

MacLeod, J. (1995 [1987]), *Ain't No Making It: Levelled Aspirations in Low Income Neighbourhoods* (Boulder, Col.: Westview).

McNeil, M. (1993), 'New Reproductive Technologies: Dreams and Broken Promises', *Science as Culture*, 3 (17): 483–507.

McNeil, M., Varcoe, I., and Yearley, S. (1990) (eds.), *The New Reproductive Technologies* (London: Macmillan).

McWhinnie, A. (1993), 'Doubts and Realities in DI Family Relationships', *Politics and the Life Sciences*, 12 (2): 189–91.

Malinowski, B. (1929), *The Sexual Life of Savages in North Western Melanesia* (London: Routledge & Kegan Paul).

Malkki, L. (1992), 'National Geographic: Rooting of Peoples and Territorialisation of National Identity among Scholars and Refugees', *Cultural Anthropology*, 7 (1): 24–44.

Marcus, G. E., and Fischer, M. J. (1986), *Anthropology as Cultural Critique: An Experimental Moment in the Human Sciences* (Chicago: Chicago University Press).

Martin, E. (1987), *The Woman in the Body: A Cultural Analysis of Reproduction* (Boston: Beacon).

Martin, E. (1991), 'The Egg and the Sperm: How Science has Constructed a Romance Based on Stereotypical Male–Female Roles', *Signs*, 16 (3): 485–501.

Mauss, M. (1966), *The Gift* (London: Cohen & West).

Miller, D. (1998), *A Theory of Shopping* (Cambridge: Polity).

Monks, J. (n.d.), 'Describing Sickness: Talk, Social Relations and Personhood Following a Diagnosis of Multiple Sclerosis', Ph.D. thesis (Brunel University, 1996).

Moore, B. (1991), 'Rossendale', *Lancashire Lives: The Lives and Times of some Interesting Lancashire Folk*, ii (Preston: Carnegie).

Muggeridge, K., and Adam, R. (1968 [1967]), *Beatrice Webb: A Life 1858–1943* (New York: Alfred A. Knopf).

Needham, R. (ed.) (1971), *Rethinking Kinship and Marriage*, ASA Monographs, 11 (London: Tavistock).

Newbigging, T. (1868), *The History of the Forest of Rossendale* (London: Simpkin, Marshall); 2nd edn. (Rawtenstall: J. J. Riley, 1893).

Okely, J. (1983), *The Traveller Gypsies* (Cambridge: Cambridge University Press).

——(1987), 'Fieldwork up the M1: Policy and Political Aspects', in A. Jackson (ed.), *Anthropology at Home* (London: Tavistock).

——(1996), *Own or Other Culture* (London: Routledge).

Okely, J., and Callaway, H. (eds.) (1992), *Anthropology and Autobiography* (London: Routledge).

Parry, J., and Bloch, M. (1989), *Money and the Morality of Exchange* (Cambridge: Cambridge University Press).

Percy, J. (1991), 'Scientists in Humble Life: The Artisan Naturalists of South Lancashire', *Manchester Region Historical Review*, 5 (1): 3–10.

Personal Narratives Group (ed.) (1989), *Interpreting Women's Lives: Feminist Theory and Personal Narratives* (Bloomington: Indiana University Press).

Pfeffer, N. (1992), 'From Private Patients to Privatisation', in M. Stacey (ed.) (1992).

Plummer, C., and Earle, J. (1899), *Two of the Saxon Chronicles Parallel* (Oxford: Clarendon).

Powdermaker, H. (1966), *Stranger and Friend: The Way of an Anthropologist* (New York: Norton).

Pratt, M. L. (1986), 'Fieldwork in Common Places', in J. Cifford and G. Marcus, *Writing Culture: The Poetics and Politics of Ethnography* (Berkeley: University of California Press).

Price, F. (1994), 'Conceiving Relations: Egg and Sperm Donation in Assisted Procreation', in D. Pearl and R. Pickford (eds.), *Frontiers of Family Law* (London: Chancery).

——(1998), 'Collaborative Conceptions: the Social Implications of Egg Donation', End-of-grant report, The Nuffield Foundation: London.

Purdy, L. M. (1996), *Reproducing Persons: Issues in Feminist Bioethics* (Ithaca, NY: Cornell University Press).

Rabinow, P. (1977), *Reflections of Fieldwork in Morocco* (Berkeley: University of California Press).

——(ed.) (1984), *The Foucault Reader* (New York: Pantheon).

Ragone, H. (1994), *Conception in the Heart: Surrogate Motherhood in America* (Boulder, Col.: Westview).

Rapp, R. (1987*a*), 'Toward a Nuclear Freeze?: The Gender politics of Euro-American Kinship Analysis', in J. F. Collier and S. Yanagisako (eds.), *Gender and Kinship: Essays Toward a Unified Analysis* (Stanford: Stanford University Press).

——(1987*b*), 'Moral Pioneers: Women, Men and Fetuses on a Frontier of Reproductive Technology', *Women and Health*, 13 (1–2): 101–16.

Rapport, N. (1993), *Diverse World Views in an English Village* (Edinburgh: Edinburgh University Press).

——(1997), '"The Contrarieties" of Israel: An Essay on the Cognitive Importance and the Creative Promise of Both/And', *Journal of the Royal Anthropological Institute*, 3 (4): 653–72.

Robertson, A. F. (1991), *Beyond the Family: The Social Organisation ofHuman Reproduction* (Oxford: Polity).

Rosenwald, G. C., and Ochberg, R. L. (eds.) (1992), *Storied Lives: The Cultural Politics of Self-Understanding* (New Haven: Yale University Press).

Rowbottom, A. (n.d.), 'Royal Symbolism and Social Integration', Ph.D. thesis (University of Manchester, 1994).

Schneider, D. M. (1968), *American Kinship: A Cultural Account* (Englewood Cliffs NJ: Prentice Hall); 2nd edn. (Chicago: University of Chicago Press, 1980).

——(1984), *A Critique of the Study of Kinship* (Ann Arbor: University of Michigan Press).

——(1997), 'The Power of Culture: Notes on some Aspects of Gay and Lesbian Kinship in America Today', *Cultural Anthropology*, 12 (2): 270–4.

Secord, A. (1994*a*), 'Science in the Pub: Artisan Botanists in Early-Nineteeth Century Lancashire', *History of Science*, 32: 269–315.

——(1994*b*), 'Corresponding Interests: Artisan and Gentlemen in Nineteenth-Century Natural History', *British Journal for the History of Science*, 27: 383–408.

——(1996), 'Artisan Botany', in N. Jardine, J. A. Secord, and E. C. Spary (eds.), *Cultures of Natural History* (Cambridge: Cambridge University Press).

Shanklin, E. (1985), *Donegal's Changing Traditions: An Ethnographic Study* (New York: Gordon & Breach).

Shore, C. (1992), 'Virgin Births and Sterile Debates', *Current Anthropology*, 33 (3): 295–311.

Spallone, P. (1989), *Beyond Conception: The New Politics of Reproduction* (London: Macmillan).

——(1992), *Generation Games: Genetic Engineering and the Future for our Lives* (London: Women's Press).

Spallone, P., and Steinberg, D. (eds.) (1987), *Made to Order: The Myth of Reproductive Progress* (Oxford: Pergamon).

Spiro, M. E. (1968), 'Virgin Birth, Parthenogenesis and Physiological Paternity: An Essay in Cultural Interpretation', *Man* (NS), 3: 242–61.

Stacey, M. (1992) (ed.), *Changing Human Reproduction* (London: Sage).

Stanworth, M. (ed.) (1987), *Reproductive Technologies: Gender, Motherhood and Medicine* (Cambridge: Polity).

Stolcke, V. (1988), 'New Reproductive Technologies—Same Old Fatherhood', *Critique of Anthropology*, 6: 5–32.

Strathern, M. (1981), *Kinship at the Core: An Anthropology of Elmdon, a Village in North-West Essex in the Nineteen Sixties* (Cambridge: Cambridge University Press).

——(1982*a*), 'The Place of Kinship: Kin, Class and Village Status in Elmdon, Essex', in Cohen (1982).

——(1982*b*), 'The Village as an Idea: Constructs of Village-ness in Elmdon, Essex', in Cohen (1982).

——(1984), 'The Social Meaning of Localism', in T. Bradley and P. Lowe (eds.), *Locality and Rurality: Economy and Society in Rural Regions* (Norwich: Geo).

——(1987), 'The Limits of Auto-Anthropology', in A. Jackson (ed.), *Anthropology at Home* (London: Tavistock).

——(1991), *Partial Connections*, ASAO Special Publication, 3 (Savage, Md.: Rowman & Littlefield).

——(1992*a*), *After Nature: English Kinship in the Late Twentieth Century* (Cambridge: Cambridge University Press).

——(1992*b*), *Reproducing the Future: Anthropology, Kinship and the New Reproductive Technologies* (Manchester: Manchester University Press).

——(1993), 'Introduction', in Edwards, J. *et al.* (1993).

——(1996), 'Gender: Division or Comparison', in N. Charles and F. Hughes Freeland (eds.), *Practising Feminism: Identity, Difference and Power* (London: Routledge).

Toren, C. (1993), 'Making History: The Significance of Childhood Cognition for a Comparative Anthropology of Mind', *Man*, 28: 461–78.

Tupling, G. H. (1927), *The Economic History of Rossendale* (Manchester: Manchester University Press).

Wagner, R. (1975), *The Invention of Culture* (Englewood Cliffs, NJ: Prentice-Hall).

Wallman, S. (1984), *Eight London Households* (London: Tavistock).

Wallman, S., Buchanan, I. H., Dhooge, Y., Gershuny, J. I., and Wann, M. (1982), *Living in South London: Perspectives on Battersea 1871–1981* (London: Gower/London School of Economics).

Walsh, S. (1989), 'Beatrice Webb and Bacup', *Manchester Region History Review*, 3 (2): 9–14.

Webb, B. (1929), *My Apprenticeship* (London: Longmans, Green).

Weston, K. (1997), 'The Virtual Anthropologist', in A. Gupta and J. Ferguson (eds.), *Anthropological Locations: Boundaries and Grounds of a Field Science* (Berkeley: University of California Press).

Whiteford, L. M., and Poland, M. L. (1989), *New Approaches to Human Reproduction: Social and Ethical Dimensions* (Boulder, Col.: Westview).

Whitelock, D. (1961), *The Anglo-Saxon Chronicles: A Revised Translation* (New Brunswick: Rutgers University Press).

Williams, R. (1985), *The Country and the City* (London: Hogarth); 1st edn. (London: Chatto & Windus, 1973).

Willmott, P., and Young, M. (1960), *Family and Class in a London Suburb* (London: Routledge).

Wolcott, H. F. (1995), *The Art of Fieldwork* (Walnut Creek: Altimira).

Wolfram, S. (1987), *In-laws and Out-laws: Kinship and Marriage in England* (London: Croom Helm).

Wright, P. (1985), *On Living in an Old Country: The National Past in Contemporary Britain* (London: Verso).

Yanagisako, S. (1985), *Transforming the Past: Kinship and Tradition among Japanese Americans* (Stanford, Calif.: University of Stanford Press).

Young, M., and Willmott, P. (1957), *Family and Kinship in East London* (Harmondsworth: Penguin).

Young R. (1995), *Colonial Desire: Hybridity in Theory, Culture and Race* (London: Routledge).

Zonabend, F. (1984), *The Enduring Memory* (Manchester: Manchester University Press).

INDEX